Brain Informatics and Health

Editors-in-Chief

Ning Zhong, Department of Life Science & Informatics, Maebashi Institute of Technology, Maebashi-City, Japan

Ron Kikinis, Department of Radiology, Harvard Medical School, Boston, MA, USA

Series Editors

Weidong Cai, School of Computer Science, The University of Sydney, Sydney, NSW, Australia

Henning Müller ⓘ, University of Applied Sciences Western Switzerland, Sierre, Switzerland

Hirotaka Onoe, Graduate School of Medicine, Kyoto University, Kobe, Japan

Sonia Pujol, Department of Radiology, Harvard Medical School, Boston, MA, USA

Philip S. Yu, Department of Computer Science, University of Illinois at Chicago, Chicago, IL, USA

Informatics-enabled studies are transforming brain science. New methodologies enhance human interpretive powers when dealing with big data sets increasingly derived from advanced neuro-imaging technologies, including fMRI, PET, MEG, EEG and fNIRS, as well as from other sources like eye-tracking and from wearable, portable, micro and nano devices. New experimental methods, such as in to imaging, deep tissue imaging, opto-genetics and dense-electrode recording are generating massive amounts of brain data at very fine spatial and temporal resolutions. These technologies allow measuring, modeling, managing and mining of multiple forms of big brain data. Brain informatics & health-related techniques for analyzing all the data will help achieve a better understanding of human thought, memory, learning, decision-making, emotion, consciousness and social behaviors. These methods also assist in building brain-inspired, human-level wisdom-computing paradigms and technologies, improving the treatment efficacy of mental health and brain disorders.

The Brain Informatics & Health (BIH) book series addresses the computational, cognitive, physiological, biological, physical, ecological and social perspectives of brain informatics as well as topics relating to brain health, mental health and well-being. It also welcomes emerging information technologies, including but not limited to Internet of Things (IoT), cloud computing, big data analytics and interactive knowledge discovery related to brain research. The BIH book series also encourages submissions that explore how advanced computing technologies are applied to and make a difference in various large-scale brain studies and their applications.

The series serves as a central source of reference for brain informatics and computational brain studies. The series aims to publish thorough and cohesive overviews on specific topics in brain informatics and health, as well as works that are larger in scope than survey articles and that will contain more detailed background information. The series also provides a single point of coverage of advanced and timely topics and a forum for topics that may not have reached a level of maturity to warrant a comprehensive textbook.

Tianhua Chen · Jenny Carter · Mufti Mahmud ·
Arjab Singh Khuman
Editors

Artificial Intelligence in Healthcare

Recent Applications and Developments

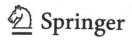 Springer

Editors
Tianhua Chen (iD)
Department of Computer Science
University of Huddersfield
Huddersfield, UK

Jenny Carter (iD)
Department of Computer Science
University of Huddersfield
Holmfirth, UK

Mufti Mahmud (iD)
Department of Computer Science
Nottingham Trent University
Nottingham, UK

Arjab Singh Khuman (iD)
Computing, Engineering and Media
De Montfort University
Leicester, UK

ISSN 2367-1742   ISSN 2367-1750 (electronic)
Brain Informatics and Health
ISBN 978-981-19-5274-6   ISBN 978-981-19-5272-2 (eBook)
https://doi.org/10.1007/978-981-19-5272-2

This Springer imprint is published by the registered company Springer Nature Singapore Pte Ltd.
The registered company address is: 152 Beach Road, #21-01/04 Gateway East, Singapore 189721,
Singapore

Preface

Artificial Intelligence (AI) was founded as a discipline in 1950s, and after several waves of attempting and discarding many different approaches, recent machine learning-based AI approaches have proved successful in many areas. Owing to the increasing availability of healthcare data and more complex needs and challenges in clinical practice, AI is also bringing a paradigm shift to healthcare sector, which increases the ability for healthcare professionals to better understand patterns of diseases and cater to rising the needs of the people. Having been popularly applied domains such as cancer, neurology and cardiology, AI has witnessed successes in different stages of clinical processes including diagnosis and detection, monitoring and prognosis, to make more informed clinical decision-making and enhance healthcare systems.

In this book, the authors present key applications in health areas where AI has had significant successes. The chapters cover a plethora of health subareas, proving credence to the versatility and effectiveness of AI advances. With a varied range of examples and various AI techniques employed, this book illustrates how AI can be capable of and how it can be applied to allow for a better appreciation of AI advances. Of the included 16 chapters, this volume starts with the discussions of AI in key emergent health areas, followed by the presentation of AI techniques in a number of high-profile domains, such as brain disorders, mental health, COVID-19, cardiovascular diseases and diabetes.

The book will be ideal for individuals new to the notion and application of AI in health and medicine, as well as for early career scholars who wish to further extend their knowledge of data-driven informatics in health. The book is also suitable as a supporting text for advanced undergraduate and graduate-level models on artificial Intelligence techniques and applications.

Huddersfield, UK
Holmfirth, UK
Nottingham, UK
Leicester, UK

Tianhua Chen
Jenny Carter
Mufti Mahmud
Arjab Singh Khuman

Contents

AI in Healthcare: Malignant or Benign?

Nathan Lloyd and Arjab Singh Khuman⊙

1 Introduction

Despite a slightly tumultuous past, the popularity and growth of Artificial intelligence are observable in every nook and cranny. AI has engrained itself within a multitude of industries as a principal tool for success, all whilst being a fledgling domain itself. Its conception can be proudly attributed to both Alan Turing [230] and the Dartmouth summer school respectively [152], kicking off the domain in a glorious fashion in the middle of the twentieth century. Although a comparatively young discipline, AI has survived many metaphorical winters, hibernating, evolving, and pivoting from one sub-field to the next. Founding researchers mistakenly promised more than they could deliver, anticipating AI to be equal to human intelligence by the end of the century [48]. This aggrandised vision of AI could not be fulfilled, causing metaphorical winters, cancellation of funds [137], and ridicule from peers. Ironically, it is likely due to this hubris that AI survived, its durability forged within the midst of overhype. Of course, with all things sensational, literature and media amplified this fanfare, perpetuating notions of killer robots and sentient AI, yet over half a century later, we are still some distance away from the singularity.

Regardless of the unkept promises and unfulfilled goals, AI has continued, becoming one of the most popular domains. Perhaps it would be fair to state that AI has entered its adolescence, sparking another golden age of research and development. In fact, AI already eclipses the earnings of many countries, receiving broad investment and maintaining a prominent place within academia [81], contributing trillions of dollars to the global economy. COVID-19 has only accelerated the adoption

N. Lloyd
School of Informatics and Digital Engineering, Aston University, Birmingham, UK

A. S. Khuman (✉)
School of Computer Science and Informatics, Institute of Artificial Intelligence (IAI), Leicester, UK
e-mail: arjab.khuman@dmu.ac.uk

© The Author(s), under exclusive license to Springer Nature Singapore Pte Ltd. 2022   1
T. Chen et al. (eds.), *Artificial Intelligence in Healthcare*, Brain Informatics and Health,
https://doi.org/10.1007/978-981-19-5272-2_1

of AI, online working as a catalyst for digital transformation, widening the horizon for AI's applicability [106]. Today's AI ubiquity has undoubtedly been determined by the unsurmountable advancements in processing power [165], this, in combination with much cheaper hardware has reduced the threshold for access, a step towards the democratisation of AI. Not only has the general hardware improved, but the development and utilisation of specialised processing units have vastly changed the AI landscape [240, 242], the domain has welcomed these advancements and since 2012 there has been a 300,000 times increase in computer utilisation [10]. Processing power alone is not the sole reason for the domain's prosperity, the age of big data has thrust cognitive-based approaches into the limelight, with terms such as machine learning and deep learning becoming common vernacular to describe AI. Whilst the media perpetuates that these terms and AI are one in the same thing, they are but part of the whole, individual components of AI.

Health and social care are much older institutions, historically maintained by militaristic or religious groups, their earliest documentation can be found within classical history. Something more akin to a hospital was developed in the mid-sixth century [222], and since then, hospitals have reformed, centralised, and employed state of the art research to deal with human health more effectively. Scientific research has propelled the understanding of human anatomy alongside the tools best suited for palliating disease. AI, like all previous advancements within modern medicine, can be utilised as an instrument to treat the sick and prevent disease. It was not long after the birth of AI until its relevance as such was realised. The symbiosis between the two was originally kicked off at Stanford in the 1960s, DENDRAL [31], a collection of systems (primarily known to be an expert system), was utilised for scientific discovery on unknown organic molecules. Like the aforementioned cognitive approaches, expert systems too are another variation of AI. Commonly referred to as knowledge-based systems, expert systems follow a deterministic rule-based algorithm to emulate the reasoning of a human expert, thereby recreating intelligence through the distillation of human knowledge. In the wake of damning reports and underfunding, expert systems flourished and distanced themselves from the publicity of cognitive approaches, edging the domain towards a profitable and commercialised future. This viability saw the development of multiple applications within healthcare, most notably MYCIN [213], which like DENDRAL, utilised a knowledge base to identify bacteria and diagnose infections. Although this form of AI has been somewhat left behind, being far from what people today recognise as AI, it notably paved the way for AI's success through branching into different industries.

But then, why the provocative title? On the surface the benefits of AI in healthcare are glaringly obvious, being an undisputed tool to more accessible and often more accurate medical assistance. Yet, like a malignant form of cancer, there are issues currently unaddressed that if left to fester will proliferate a system of inequality, doing more harm than good. To unpack these issues, it is important to explore the where's, the how's and the who's of AI healthcare, consequently if these issues remain untreated, their impacts on society may be irreversible. It is important to note that these issues are not exclusive to AI in healthcare, in fact, they are at the very core of AI, being its strength and its greatest weakness. These questions tackle ownership, its application, the rights of patients and the accuracy of AI in making life-changing decisions. Although this may paint a doom and gloom picture for the domain of AI, all hope is not lost, through a crucible of scrutiny and the correct treatment, AI can make a full recovery becoming stronger than it had ever been before. To uncover these ailments a deep dive beneath the metaphorical membrane of AI is required, permitting the exploration of the guts of AI healthcare within the life-death cycle.

2 Prevention

The proverbial saying, "Prevention is better than cure" is arguably the most idyllic pillar of healthcare. Often, prevention is envisioned as a health service firewall, protecting humanity from all manner of disease. The prevention of illness, however, goes far beyond health services, and truly must be observed through a socioeconomic lens. Research suggests that a low socioeconomic standing increases the likelihood of contracting non-communicable diseases [217]. Modern diseases do not solely originate within biology but appear through the circumstances in which people lead their lives. These socioeconomic factors encapsulate education, income, and type of occupation, each arguably responsible for lifestyle choices such as drinking or smoking. The health disparity is most notable between the richest and poorest among society [231], and so, the democratisation of AI opens a wealth of opportunities to minimise this gap. Perhaps one of the most noteworthy implementations would be to tackle environmental degradation, a process which the poorest bear the brunt of [254].

2.1 AI as a Tool to Change the World

It is estimated that 40% of global deaths are a result of environmental factors [187], with deaths from pollutants, malnutrition and contaminants at the forefront of increasing disease. Mitigating these preventable deaths is what many would argue is the noblest application of AI, a utilitarian approach affecting everyone on Earth. Necessity is the mother of invention and prominent research has already established AI's feasibility in these areas. The poster child of AI, machine learning, is spearheading a majority, tackling climate change [198], clean water [43], air pollution [6], food contamination [136], and improvement in agriculture [235]. The beauty of these solutions is their broad impact, able to solve the root problems, rather than the on-branch symptoms that currently plague the worlds healthcare systems. They have the potential to benefit the many, and not just the few, solutions which will undoubtedly aid in a greener and healthier future. However, once the rose-tinted glasses have been set aside, the irony becomes obvious. The current means of acquiring power, and AI's insatiable demand for it, will inevitably cause more pollution [115]. A study conducted by the University of Massachusetts found that training numerous large AI models for natural language processing produced over 626,000 pounds (approx.

284,000 kg) of carbon dioxide [219]. The findings highlight the stark financial cost, and more importantly the carbon footprint that is left behind when utilising state of the art tools. But even here, AI can be applied to increase the efficiencies of electricity use, providing forecasting for supply and demand [53], or the discovery of new energy sources entirely [198], only time will tell if a balance can be struck and environmental causes of death can be minimised.

Education, like the environment, is a prime contributor to health, with those at the highest levels of education by the age of 30, expected to live four years longer than those at the lowest level [175]. Further studies have observed similar findings, noting education level to be a key indicator of an individual's health [248], a factor that limits access to the labour market, which in turn exponentiates the effects upon a person's health. With such an apparent impact, education appears to be an obvious domain for the utilisation of artificial intelligence. One such proposed application is streamlining the learning process. Artificial intelligence can tailor the learning experience through leveraging machine learning: previous test scores, engagement and goals can all be quantified to recognise weaknesses, spot trends, and automatically adjust content accordingly. AI-driven personalised teaching could feasibly provide lifelong learning partners [145], able to automatically utilise specialised knowledge, enabling users to make informed decisions throughout their life. Content curation is but one of many applications within the sector aimed to reduce the overhead for teaching, automation of administrative processes is another that has seen plenty of success [37]. Such mechanisms provide staff with the opportunity to utilise their time elsewhere, perhaps prioritising student needs or taking advantage of vastly reduced workloads to improve their well-being and halt burnout. Whilst these examples are a clear detour from obvious preventatives, not a single surgical knife in sight, it was important to highlight that the factors that contribute to disease, can be uprooted through AI, treating the disease and not the symptoms.

2.2 Governance, Laws and Ethics

Although individuals within society possess the ability to harness artificial intelligence, eradicating the determinants of poor health is a matter of policy. This responsibility is bore upon the collective authorities who wield such power, able to cap the causes or mandate the use of AI as a tool for good. Currently, there is no single AI authority, nor is there standardised legislation to define artificial intelligence and how to control it. The last decade exhibits this lawlessness, a time that is unofficially dubbed as the wild west of AI [76, 122], a place where fame and infamy steer public opinion and do little to motivate legislation. Perhaps an era of lawlessness is disingenuous, hyperbolic at the very least, but in the absence of AI-specific laws, the prospecting of data, the rights of the public, and the question of ownership and blame are legal grey areas. New laws are evidentially required, but movement in this regard has been agonisingly slow. The media has done very little to help, obfuscating today's facts with tomorrow's killer robots, sensationalising events and masking the essential nuggets of truth. Naturally, a hyperopic view of AI has followed, discussions of humanities perilous future rather than the issues of today. This outlook is an obvious lapse in judgement considering self-driving car deaths [39], racist chatbots [236], and tremendous breaches in privacy [112]. Assumably, such incidents would set precedent, motivating change at an accelerated rate, yet due to the difficulty in explaining AI, many of these problems remain unchecked.

Like many technologies, artificial intelligence is somewhat mystified, shrouded behind complex terminology, comparable to alchemy for those outside of the loop. Ironically, for those who reside in the world of AI, not much is clearer. AI is a field composed of confusing Blackbox technologies and divisive subdomains, each with its vision for, and definitions of, artificial intelligence. Buiten discusses this problem in great lengths [33], highlighting that many definitions are too subjective or vague for legislation. The definition of AI and its infinitely many applications are just the tip of the iceberg, one of the most pressing concerns for machine learning is explainability. A term coined to contrast Blackbox approaches, explainability allows solutions to be unpacked, interpreted, and scrutinised. These qualities are essential not only within healthcare, where applications may determine an individual's life expectancy [199], but so too within AI-assisted insurance policies, job hiring or again within autonomous vehicles. Explainability allows researchers to peer into the looking glass, to comprehend and verify the model, in short, it's about trust and transparency. There can be no argument that research in the last decade has revolutionised the domain, if not the world, yet with each advancement, AI appears to be regressing towards alchemy [105]. Like alchemists, AI researchers have developed plenty of useful tools, they are, however, muddied by a domain saturated in innovation, often lacking good laboratory processes [121], or complicit in the utilisation of tools that are not fully understood. In such a messy domain, it is evident why there are discrepancies between experts and even clearer how these issues stack up, amplifying the difficulty of cohesive definitions. Compounding the complexity within the domain is the ignorance of decision-makers, the comical display at the US congress is evidence of such [224]. Whether the digital divide is to blame, the media or explainability, it's unsurprising to see legislation lag within a nebulous cloud of confusion.

All hope is not lost, however, the days of AI cowboys are numbered as the sun sets on lawless AI [122]. The European Commission has proposed rules to enforce trustworthy AI, developing new legal frameworks [2]. Through the proposed framework, risk will be categorised through the expected impact to human life, with high attributed risk requiring further assurances, all but in name championing (F, A, T, E). Fairness, accountability, transparency and explainability are what many believe to be the core principles for ethical AI, pillars expected to be standard practice within healthcare. It is important to distinguish the difference between ethical AI, which is defined by objective standards, and moral AI which typically originates from a groups culture, religion, or environment. Without such a distinction, attempts at defining and attaining fairness would otherwise be subjective, permitting the discrimination of groups or impeding upon an individual's privacy. China's handling of the COVID-19 pandemic presents an exemplary case study of moral AI. One that is successful [260], yet vastly different to the moral considerations of the West. A prime mover

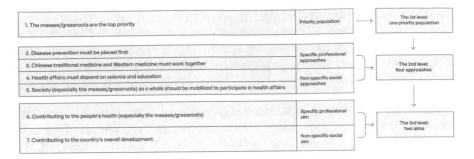

Fig. 1 Logical structure of China's National Health Guiding Principles

of China's success is its cornering of the market for facial recognition [259], and its contrasting outlook towards individuals and society. [262], discuss Chinas approach to healthcare, summarising the overwhelming focus upon the population, rather than any individual,see numbered in Fig. 1.

China's healthcare reflects the communist ideals from which the country is governed, leveraging its healthcare data for the masses [197], a contrast to the West and its fixation upon personalised medicine [173]. This simple, on the surface comparison, highlights one of the most difficult aspects of distilling ethics within a machine, highlighting how variations in culture and moral values drastically change the implementations of AI and its subsequent regulations. As a preventative measure, China's utilisation of facial recognition for tracking and quarantine is most effective, its implementation, however, goes far beyond healthcare. Alongside facial recognition, China is leading the way in digital authoritarianism [124], utilising its wealth of data and variety of tracking mechanisms, to endlessly support a vicious cycle of surveillance capitalism. When combined with China's social credit system, it is clear to see how the lack of regulations within China has permitted technological tyranny [240, 242]. Evidently, AI has unleashed a beast, a power that allows for the unabated oppression of ethnic minorities [167], the impediment of free speech, and the punishment of political dissidence [15]. Such a system penalises the mentally ill and those who are born into less-than-ideal circumstances [258], enabling the perpetuation of disparity between social groups, disregarding the socioeconomic factors that cause the punished behaviours.

Citizens are monitored and scored throughout their cities, work, and home, with their social standing gamified as a method of control. Bentham's panopticon is the perfect metaphor for this form of surveillance [25], "becoming almost synonymous" with its definition [83]. Originally proposed for prisons, the panopticon allows for inmates to be monitored by a singular and often unseen watchman, acting as both a deterrent for and observer of, any crime or dissidence. Facial recognition and surveillance capitalism takes this one step further, ushering in an Orwellian future, evoking a dystopian world with an authoritarian rule. The counterargument is to point out the overestimations of the current credit system [5], with common misconceptions of a singular central score and omnipresent sensors. China's lax regulations in security and privacy, and its history of punishing political journalists, do little to soothe the existing worries [103, 197]. The China case study displays the duplicity of AI, its potential for malignancy, and the fine rope that must be walked for its utilisation. Fortunately, since 2019, Chinese companies, universities, and authorities alike have strived to make progress in the development of regulations, mimicking the qualities observed within the European Commission. A noteworthy example of the ethical collaborations between institutions, is the Beijing AI Principles [22], a schema that outlines the requirements for an increase in ethical design, whilst still maintaining the collectivist ideology found within Chinese governance; aiming to benefit the masses and not the few. Such declarations are promising to see, as, without adequate protections, good intentions would undoubtedly pave the proverbial road to hell.

2.3 Touchless Control Preventative Healthcare in COVID

Away from the existential dread of a dying Earth, societal disparities, and the lack of adequate legislation, the sunnier side of preventative AI healthcare can be displayed. Although the detour through ethics and law may paint a doom and gloom future for AI, there are plenty of technologies that do not entirely uproot society... but this does not infer perfection either. In the efforts to explore the breadth of AI without forming an exhaustive list, the initial examples will touch on how preventative AI has been applied within the pandemic. An exemplary use is within natural user interfaces. NUI's are methods of interaction that utilise existing competencies and modalities, facilitating natural and simplistic control. The most notable examples of NUI's are touch, speech, and gesture, all of which can be built from a variety of AI techniques. The COVID-19 pandemic has highlighted the associated risk of computer interaction through physical contact, with frequently touched surfaces increasing the risk of transmission; risks routinely advised against [207, 256]. Such risk has incited the adoption of AI techniques to revolutionise existing practices, with efforts to maximise public safety. With the predicted continual growth of touch screens [108, 223], the development of alternative touchless interfaces emerged as a necessity in a post COVID world [110]. One such alternative is the 'predictive touch' system [84], a method which not only reduces interaction effort and time by 50% but crucially eliminates the requirement for physical contact. Similarly, AI-powered voice and gesture recognition provide similar benefits, albeit through a different medium of control. It is promising to observe a multitude of AI-based solutions for a single problem, especially where individual methods of interaction may be inadequate for specific disabilities,a catalogue of solutions thereby providing accessibility. Although the pandemic has unquestionably magnified the matter of hygiene and disease transmission, existing research has found bacteria spread from the gut, nose, mouth, as well as faecal matter, on touch screen devices prior to the pandemic [157]. One could hypothesise that the pandemic will symbolise a landmark for touch-based control, ushering in further research for touchless interfaces that could be implemented in mass, even from the front door of a user's home [118, 156].

2.4 Personalised Medicine: The Bridge Between Prevention and Diagnosis

Bridging the gap between prevention and diagnosis is that of personalised medicine, health care that is tailored towards the user rather than the disease. Personalised medicine has been heralded as the "future" [226], but as to be explored, this future is in fact reality. The partnership between these two overarching healthcare functions has been realised through the age of big data, propped up by the abundance of mobile sensors, many of which are discretely included within wearables and phones. Discrete may connote a hidden and malicious sensibility, rather it simply highlights the dramatic reduction in the size of sensors, their decreasing cost, and their mass implementation (IoT, many of which can be found at the forefront of highly personal and commercialised products. This extends to the sensors found within the common wearables: Fitbit, Samsung watch, Apple Watch, each empowering self-monitoring and tracking, technologies which would have required a separate tool and professional help but 20 years ago. These watches alone display the variety of data available for collection: distance moved, exercised minutes, calories burnt, heart rate, O_2 levels, quality of sleep, time spent sedentary, menstruation cycle and even fall detection; with many offering alerts in the case of worrisome figures. Throughout the chapter, the democratisation of AI will be highlighted, but it's the democratisation of technology and the willingness to use it that have made personalised medicine a reality. Like many of the suggested preventative measures, much of personalised medicine can be done without the need for expert help in shallow ways outside of healthcare institutions; deep personalised medicine, however, requires both in tandem.

Despite taking a small liberty of including diagnosis-based tools within prevention, it is often the case that a disease has been identified and informs a response. Personalised medicine can somewhat blur this distinction, providing risks and likelihoods of future disease rather than existing issues, although as discussed within the diagnosis section, it is more than capable of that too. Naturally, personalised medicine requires personalised data, and when recorded continuously, an unthinkable mountain of data makes analysis too difficult to do by hand. Fortunately, machine learning is built to wrangle large quantities of data, able to discover nuanced health insights, permitting prevention and intervention at an expediated rate. Schork highlights the harmony of AI preventative personalised medicine [205]. Discussing the potential for pairing AI-driven 'polygenic risk scores' with AI-empowered analysis, arguing that such a pairing could potentially stop diseases in their tracks. Personalised medicine goes far beyond disease management, Segal and Elinav suggest personalised diets [208]. Their shared body of research challenges the dogmatic diets and health fads, understanding that like unique genomes and subsequent personal risks, a diet too, is extremely personal.

To this end, AI has been utilised as a method of delivering personalised food plans. A noteworthy example is Heali [99], an app that allows for tailored nutrition, recommending food around a user's medical conditions such as IBS and diabetes. AI-based meal planners are built to scour existing diets, publications and user feedback to tailor menus for specific needs, eradicating the necessity for 1–1 nutritional advice or extensive individual research. A study explored the perceived success of health apps by their users, noting that a limiting factor was the required time to manually enter data [241]. Alongside planners, 'smart calorie counters' are utilising AI-based tools to reduce the knowledge threshold and effort required even further. Underpinning these applications are image classifiers and natural language processing, both of which enable the automatic logging of calories, nutrients, and macros. Likely the most tropic advice within dietary healthcare is to maintain a healthy diet, it is promising to see the use of AI in facilitating this core pillar of preventative health, made abundant through a wealth of wearables and other sensor-based technologies. AI is not integral to these practices, but the tools are able to reduce the effort required for users whilst also providing educational benefits which naturally provide a positive feedback loop into an individual's investment in their own health. The benefits notably transcend dietary diseases, the management of eating disorders can also be tracked through such applications, yet the effectiveness of health apps is up for debate [161]. Alongside the questionable effectiveness of individual care, comes with it the potentially detrimental impact of an ever-increasing deluge of data,a topic discussed within the care section. Without leaving this point unfinished, and to leave a nugget of truth ahead of the upcoming section: the irony of personalised care, is the inevitable removal of empathic 'care', as health professionals shift to data scientists [14]. To briefly mention the creativity of AI on the theme of diets, welcomes the discussion on digital chefs and AI-created nourishment. Perhaps a poor example, on the topic of health, would be to highlight the world's first AI-created gin [164]. Despite alcohol being a nonsensical choice for healthcare, Monker's Garkel highlights the power of neural networks and their creative ability. One definition of creativity is "the production of new knowledge or artefacts from what already exists" [160], neural networks are aimed to emulate human cognition, and like humans who may be inspired by existing material, AI can utilise data to return new concepts, combining or transforming established recipes. Digital chefs, like plant jammer [188], utilise this notion to personalise meals, removing allergens and inaccessible products whilst maintaining the expected final taste. It is exciting to see the various ways in which AI is utilised as a tool to enrich people's lives and improve their well-being, many of which enable passive augmentation rather than hands-on user-driven tasks.

Briefly discussed are a multitude of avenues for the prevention of disease through AI. Some of which drastically impact society, whereas others are relatively harmless and provide local benefits. However, in the absence of sufficient legislation, trusting AI to make life and death decisions is one of increased risk. Fortunately, legal and ethical guidelines are being constructed to ensure the rigidity of AI systems, minimising the potential risk albeit at an agonisingly slow pace. The difficulty in regulating AI is its likeness to a Swiss army knife, it is a domain much like the tool, encompassing many practices each with its methodologies and frameworks. The inner complexities combined with the reactivity of governmental regulation often infers a very long time to get 'things' moving [251]. Away from regulating its use within healthcare institutions, AI can boost the faculties that directly impact one's socioeconomic value, naturally providing osmosis-like benefits through the modification of the core functions within society. Healthcare that prioritises prevention and well-being is thereby a vicarious form of care. Unlike social care, which is intense and directed, humans' profit from preventative measures passively within everyday life. The availability of technology and AI has permitted these tools to take root, allowing users to become more informed about their health and become paraprofessionals through AI-assisted planning tools and the ability to constantly self-monitor. Despite the clear upsides to this approach, many healthcare institutions provide lacklustre funding, the NHS explicitly spending <5% of its budget on preventative measures [8]. Although more could be done to utilise artificial intelligence within preventative care, it is important to reaffirm that prevention goes beyond healthcare institutions, with many AI preventative tools lying outside of healthcare institutions. Regardless of funding and politics, AI is most certainly able to stimulate the focus from sick care to well-being through prevention.

3   Diagnosis

3.1   History

Medical diagnosis is likely the application that many have in mind for artificial intelligence in healthcare, after all, one of the original collaborations between healthcare and AI was the aforementioned MYCIN [213]. MYCIN was an expert system developed to diagnose bacterial infections but struggled to be adopted in practice, being only slightly better than humans and incredibly difficult to integrate into established workflows [54]. Despite the limited success, artificial intelligence and medical diagnosis have been intertwined since, displaying a rich history where state-of-the-art techniques are utilised. Over the last half-century, these adopted techniques have changed drastically, initially shifting from well-defined heuristics to fuzzy logic and belief systems, an attempt to handle the uncertainties and inaccuracies within diagnosing disease [159]. These augmentations of rule-based systems did little to quell the underlying issues, primarily the exhaustive process of constructing and maintaining large rule bases. Knowledge base systems, alongside symbolic approaches, excel within static problems, where specialist knowledge allows for narrow intelligence and reasoning. The reality, however, is dynamic, and such systems struggle to keep up with the discovery of new knowledge and disease, incrementing the difficulty of creating a general all-purpose system. A paper from 1993 that evaluates Dendral, understands these limitations as a lesson for expert systems:

that it is possible to select problems of modest complexity that nonetheless baffle the novice, and to reduce these problems to some order, resulting in a problem-solving system that lends needed assistance on human intelligence. By lowering one's sights from solving broad, general problems to solving a particular problem, by applying as much specific knowledge to that problem as can be garnered from human experts, and by systematizing and automating the application of this knowledge, a useful system can be produced. [138]

Whilst still relevant today, expert systems are somewhat eclipsed in the name of machine learning, despite being a domain also known to be currently relatively narrow. Machine learning's dominance has been perpetuated due to one key factor, its ability to automate the knowledge acquisition and representation steps: learning bottom-up from data. Healthcare institutions, like many others, are seated upon mountains of data, data that can be efficiently integrated and utilised within machine learning [146]. Before continuing, a distinction between machine learning and its subdomain of deep learning must be made. Whilst both approaches utilise data, deep learning is about the use of deep neural networks, a type of model that is inspired by the biological brain,commonly referred to as "Artificial Neural Networks". Neural networks are comprised of nodes and layers, the number of layers being the determining factor to constitute the label of "deep", though the two terms are frequently used interchangeably. Both approaches can be utilised to complete many of the same tasks, but the complexity afforded to neural networks permits an increasing catalogue of applications, albeit at the cost of computational power and time. Displayed in Figs. 2 and 3 are visualisations of how these approaches gel together. Ironically, Miller [159] highlighted the use of neural networks within medical diagnostic as early as the 1980s but noted the lack of meaningful datasets as a prime limitation. Since then, the cost of digital storage has plummeted, making health records and compliance documents readily available for healthcare organisations [189]. With the potential unlocked for machine learning approaches, and expert systems already well established within healthcare, the metaphorical training wheels can be removed from AI diagnostic tools.

3.2 Fuzzy Diagnosis

Although machine and deep learning algorithms have garnered much of the attention and will naturally comprise a larger proportion of the discussed AI tools, it is important to note the prevalence of other AI techniques. A revival of fuzzy logic has gained traction within medical diagnosis over the last few years [119]. As discussed, fuzzy logic enables uncertainties to be captured, handled, and reasoned, turning imprecision into a feature rather than a detriment. The success of a fuzzy system is derived from its ability to handle a diverse range of data, able to combine subjective observations with a range of quantitative data,much like a human clinician. Through its rules, memberships and processes, these approaches can turn uncertainty into crisp and interpretable values, and in a domain where inaccuracy and imprecision are in abundance [16], accentuating the scope of its application. Ahmadi et al. [4], displays

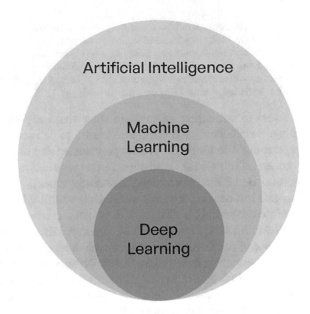

Fig. 2 Layers of AI & ML

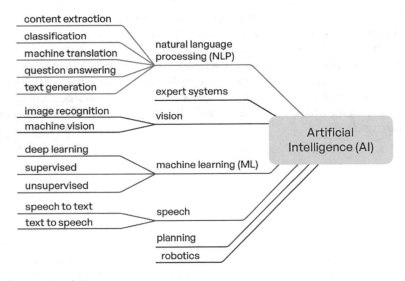

Fig. 3 Domains of AI

the wealth of fuzzy approaches within medical diagnoses, conducting metanalysis and finding 90% of the studies to have found a positive impact, many discovering their model's ability to lead to an early diagnosis, preventing the progression of complex disease. Whilst Ahmadi et al.'s review displays a general increase in literature from

2005 to 2016, the year following spotlights a substantial decline of 62%. An assumed justification can be made with 2016 being the year that deep learning "took over" [158], revolutionary innovations and media alike diverting attention away. Before discussing the elephant in the room (machine learning approaches, the hybridisation between machine learning and fuzzy systems can be discussed,an example of the partnerships seen between cognitive and symbolic approaches. A notable instance is a hybridisation within an early detection system for a stroke [234]. Two algorithms completed this task, one dedicated to modelling human activity through a genetic fuzzy finite state machine, able to learn and optimise its rules to the training data, with the other, principal component analysis able to detect the onset of a stroke, the combination of which enabling alerts to be triggered if the movement of an individual differs from their established norm. To highlight the symbiosis are examples within deep learning, able to detect coronary heart disease [12], breast cancer [120] and liver disease [70], with others hybridising once more with additional computational intelligence methods [190]. These combinations not only permit a reduction in effort with self-learning and adaptive rule sets but through the maintenance of symbolic qualities, interpretability is upheld, a quality typically in short supply within deep solutions.

3.3 NLP and Diagnostic Chatbots

The sheer quantity of electronic health records heavily favours machine learning approaches, but it is not solely due to their medical contents, rather their function as a logging tool able to record patient interactions as time-stamped events. Choi et al. suggested that modelling temporal relations between these data points can be utilised to improve upon model performance when predicting heart failure [42], a consideration argued to be absent from established techniques. Predicting future medical conditions once again highlights the large overlap between preventative personalised healthcare and diagnostic methods, evoking thoughts of a medical 'Minority Report', stopping disease before it happens. Substantial research has been diverted into developing such tools, able to predict future clinical events such as treatment trajectories, recovery and future diagnoses [41, 61, 65]. *Evidentially, advanced diagnosis and future predictions can facilitate the clinical decision-making process*, capitalising on an individual's historical patient data is not only intuitive, but it also follows a procedure much like a clinician where context is established through patterns over time; the present is dependent upon the past as is the future to the present. Historical context is frequently modelled through recurrent neural networks, a deep learning architecture specialised in modelling sequential data, most notably applied to time series data, audio signals and language data. Unlike typical feed-forward neural networks, recurrent neural networks are dynamical systems that allow states to be stored at a specified time, permitting a different output given the current state. Although RNN's excel within time series analysis, they're typically associated with modern natural language processing, a domain that has strong roots within all pillars of healthcare [111].

NLP has a variety of applications within medical diagnoses, often appearing within niche tools enhancing processes and assisting in ways that are often overlooked. Some of the most popular applications are within conversational AI, commonly referred to as chatbots. Chatbots are not exclusively utilised within medical diagnoses and will appear again within the care section, but in the context of medical diagnoses, they are frequently used as a preliminary service before human interaction. Much like personalised healthcare, which has been referred to as a bridge between prevention and diagnosis, chatbots often facilitate a bridge between diagnosis and care, emulating the conversational and investigatory practices of clinicians whilst simultaneously providing a para-social relationship between patient and machine. With a global increase in population [227] and human life expectancy following suit [176], the hypothesized future is one of more disease and a much higher demand for healthcare services. Chatbots can reduce the stress upon healthcare services by providing a familiar, albeit automated diagnosis procedure, acting as the first point of call, greatly improving access whilst also reducing healthcare costs [215]. A great example to spotlight is Geppetto Avatars [44], a company developing virtual doctors with the preliminary aim of tracking asthma conditions for young people. The application utilises various state of the art techniques, most notably analysing the contents of speech through voice to text, followed by sentiment analysis, both of which are at the core of NLP. Away from health monitoring and the explicit act of diagnosis are the tools that provide auxiliary benefits. Once again, NLP is front and centre of these tools, with chatbots developed to fulfil the role of a patient, flipping the interaction entirely and seeing doctors trained by a virtual agent to provide a higher quality of care and diagnosis [212]. Away from chatbots, NLP has been utilised to decipher medical jargon, translating complex terminology into lay speak [40], enabling paraprofessionals, patients, and non-domain experts' insight, bridging knowledge gaps entirely. With an ageing and ever-increasing population, providing superficial access to diagnosis through chatbots and boosting auxiliary practices might not be enough, a much more detailed diagnosis is required.

3.4 Medical Imaging

One of the most discussed AI-supported domains is medical imaging [113], an integral tool for clinical diagnosis [261]. A tool that has been revolutionised through the advent of convolutional neural networks as a computer vision technique. Deep learning is to thank, or blame, for this notoriety, becoming a state of the tool within medical imaging since the ImageNet challenge [130], motivating an abundance of research within medical imaging alone, propelling the claims of equal or better skill than their expert human counterparts [140]. A dramatic increase in publications between 2007 and 2017 within radiology hints at the power of convolutional neural networks, with MRI's accounting for more than 50% of the articles [186]. Magnetic resonance imaging is a scanning device that utilises magnetic fields and radio waves, producing detailed images of the inside of a body [172], frequently utilised to example the bones, breasts, and internal organs. The high-resolution, high contrast images produced by MRI synchronise extremely well with machine learning techniques, providing both quantity and quality data. MRI has been singled out due to QuantX [181], the first FDA approved AI tool for the diagnosis of breast cancer. The results obtained from its clinical trial found a 39% reduction in missed cancers, 20% improvement in diagnosis and 4% increase in sensitivity [114], a tool marketed as enhancing the arsenal of a trained radiologist. AI is evidentially reshaping the radiologist industry [62], and as discussed, the steady growth in literature only broadens the horizon of AI imaging techniques. The symbiosis of AI and MRI can be seen with a variety of disease diagnoses, a recent review compared the bounty of artificial intelligence techniques for the diagnosis of Schizophrenia [202], finding that many applications are able to assist practitioners in making accurate diagnoses. The review did note, however, that there are a limited number of datasets available for accurate Schizophrenia diagnosis, an unsurprising statement given the stigma around neurodegenerative disease and mental illness, compounded by the technical issues of lacking obvious biomarkers.

Whilst deep learning has definitively changed AI imaging techniques, a variety of classical machine learning approaches are frequently used within a variety of image-based problems. Jian et al. discussed the multiple approaches available for diagnosing a stroke through MRI data [113], one utilising a support vector machine for 87.6% accuracy [195] and another utilising Naïve Bayes [93], results of which were comparable to a human expert. Lee et al. conveyed the wide applicability of machine learning techniques for the same problem [134], providing an additional solution utilising a support vector machine, another through logistic regression and a final utilising a random forest. With plenty of cheaper solutions for medical diagnosis, it is important to understand why deep learning has taken precedence over many tasks. Mahapatra suggests that deep learning is superior on more complex problems, and problems that require more data, but more importantly its beneficial for developing solutions that require less domain knowledge, requiring less feature engineering [148]. In many ways the need for expert knowledge has become superfluous, snowballing the democratisation of AI further. This has naturally bled into personalised healthcare, with smartphone applications explicitly marketing AI tools for self-managed healthcare. Typical examples are the dermatological medical image classifiers, assessing the qualities of moles to determine whether it is malignant or benign. Applications like [214] provide a pocket-sized "personalised skin health journey", allowing users to detect signs of melanoma, albeit at a premium price. The irony of democratised healthcare behind a paywall is not lost on a Brit who has access to the NHS, perhaps some naivety would expect such systems to boost accessibility like some media has claimed [183]. The moral pit of profit healthcare aside, many would expect the premium features advertised and allowed upon app stores would be fit for purpose, well… no, not exactly. A study conducted by Freeman et al. [80], aimed to assess the validity of studies that examine AI-drive smartphone melanoma detectors. In three of the studies, SkinVision was highlighted as an application that performed poorly when compared to experts, with many of the studies displaying poor academic research.

3.5   *Mental Health*

So far, the discussed diagnostic tools have been focused upon physical disease, a focus that is also present within the literature. A Google Scholar search, adjusting the terms: "AI Diagnosis for… mental health/physical disease", highlights the disparity. The focus upon physiological disease comparative to mental illness is unambiguous in the context of stigma, the difficulty in obtaining data, and the often-subjective terms used to describe mental illness. Thankfully, Fig. 4 highlights a recent shift in the literature, research undeterred by such obstacles.

Unlike many other fields within biology and medicine, the mind remains an elusive idea, muddied by varied metaphysical views and limited understanding of consciousness. Whilst the mind remains a mystical term, human understanding of the physical brain and neurochemicals has continued to develop, knowledge which has allowed some insight into neurodegenerative diseases and the ability to assess damage to the brain. Whereas physical diseases are often measurable and quantitative, mental illness, feelings and moods are quite difficult to record due to a tacit understanding. Yet there are surprising forms of diagnosis away from the run of the mill methods. Diagnosis is often completed through tools that have been tailored towards the environment, observing characteristics, actions, tones or even posture to gain insight on an individual's mood or mental illness, diagnosing through symptomatic expressions; much like a psychiatrist. A study conducted by Cao et al. [36] aimed to discover how expressions of mental illness can manifest through the use of a mobile phone. By providing their participants with a modified smartphone that was able to collect

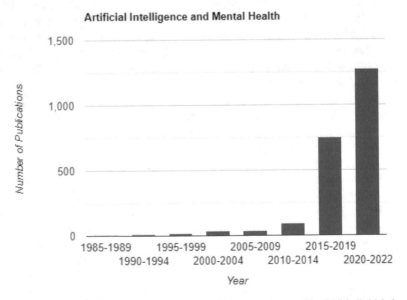

Fig. 4 Frequency of publications for "artificial intelligence and mental health" in PubMed

keystroke metadata, the model, dubbed DeepMood was able to achieve 90% accuracy for predicting a user's mood. Similar projects assess mental illness through their interaction with technologies, many of which are centred around social media use. Schwartz et al. [206], aimed to predict a Facebook users' degree of depression through their written posts, modelling through regression to enable predictions over time. Shwartz et al.'s input features indicated that the number of words, topics, and lexica were integral measures for diagnosis, and by continuing modelling through regression, they propose that predictions could be made for the ever-changing mental states of individuals. It is commonly accepted that an individual's mental health lies upon a spectrum [3], and so, a continuous scale (regression) is suitable for modelling such conditions. Within the literature, however, there is a tendency to gravitate towards binary classifiers [91], favouring model parsimony over mental illness severity. Unfortunately, there is a disconnect between the methodologies within AI and those within psychology, hinting at the underlying issues within AI. An alternate method of assessing mental health conditions is through speech recognition and acoustic features, a method of diagnosis established long ago in psychiatry, Emil Kraepelin noted factors such as tone, cadence and pitch could be utilised in diagnosing depression [128]. A variety of techniques exist for assessing mental health through voice, Tasnim and Stroulia highlight machine learnings vast applicability in such tasks, applying a variety of algorithms across two individual datasets [221]. Within this study, the two approaches of binary classification and regression were assessed, finding deep methods to be superior within binary classification and the dominance of a classical machine learning algorithm: random forest, for the regression task. Although depression is the most common illness investigated [91], a wide variety of mental illnesses and neurological diseases are captured through modelling voice inputs, successfully applied to Alzheimer's [79], bipolar and schizophrenia [13], and suicidal ideation [88]. These tools provide benefits to medical professionals, like psychiatrists, who may benefit from a method of quantifying the complexity of human language as a method for diagnosis [46].

3.6 Problems with AI Diagnosis

With self-reported supremacy and the mesmerising performance metrics posted within abstracts, it is all too easy to be carried away in the commotion, forgetting the incompleteness of AI diagnosis. Frequent are the titles that declare AI supremacy [135, 239], many citing deep learning algorithms that can outperform specialists. Whilst Liu et al. does not deny the claims of matching or surpassing clinician accuracy [140], it is argued that the research methods often undermine the findings. Through conducting a meta-analysis, they found human to AI tests that there were unrealistic, many of which utilising artificial data, and a number more who failed to report their performance metrics, highlighting the unreliability of such claims. Unrealistic testing is one seen throughout the body of literature, so too within mental health speech diagnosis is there a noticeable lack of clinical trials [142], with many omitting held out test sets to validate accuracy. As one may expect, considering the last two years, recent literature has focused upon diagnosing COVID-19 through AI, with many expecting machine learning to be able to help clinicians make informed decisions [101]. Heaven notes that many studies have found evidence to the contrary, finding that none of the numerous tools created are fit for clinical use, providing minimal, if any, benefit. Heaven suggests that the primary issue across each of the studies was the lack of quality data, most of which was taken from public datasets that included mislabelled, unlabelled, and unintentionally noisy data, many datasets originating from unknown sources. An axiom of machine learning is better data beats more data [96], and so, many of these projects were doomed from the start. To play devil's advocate, and naively believe the superiority of machines, it is then important to question the use of AI, and it is all too clear to observe the consistent failures. Often, it is the simple things that are left out of the discussion, for example, a common motivation for the development of AI-based diagnosis is the lack of specialists; through automation, the lack of labour is circumvented. The irony of this motivation is the paradoxical outcome, by displaying any field as automatable, the human counterpart will be less likely to pursue a career there [169]. Alternate research states that AI won't replace human specialists, but human specialists with AI augmentation will replace those without [132]. If it is proposed that the two work in tandem, then a notable factor is automation bias, a bias where people are more likely to trust an automated decision rather than one generated by a human [86]. In the grand scheme of things, how is this any different from replacement? So then, when things go wrong, who is to blame? Is it the developer responsible for creating a faulty tool, or is it the practitioner for relying solely upon the judgement of the AI system? The European Parliament believes the responsibility should lie with the professional [66], urging education to best inform the human specialist upon the limitations and appropriate use of AI. But with the rhetoric of "AI that is better than humans", and the subsequent automation bias, is it truly that simple? Clearly, AI informed specialists would remediate the potential for negligence, but developers can contribute to more secure and trustworthy AI.

As briefly discussed in the prevention section, a compounding factor to many failures of AI is the absence of explainability, a common absence within machine learning and deep learning approaches. Currently, automated decisions through black-box techniques leave no room for back-and forth-discussions to deliberate upon how a conclusion was reached [85], dissuading scrutiny and allowing automated recommendations absolution,a questionable factor given the potential for life and death decisions to be made within healthcare. Rudin and Radin [199] advise against blackbox techniques, stating the profound implications for their use within highly sensitive areas like healthcare, arguing that interpretable models can be constructed, but the community has not been trying. This is probably too harsh a critique for AI, a whole field is dedicated to stripping away the walls of black-box techniques, offering interpretability and explainability. Explainable AI (XAI) has recently boomed to fill this existing failure, offering many discussions [38, 58, 60, 168], with solutions specifically proposing frameworks for healthcare. One such proposal is to extract clinician knowledge as a way of evaluating a model's performance, whilst also utilising clinicians to generate explanations for correct decisions [185]. It could be argued that there is a notable irony to the high demands imposed upon AI when compared to other medical practices like prescriptions drugs, where they too are often unexplained [228]. This is an issue about trust, whereas the medical fields have centuries of literature and public exposure, AI is a relatively new domain, plagued by hype and mysticism, obfuscated by probability. But AI is often reported to be just as good as clinicians, with literature promoting "better than" accuracies, so what is not to trust?

Unfortunately, blurring most of AI's success within healthcare is a variety of coded biases. A noteworthy affliction of machine learning is its ability to reproduce human bias through poorly collated datasets and obviously biased features. In worst-case scenarios, the result is a breach of civil rights, and at best, a reduced performance upon specific demographics; both of which are unacceptable outcomes. General research has discovered the limitations of commercial AI systems, most notably affecting women, and individuals with a darker complexion [34]. Perhaps an assumption would be made, that such bias would not exist within existing AI health systems, regrettably, this is not the case [174]. In the absence of the aforementioned legislation, ethical design principles such as inclusivity and fairness are not at the forefront of development. The disparity between accuracy when skin colour is variant is an incredibly dangerous bias, nowhere more dangerous than in healthcare where poor results may misdiagnose or infer the wrong treatment. Deep learning techniques may enforce racial disparities further. Banerjee et al., displayed the ability for deep learning models to easily learn and recognise race through x-ray and CT images [18], potentially compounding the existing imbalance in medical care. Similar biases can be observed through the lens of sex, often imbalanced within medical data and wrongly referred to as gender [133], again, reinforcing researcher bias. Class imbalances and poor representation within data is a problem that was discovered in the publicly available datasets for ophthalmology [123]. The findings highlight skewed data and uneven distributions across countries, impeding the generalisability of any inference from machine learning models, noting this imbalance as a form of data poverty. Despite a worrying trend of bias, it would be unfair to unequivocally ridicule artificial intelligence as a lesser tool when compared to human diagnosis. The findings are not exclusive to AI, such qualities are noted to be an institutional problem, a problem that has been equally detected within human facing healthcare [141, 151, 155]. Naturally, it is human prejudice that informs the bias within data, whether done maliciously or ignorantly, the social issue bleeds into machine learning. Whereas health institutions have had centuries to ensure ethical practices are followed, artificial intelligence is just beginning in this regard. Perhaps at the cost of injecting some optimism, one could argue that the development of more rigorous systems, as a consequence of more stringent laws and ethical guidelines, would inevitably remediate the bias completely,superseding human prejudice entirely.

4 Care

4.1 The Problem with Current Care

Care is quintessential to medical professions, metaphorically and figuratively at the core of social care and healthcare, it is a quality often expected, yet seldom given; "care is missing from healthcare" [229]. Whilst clearly a broad generalisation, it is not difficult to observe this statement when surveying the underpinning factors behind patient satisfaction. Ng and Luk [171], argue these attributing factors to be: the providers' attitude, their competency, alongside the accessibility and efficacy of treatment. Each of these integral qualities of care can greatly be improved through the utilisation of technology, more specifically AI. Returning to Topol, he argues a current absence within the former, a "palpable lack of compassion", a troubling factor when evidence suggests that a patient may prefer empathic qualities over technical competency [264]. Within the medical industry, empathy is recognised as a universally beneficial quality, it is necessary for understanding a patient's concern, and acting in a manner to reduce their anxiety,it's a quality essential to building rapport. Whilst empathy and attitude are essential to establishing a sound relationship, research suggests that it can be detrimental, bringing forth an inevitable increase in emotional exhaustion for the practitioner, alongside attachments that may impede objectivity [102]. Aggravating these negative impacts upon a practitioner is the sheer demand for primary healthcare around the world, this demand bleeds into patient satisfaction becoming a negative impact through an increase in wait time and a decrease in consultation time [98]. The issue is evidentially complex, practitioners are burnt out, depressed and are outspoken in their shared low morale [27, 107], whereas, patients are receiving a perceived reduction in care, preferring a more personal and time-consuming relationship [166, 178], which current institutions cannot provide. The high demand and even higher expectations have become a vicious cycle for practitioners, a cycle of depression and burnout, which in turn leads to mistakes and poor practice; a negative feedback loop [182], It is clear to see why techniques of detached concern are employed to manage stress and time, all but avoiding the emotional exhaustion altogether [97]. But as discussed, this impedes the quality of care, fortunately, many believe AI can help break this cycle!

Like AI's potential effect upon teachers, medical professionals can also benefit from a reduced workload. The potential for AI automation not only includes primary care but can also be sufficiently applied to emergency departments alike [26, 162]. The potential should be unlocked to level up the patient care process, greatly reducing time and effort whilst maximizing effective treatment. To restore care, a feasible application would be automating the administrative duties that worsen productivity, increase stress, and reduce the time for clinical work [179]. Studies completed within the USA found that on average, between 16 and 55% of total working hours were dedicated to administrative tasks [253], most of the time taken up scouring over electronic health records. Compounding the overwhelming time spent on these perfunctory tasks is their perceived burden [210], a burden that undoubtedly contributes to the self-reported excessive workload [35], explaining why many rely upon inaccurately copying and pasting common templates and terms. Automating these administrative processes is a highly discussed application within AI literature, a method to improve practitioners well-being alongside cultivating a more efficient and robust health system, absent of the risks carried through carpet-bombing copy and pastes [244]. One such application is the use of voice recognition and natural language processing to extract and interpret conversations between doctors and patients, automating the documentation process within clinical encounters [126].

Furthermore, Deliberato proposes an AI system that would automatically unpack, sort, and formulate medical records from relevant sources, expediating knowledge discovery for practitioners [55]. The system would seamlessly integrate a catalogue of inputs, such as electronic health records, wearable data, and vitals to assemble sufficient reports, greatly increasing the speed of document creation. The system would utilise machine learning and its wealth of sources to learn what data to prioritise, instinctively searching and emphasizing the appropriate data. Deliberato recognises that such a system cannot exist without exemplary data points to begin with, which as discussed, will be hard to locate with the frequency of copy and paste jobs, reflecting the old idiom, of garbage in, garbage out. Naturally, these AI-driven solutions highlight the potential in automating the tasks that were otherwise completed by practitioners, reducing the administrative overhead, and affording practitioners time that can be best spent elsewhere. When these tasks are so frequently required and extremely well structured, it is clear to see why AI is fit to automate the most monotonous and disliked aspects within the medical field; a change that could feasibly re-establish the patient-doctor relationship, or at the very least, reduce burnout. Yet, despite these applications and their noble aims, it is argued that the technological imperatives repeatedly neglect the complexities and uncertainties within healthcare systems [250]. It is important to navigate these problems and solutions with care, understanding that whilst AI symbiosis may be feasible, it may not always be the most logical or effective choice; it is not the panacea for healthcare [55]. Alternate solutions away from automation already exist, a common example growing in popularity is the use of paraprofessional scribes [87], another symbiotic solution that instead averts the problems innate to artificial intelligence through good old fashioned human employment. This mantra will be continued throughout the section, and whilst in theory, AI could feasibly be used for each of the following problems, the question is, should it be? A question that alludes to the myth of the technological fix [177].

4.2 Mental Health Chat Bots

Oelschlaeger's statement questions whether humans are attempting to solve fundamentally social issues with technology. When considering AI, this becomes an increasingly complex topic, with solutions becoming ever similar (at least in narrow ways) to human capabilities. It is important to focus upon these critiques as they can dispel some of the absurd idealism surrounding AI within healthcare, yet it is hard not to be optimistic and blinded by the fanfare. One of the prime motivations for overhauling professions is the current systemic failures within a variety of industries and occupations. Healthcare is no different. Susskind and Susskind point out six ways in which the professions are limited: economically, technologically, psychologically, morally, qualitatively and their inscrutability [220]. Both father and son discuss the exclusivity of professions, their proclivity towards quacks and their and paywalled services. The product or service for many professions is the knowledge base they hold, but as the theme continues, AI can democratise many of these knowledge bases. Continuing with the restoration of care, another question can then be asked, what if, instead of reinstituting care, it could be emulated and replaced through AI? The question is perhaps a richer topic of discussion, covering whether professions should be replaced and whether the supposed replacements should be trusted. With the current state of AI, it should go without saying that the rhetoric often spouted by media should be filtered from the answer, and of course, no blanket statements should be made. Nonetheless, through exploring exemplary subdomains, at least a part of the future can be envisioned.

When thinking upon care, it noticeably extends far beyond the consultation and emergency rooms, thoughts are evoked upon rehabilitation, counselling, palliative, elderly and end of life care, increasingly intimate and personal domains of healthcare. Likely the most contentious use of artificial intelligence, is the replacement of humans within these scenarios, removing humanity from overwhelmingly social issues. These therapy-based domains rely heavily upon empathy and compassion, qualities, that as established, are deemed to be in short supply.

A pair of questions should then be proposed: *"Can a machine empathise, and should it?"*.

Here lies the first stop in the AI replacement for care-based services. As discussed within the diagnosis section, and contrary to the traditional methods of evaluation, AI can be utilised to detect mental health disorders and predict the user's current mood given some input. But AI can go one step further, a possible future exists where diagnosis and treatment can all be completed within an enclosed loop [229]; pocket psychotherapist if you will. Through a variety of sensors, most of which are non-invasive, AI can democratise therapy, a benefit that cannot be understated given the stigma around mental health. Despite the efforts to reduce the stigma, it remains a prevalent issue within countries [243], racial and ethnic minorities [67], and the vulnerable alike [94, 100, 203]. For many, mental health remains a taboo topic, going unspoken and perceived as a weakness, a troubling statement when in 2017, estimations saw 800 million suffering from a form of mental health disorder [52], a figure which can only have increased during the pandemic [150]. The lack of accessible care is rife within the domain, enormous waiting lists [11] are compounded by a global 13% rise (between 2007 and 2017) in mental health conditions [255]. An additional barrier is the personality of the therapists, a simple, yet integral quality for those who seek therapy [19]. Aggravating the lack of access and stigma is the finding that mental health conditions often contribute to job loss, and when referring to the socioeconomic values that underpin an individual's health, the ability to spiral out of control is all too clear [216]. Education and policy are integral for removing the stigma, but there is room, and demand for AI to be used as a method to ensure these services are more accessible, removing the need for face-to-face interactions altogether. Enter conversational agents.

Conversational agents, often called chatbots, are AI-empowered tools becoming increasingly popular for online mental health platforms. In place of human-led cognitive behavioural therapy sessions, with a licensed therapist, users interact with agents who emulate humans, providing the users with *someone* to talk to and unload, with select platforms providing 1–1 coaching for specific mental health disorders. This application of AI is not new, the idea of a chatbot therapist can be traced back to 1966 with the development of ELIZA [245]. ELIZA was able to simulate human understanding through following pre-defined rules that allowed for pattern matching, and, when combined with scripts that would define the context of the conversation, ELIZA would act as an interpreter between the user and the script. In Weizenbaum's paper, the script found within the appendices is none other than "DOCTOR", a script which simulated Rogerian psychotherapy, famous for repeating back key words from a user's statements within a new question; simulating an attentive attitude. Despite being unable to contextualise events and relying upon predefined scripts, when tested upon humans ELIZA (running DOCTOR) was able to fool others into believing they were speaking to a human, noting a "striking form of the Turing's test". Fast forward to today, natural language processing has moved away from simple heuristics, being dominated by machine learning and deep learning, the utilisation of which has cultivated more sophisticated outputs. These advancements have enabled chatbots to understand intent, analyse sentiment and respond in a more dynamic, natural, and human way. Since ELIZA, there has been plenty of chatbots, but the last decades' developments and the demand for mental health services have culminated in a number of these tools developed explicitly for therapeutic reasons. Woebot [252], Wysa [257], and Xiaoice [263], to name the most heavily discussed within this niche. The wealth of options and the variety of supported languages reiterates the demand for mental health chatbots across the world.

A recent review by Kretzschmar et al. compared the initial three listed chatbots [129], the review aimed to spark an ethical debate on its application and looked towards its application with young demographics. Not only are young people more likely to use this technology due to factors such as the digital divide, but a large proportion of mental illness can be accounted for by younger populations [184]. Within the review, multiple barriers within traditional mental health services were addressed, recognising the internal and external factors that impede a solid relationship between human actors. Common, is the fear of rejection, the difficulty of trusting humans in remaining impartial, trusting humans to uphold confidentiality and the perception of inadequacy within human counsellors, factors which are well established within student counselling [246]. A study conducted by [74], found that these barriers appear to be almost non-existent when testing Woebot on 18–28-year-olds, finding a statistically significant decrease in self-reported depression levels when compared to a control group over 2 weeks. Darcy argued its success was due to it being a bot, not despite being one [19]. A statement that is ratified by further studies, one of which finding users were more likely to disclose personal information to a bot than a human [144], and another that found a lack of judgement from bots as an integral quality [17]. Interestingly, the comments provided by participants within the Woebot study, answer the first question. Many of which remark upon Woebot's perceived empathy and personality, choosing to anthropomorphise the bot, calling it a "friend" or a "fun little dude". Clearly, despite the current limitations, the human characterisation highlights the success of AI in replicating empathy and companionship. And whilst neither of these bots have passed the infamous Turing test, a tool for assessing whether AI is indistinguishable to a human, it appears that for some, the disconnection from being 'totally' human, is better than the real thing.

To ask whether empathy is necessary for chatbots is a much more difficult question. The lack of large-scale rigorous studies [73], and the individual differences between each user, make it, at least the moment, incredibly difficult to determine. Whereas no sweeping statements can be made, a study conducted by Liu and Sundar notes that the inclusion of sympathy and empathy were perceived as more supportive than solely given advice [139]. It is important to note that these services do not have to completely replace human-led therapy, especially as bots are still unable to recreate the proficiencies of face-to-face contact with trained professionals, being some way away from human-level responsiveness and empathy. But where these bots lack, they more than make up for providing an accessible route into more traditional methods of help [73], reducing the barriers of accessibility through a variety of languages, their scant use of mobile data [238], and ability to be used in parallel with face-to-face therapy [225]. The use of embodied conversational agents does not stop there, with recent proposals suggesting their use for general well-being and self-reflection for users who have been forced to work from home during COVID-19 [131], highlighting the effectiveness of chatbots within the contexts of diagnosis and care. Before discussing the ethical and societal implications for their use, further avenues can be explored in the emulation of care, more specifically companionship.

4.3 Companionship for the Elderly

Whilst chat and companion bots are equally deserving to be placed within the preventative category, for their general wellbeing qualities, the distinction of care was necessary given its aforementioned absence. As discovered by the human characterisation of chatbots, companionship is one of the areas in which AI can be utilised to provide care, and, when combined with prompts and routines, it is clear to see its application within social care. The requirement for social robotics within this field is all too evident within England. A vast shortage of social workers has been exacerbated by the pandemic [95], multiplied by the continuously low wages within the sector, and its heavy reliance upon migrant workers will undoubtedly prove to be a casualty of Brexit [104]. Like the increase in mental health disorders and the demand for mental health services, the increasing elderly population within England (and the UK) [180], highlights the demand, and market for AI's use within social care.

First, a brief distinction should be made between socially assistive robotics [72], those which are companions and fit the theme of empathy and care, in comparison to those that solely provide physical help. Looking into the market leaders within the socially assistive robotics field, it is clear they offer similar qualities to the mental health systems, daily check-ins, breathing exercises and a personal relationship at the centre of the experience. ElliQ [63], 'a personal care companion' does much of what may be expected within Alexa or Siri, but appears to be tailored to the requirements of social care offering reminders of scheduled medicines and tests and appearing attentive to the users [64]. It would be fair to assume that older members of society would be the least likely to adopt new technology, yet those who lack companionship are incredibly open-minded in the face of automated friends [163]. This unlikely pairing necessitates the development of companion bots to be tuned into the requirements and wants of the elderly, a recent study found that the emulation of human behaviours was paramount, eye contact and the ability to talk [30], were key. The study highlighted the perceived importance of features between the elderly and roboticists, showing the naïve assumptions from developers, some of the most favoured qualities were that of comforting factors, soft fabrics akin to the fur of pets were in high demand. Paro, one of the most notable entries within this field, is just that, a robot designed to look like a baby seal, found to improve social interactions and reduce stress within elderly adults who have dementia [201]. Evidently, emotive bots are suited to the task of companionship, another study [1], testing the humanoid Ryan companion bot [59] found that 'Ryan' was able to establish a deep connection between elderly participants, notably boosting the mood of those who were diagnosed with depression. The study concludes with a statement that may appease the worries of human obsoletion, with each participant recognising that whilst Ryan is a great companion, it is not enough to replace human relationships. Even as this technology advances and empathic AI becomes more realistic, this sentiment appears to be steadfast, many experts believing that companion bots will not replace human-led care [163], rather such technologies will fill the gaps that humans cannot, allowing those in care to live more fulfilling, less lonely lives.

4.4 Sex Bots

Tangential to the development of mental health bots and companions, a considerable amount of contention can be noted within the sex bot domain. Like other 'bots', sexbots have harnessed artificial intelligence to empower speech, text, and visual recognition, with aims to provide lifelike qualities [191, 193]. Whilst this section will explicitly focus upon the embodied sex bot with humanoid qualities, it is worth stating that sex bots can exist void of anthropomorphic qualities, as well as function within an exclusively virtual space, or a hybrid with haptic technologies [51]. The level of contention has been garnered through a wide array of factors, most notably the lacklustre ethical guidelines, the focus upon market rather than research, and the highly disputed "psychological aspects" [90]. At its core, the division stems from opposing moral values and the current legally grey areas that permit the reinforcement of detrimental behaviour. It is important to note that AI isn't the cause for many of these issues, many are upheld just by including a humanoid form, but the inclusion of AI is gasoline to the fire. The problems are made increasingly complex through the unavoidable conflation of mental health and sexual health, Matt McMullen, CEO of the company behind the AI-empowered Harmony, suggests that to some, his creations are not simply just sex bots, they are companions [109]. Whether credible or not, the testimonials from their site affirm Matt's point of view [192]; owners of dolls naming them as 'actual girlfriends', with the renowned robosexual 'Davecat', going as far as marrying his doll [23]. The moral issues begin here, whilst the current variations of sex bots are mere simulacrum, akin to animatronic puppets, their inability to hold true emotion does not stop their ability to evoke it in humans [153]. With the onus upon becoming as similar to the 'real thing', sex bots lie within a realm of subscribed deception, setting up a disingenuous one-sided relationship, skewing the reality of sex and companionship alike. Mackenzie highlights the contradiction between wanting an intimate companion and a customised sexbot [147], the two don't appear to pair.

In Kleeman's investigatory book, Kleeman [127], Matt argues Harmony (and sex bots) as a force for good: a therapeutic tool for the bereaved, disabled and socially awkward. Yet, one of the most noteworthy oppositions to sex bots is their inability to solve any underlying issues, treating the symptoms of mental and sexual health, rather than the cause. For example, there is an obvious irony in remediating loneliness through robots, which, as a by-product, will keep the user at home and increase social isolation [68]. A common suggestion, again, highlighted by Kleeman [127], is the use of a sex bot as a training tool for the real world, for users to first become comfortable and confident in themselves. However, AI's ability to learn, adapt and in some cases, be manually controlled, would allow an echo chamber affect, it would enforce confirmation bias and distort the perception of human relationships, all but making this task impossible. This is especially dangerous for users where the line between reality and fantasy has been blurred, a line that will increasingly distort as sex bots become more realistic and responsive through AI. Within this problem alone, a plethora of societal issues can be explored, most notably the male hegemony of sex bots [92], the objectification of women [47], and the reflection of societal issues such as: toxic masculinity, rape culture and the reinforcement of gender stereotypes [247]. Designer bodies and echo chamber AI exacerbate these factors, permitting unrealistic expectations and allowing users to treat 'things' as humans, which may lead, to users treating humans as 'things' [147]. Furthermore, the danger of suggesting sex bots for well-being and mental health issues without the consultation of a trained professional is not only irresponsible, but it highlights the focus upon the market and the user without sound research, especially when it is unproven that intimacy needs can be fulfilled by sexbots [24]. Such statements run the risk of reducing care further, inferring sex bots are to sexual and mental health, the same as anti-depressants are for anxiety and depressive based disorders. If such issues are to be solved, they surely cannot be done so alone without care, more specifically, therapy. Despite the lack of evidence for intimacy, it would be unfair to unequivocally discount its application, further research is required to evaluate its performance in this regard.

Whereas evidence is limited for companionship, there has been a significant investment into its application to treat sexual deviancy, most notably paedophilia. Again, this presents an entirely new moral discussion about whether protecting children from sexual predators, through robot alternatives, is acceptable [21]. Morals aside, the ethics behind this application is logical, equivalent to providing methadone for recovering heroin addicts. After all, paedophilia is a mental disorder that could be treated [9], or at least harm could be minimised through use within a controlled environment alongside psychotherapy. What is worrying, however, is AI's ability to increase the lifelike aspects, it is questionable whether this will help reduce the problem of child sexual abuse or increase it [200]. Moreover, the controlled environment needs to be emphasised within therapeutic child sex bots, not only have these devices been found on sites such as Amazon and eBay [56], but they have also been programmed to simulate rape [89], which is beyond unethical. In the aim to avoid sounding like a broken record, further research is required for the robotic sexual-companion relationship, such research will be integral to inform desperately needed regulation and legislation. To end the discussion of sex robots on an optimistic note, Frank and Nyholm's discussion of loving relationships indicates the dream of robot companionship [78]. Their vision is a world where the love gained from a machine improves the psychological and physical state of the users, who would then, in turn, live more peacefully and improve the lives of those around them.

4.5 Summary and Problems

Frank and Nyholm's view is one of optimism, a utopian world where all are made happy through their robotic companions. Each of these applications highlights how AI does not have to be a cold and calculating computer, to the contrary, they display how people are extremely happy in finding meaning and comfort within their devices; improving their mental health and wellbeing. This, however, in retrospect may turn to be nothing more than blind optimism, beneath each of the empathic and companion-based bots are issues that distort the potential of a happy ending. Returning to Oelschlager's myth of the technological fix, it is apparent that these solutions, putting their unquestionable positives aside, are attempting to solve predominantly social issues with technology, replacing humanity with a machine. On the surface, this statement alone appears to be incredibly callous, the thought of replacing human interaction with a machine is somewhat unsettling. Yet, in the face of the existing issues: lack of carers, poor mental health services, and social isolation, perhaps these AI applications can provide the support that is currently unavailable from society; especially to those on the fringe of communities that may not receive assistance otherwise. Whilst Oelschlager's statement questions the moral implications for companionship bots, one of the worries lies within its deployment, and again, the lack of protections and legislation. Each type of bot has the potential to impact a multitude of vulnerable demographics, people that require further guarantees of safety and protection. Without the expected ethical rigour and legislation, it is unfortunately too easy to see how these protected groups may be exploited. The worry here is that these tools become a business model rather than medical tools, forgoing ethical duties in favour of a market focus. One indication of this can be found within Woebot's deployment on Facebook, where Facebook's policy allows for data sharing with 3rd parties [69]. 3rd parties worryingly include advertisers and partners who offer goods or services, a potential breach of ethics would be gathering data on vulnerable people and marketing goods which could exacerbate their conditions, i.e., alcohol to a depressive alcoholic. Kretzschmar et al. suggest minimal ethical guidelines for mental health applications [129], but these too extend to companion and sex bots; confidentiality, anonymity, transparency and accessible/frequent reminders of the TOS and data policies to ensure users are informed. Privacy arrangements and legislation must be at the forefront of companion and empathic AI, especially when targeted users are the most vulnerable in society, or more importantly when the most vulnerable in society are the product itself [45]. Finally, whilst efforts to protect the users are imperative within each of their respective domains, protecting the product from societal bias is as equally important. Through sexbots the market focus has highlighted a male focus which has unfortunately exacerbated stereotypes of women, developers must ensure both the hardware and software do not become a detriment to the existing societal issues; ethics and gender must be at the forefront of design [90, 247].

5   Cure

5.1   Discovery

The final pillar in the whistle-stop tour of AI-augmented healthcare is the 'cure'. Again, a few liberties will be taken to condense a variety of technologies down into a single category, but each implementation of AI will be assisting in the repair of the human body. Whereas the section upon care focused on how technology may change the fundamental principles of society, cure, at least for now, is much more concerned with how technology can change the individual, improving their health or restoring lost function. One of the most notable applications of AI is within knowledge discovery, and like diagnosis, the best place to start is the beginning. To recap the introduction, Dendral is considered the first expert system, tasked to mimic the decision-making process of organic chemists, aiding in knowledge discovery and hypothesis formation. Dendral is better described as a collection of complementary and interlocking systems, with its fame as the "mother of expert systems" [32] eclipsing one of its core components. Meta-Dendral is the frequently shadowed machine learning system responsible for hypothesis generation, it is interesting to see, despite the dogma between symbolic and cognitive approaches one of the most famous AI systems used both in tandem. To return from the digression, in a self-review of the success of Dendral [71], Feigenbaum noted that machine learning was integral to meta-Dendral and its hypothesis generation, favouring learning of knowledge rather than the process. Feigenbaum continues, noting that whilst Dendral found no application within industry, its success was not limited, discovering new mass spectral fragmentation rules for a chemical family [32], being the first AI system attributed within assisting in scientific discovery. Like MYCIN, Dendral belongs to a different age of AI altogether, yet the goal of automatically generating and testing its hypothesis has remained.

Adam [125], dubbed the 'Robot Scientist', was the first machine to ever discover original scientific knowledge, identifying the function of a yeast gene [232]. As a robot scientist, Adam is programmed to complete cycles of experimentations, the results of which iteratively update the hypothesis or infer a change in the type of experiment. King et al., believes that robotic scientists are equal to human scientists in their capacity for work, the difficulty of scientific investigations being arguably fairly linear. The same team behind Adam later developed Eve [249], an AI system with the same objective, updated to fulfil the need for cheaper and faster drug discovery. In Williams et al., they identify the need for expedited discovery, with new drugs and treatments typically taking more than 10 years to discover and costing billions to develop. Due to the associated costs, many diseases are often pushed aside, yet Eve's ability to screen more than 10,000 molecules a day, enabled this robot scientist to be set upon the discovery of treatments for tropical diseases. Eve would go on to discover triclosan, an antibacterial and antifungal agent present in toothpaste and soaps, as a potential treatment for drug-resistant malaria [28]. Both creations utilise robotics for physical interaction and machine learning to interpret the experimental results, a combination that is much more efficient than the human hand, allowing for more tests and a wider scope of experiments, simultaneously freeing up the human mind to ponder on more difficult problems [143].

In 2018, Fleming assessed the current landscape, observing the emergence of biopharmaceutical companies that are utilising AI's power to rapidly enhance the drug discovery process [75]. Within the publication, many leading figures within the domain were discussed, most notably BenevolentBio, an AI tool that draws in data from a variety of sources, creating representations and relationships between biological artefacts; fulfilled through a cognitive and symbolic partnership [209]. Despite showing the promising applications of AI, Fleming's conclusion is one of uncertainty, highlighting the hype from vested commercial interests, echoing that the truth will be unveiled within the coming years. In a recent report this statement is unintentionally addressed, a review by Savage listing but a few of the many companies harnessing AI for drug discovery [204]. Displayed in Table 1, each entry from Savage's collection shows vast investment, varied problem scopes and the type of product, one of the most notable being Exscientia and Evotec. Evotec is a biotechnology company that has recently discovered an anti-cancer molecule, which is estimated to have taken 4–5 years was done in 8 months utilising Exscientia's AI platform; a platform that was previously discussed by Fleming with its use to locate metabolic-disease therapies. Exscientia's platform appears to be leading this wave, having three distinct

AI-discovered molecules entering trials, with another aimed at treating psychosis for those with Alzheimer's and another to treat obsessive–compulsive disorder. Flemings conservative conclusion was well justified given the history of hype within AI, but from Savage's juxtaposing conclusion, it is evident that many now believe that AI will be an integral tool within the design and development of new drugs by the end of the decade, noting the efficiencies to be just too good to ignore. Alongside the biopharmaceutical giants is the now freely available AlphaFold [116], a model developed by DeepMind (Google), that is able to find the shape of a protein from its amino acid sequence. Parallel to the model is a free largescale database containing exemplary protein structures, with the model able to analyse the structure of 98% of the proteins found within the human body and many thousands more from a variety of other organisms. Underpinned by AI, AlphaFold has been heralded as a breakthrough, utilised within COVID-19 analysis [117], and much like Eve, AlphaFold has been targeted towards the forgotten and neglected diseases [49].

Table 1 Financing of AI drug discovery [204]

Company	Date	Headline
Schrödinger	February 2020	Drug discovery software company closes $232 million IPO backed by Bill Gates and David Shaw
Insitro	May 2020	Insitro raises $143 million in Series B funding, to help drive its machine learning-based drug discovery approaches further
AbCellera	May 2020	AbCellera raises $105 million in Series B funding round to expand its antibody drug discovery platform
Relay therapeutics	July 2020	Relay Therapeutics, which focuses on understanding protein motion to design drug candidates, closes $400 million IPO
Atomwise	August 2020	Sanabil Investments co-leads $123 million Series B funding round for Atomwise to support the development of its molecule identification software
…	…	…
Exscientia	March 2021	Exscientia completes $100 million Series C financing, with investors including Evotec, Bristol Myers Squibb and GT Healthcare
Recursion pharmaceuticals	April 2021	Recursion completes $436 million IPO
Exscientia	April 2021	Exscientia secures additional $225 million in a series D round led by SoftBank Vision Fund 2

5.2 Prosthetics, Implants and Exoskeletons

Although a cure is an overstatement for prosthetics and exoskeletons, their ability to restore function is deserving of a mention and a subsequent shoehorn into this section. The collection of these mobility enhancing technologies enables many disabled people the opportunity to complete daily activities, providing the disabled with the means to remain independent. AI and robotics have shared a long overlapping history, with literature and media perpetuating imagery of the automaton, cyborgs, and the dreaded terminator. Their mutual partnership has been spurred on by the advancements across the board of technology, with some of the same advanced sensors that were discussed in personalised preventative healthcare lying at the core of modern robotics. One of the partnerships between AI and robotics within healthcare is that of prosthetics. Highlighting the potential for technology to restore lost function is the number of people living with limb amputation, in 2017 this was found to be 57.7 million people [154]. Many prosthetic solutions have been developed without AI, but as discussed, the prevalence of data-rich sensors and machine learnings ability to handle large quantities of data, an obvious partnership exists. Electromyography, commonly abbreviated to EMG, measures the electrical activity in response to muscle stimulation from the brain, a simple and fun demonstration of EMG's power can be found with Gage's TED talk [82], a demo where one human can control another's arm.

The same notion can be carried forward to prosthetics, where instead of controlling another, the processed signals motivate some combinations of actions that modify motors. Researchers from Aston University recently utilised the Myo Armband [7] to develop a voting machine learning classifier that was able to classify 4 gestures in real-time from EMG data [57]. Although the research was targeted towards human–computer interaction, it is clear to see its potential application as a control for the prosthetic components, classifications determining prosthetic poses. A notable, yet understandable limitation within the paper is the requirement for calibration, with each user having slight individual differences, however, once the calibration process was completed, the model's performance increased from 68 to 92%. Unlike prosthetics which function as a replacement for a body part, exoskeletons exist to augment or restore human performance, being wearables that support the human body. Much like a prosthetic, exoskeletons can provide functionality that may be unachievable otherwise, equally promoting independence for those who lack mobility. Where exoskeletons differ, is their potential breadth of application across multiple industries for non-disabled and disabled alike [29]. AI is frequently at the forefront of exoskeletons, and its use as a rehabilitation tool is one application that makes use of AI [233], an application where the use of AI provides improved results when compared to classical control strategies. As discussed by Joudzadeh et al., the exoskeleton also deserved an honourable mention within the prevention section, highlighting many tools that were intended to provide support as a preventative measure against injuries during heavy lifting.

A majority of research has been aimed towards amplifying signals, stronger signals inferring reduced noise, which in turn allows for more precise and fine motor control. In a recent publication, a new method to control prosthetics was discussed, this technique utilised a regenerative peripheral nerve interface, a process where small pieces of muscle are bound to the end of a severed nerve [237]. The boosted signals provide a more reliable method of predicting movement in real-time, there is, however, a key limitation. The current method requires the user to be close to a computer due to the difficulty and expense when using intramuscular EMG technologies (implants). Tech implants is another field where AI will likely rear its head, completing its function locally with its sensors at the edge, rather than at a desktop or through the cloud. A variety of interesting implants are gaining popularity, likely the most hyped would be Neuralink, an implant that gets closer to the source (brain) than non-invasive EEG [170]. Although nothing has been declared of how brain data will be decoded, it is quite probable that due to the large quantities of data, a machine learning algorithm would be employed. Neuralink and Musk have made a variety of claims which make this an interesting technology to discuss, statements of curing depression and addiction [50], curing blindness [194] and again, the ability to control prosthetics. These bold claims are mockingly called "neuroscience theatre" [194], building expectations that are incredibly hard to live up to, yet the partnership between AI and a brain-computer interface has already established control over a wheelchair [149]. Neuralink and other brain-computer interfaces have been posed as technologies that can enact a technological utopia [218], however, issues over privacy and security, with direct access to brain data, make this a much more worrying area, even in the face of its supposed applications.

For an amputee, prostheses are not only a crucial tool to restore an integral human function, but often they are requested due to the stigma behind physical disabilities [196], a stigma that unfortunately remains within the current culture [20], but here in lies a problem. Each of the discussed applications that are aimed to provide mobility is designed to change the individual and not the environment [211], often treating disabilities as a project to cure or fix. Shew argues that in spite of the good intentions of technologists, the rhetoric of being liberated from a disability causes more damage than good, enforcing ableism and detracting from social issues such as wheelchair accessibility. This is an issue that is discussed within care, techno solutionism can enforce bias and de-humanise the disabled and the elderly, reinforcing stigmas of the 'normal' body and mind. Shew argues that many of these solutions are born from convenience, convenience not for the targeted user but all others, an idea validated by the discussed lack of user-centric design for companion bots. It is an uncomfortable position to discuss, the blind optimism of many good-intentioned developers has got ahead of itself, ultimately hindering the communities that they claim to serve. The language of many articles and reports is the most damning, reinforcing ableist tropes and an unrealistic vision of supercrips [77]. To inject some personal bias, the belief is held that it is important to consider qualia, the qualitative properties of an experience. Many experiences are informed through sensory stimulation like touch, sight, and sound, as such, 'solving' a problem that enables another to achieve a more fulfilling experience is believed to be a noble goal. Evidentially, a balance must be struck, such technologies will undoubtedly cost a small fortune, they will do little to eradicate stigmas around disability, and they will also take the limelight away from more pressing issues such as the lack of accessibility.

6 Conclusion

This chapter aimed to discuss the areas that often go overlooked within media, the malignance at the root of AI and AI research, that if left to fester will undoubtedly do more harm than good. It is important that whilst the opportunity exists, actions are taken to remedy the ailments of AI, to wrangle the questionable practices, to ensure medical data is sanitary, and to observe the bigger societal pictures. Not many would argue against the statement that "AI has revolutionised healthcare", augmenting existing practices and discovering new methods of diagnosis and treatment entirely, truly the technological representation of a Swiss army knife. In the face of this, it is difficult to be pessimistic, but it is imperative to remember that AI is in its adolescence. For this, AI commonly breaks rules, does things it shouldn't, all whilst constantly changing, discovering new areas to be adopted into, and adapting to fit established industries at an alarming rate. Herein lies the danger of AI, as a multi-tentacled beast [76], it is incredibly difficult to blanketly define, a quality that makes the development of legislation and ethical guidelines extremely difficult. Naturally, innovation-focused research and media sensationalism has almost mythologised AI, obfuscating the reality, bringing about a disconnect between the perception in public and legislators alike. This is not to say that the developments have been useless, with many stakeholders benefitting from a higher quality of treatment, with AI providing avenues of care that were not possible before. As discussed throughout, many of the issues are grounded in the lack of considerations for the who's, where's and why's of AI, the motivations for its use, and the morals and ethics that guide its application. Many solutions appear to be developed out of convenience rather than necessity, forgoing user-centric design and overlooking clinical testing as a form of expediated research. These are the cancerous qualities behind AI-driven healthcare, and whilst this chapter does not intend to be overly critical of AI, with many of the discussed solutions granting an optimistic outlook, it is this same optimism that will otherwise blind the world to a dangerous future.

References

1. Abdollahi H, Mollahosseini A, Lane JT, Mahoor MH (2017) A pilot study on using an intelligent life-like robot as a companion for elderly individuals with dementia and depression. In: 2017 IEEE-RAS 17th international conference on humanoid robotics (humanoids). IEEE, pp 541–546
2. A.I Act (2021) Proposal for a regulation of the European Parliament and the Council laying down harmonised rules on Artificial Intelligence (Artificial Intelligence Act) and amending certain Union legislative acts. EUR-Lex-52021PC0206
3. Adam D (2013) Mental health: on the spectrum. Nature News 496(7446):416
4. Ahmadi H, Gholamzadeh M, Shahmoradi L, Nilashi M, Rashvand P (2018) Diseases diagnosis using fuzzy logic methods: a systematic and meta-analysis review. Comput Methods Progr Biomed 161:145–172
5. Ahmed S (2018) Credit cities and the limits of the social credit system. AI, China, Russia, and the global order: technological, political, global, and creative, p 48
6. AirQo (2018) About|AIRQO. Airqo.net. https://airqo.net/about. Accessed 17 Aug 2021
7. Aleem IS, Ataee P, Lake S (2019) Systems, devices, and methods for wearable electronic devices as state machines. U.S. Patent 10,199,008
8. All Party Parliamentary Group for Longevity (2020) The health of the nation: a strategy for healthier longer lives
9. American Psychiatric Association (2013) Diagnostic and statistical manual of mental disorders: DSM-5, 5th edn. American Psychiatric Publishing, Washington, DC
10. Amodei D, Hernandez D, Sastry G, Clark J, Brockman G, Sutskever I (2019) AI and Compute. OpenAI. https://openai.com/blog/ai-and-compute/. Accessed 13 Aug 2021
11. Anderson JK, Howarth E, Vainre M, Jones P, Humphrey A (2017) A scoping literature review of service-level barriers for access and engagement with mental health services for children and young people
12. Ansari AQ, Gupta NK (2011) Automated diagnosis of coronary heart disease using neuro-fuzzy integrated system. In: 2011 world congress on information and communication technologies. IEEE, pp 1379–1384
13. Arevian AC, Bone D, Malandrakis N, Martinez VR, Wells KB, Miklowitz DJ, Narayanan S (2020) Clinical state tracking in serious mental illness through computational analysis of speech. PLoS One 15(1):e0225695
14. Armstrong S (2017) Data, data everywhere: the challenges of personalised medicine. BMJ 359
15. ArSène S (2019) China's social credit system: a chimera with real claws. Institut français des relations internationales
16. Awotunde JB, Matiluko OE, Fatai OW (2014) Medical diagnosis system using fuzzy logic. African Journal of Computing & ICT 7(2):99–106
17. Bae Brandtzæg PB, Skjuve M, Kristoffer Dysthe KK, Følstad A (2021) When the social becomes non-human: young people's perception of social support in Chatbots. In: Proceedings of the 2021 CHI conference on human factors in computing systems, pp 1–13
18. Banerjee I, Bhimireddy AR, Burns JL, Celi LA, Chen LC, Correa R, Dullerud N, Ghassemi M, Huang SC, Kuo PC, Lungren MP (2021) Reading race: AI recognises patient's racial identity in medical images. arXiv preprint arXiv:2107.10356
19. Barras C (2019) Mental health apps lean on bots and unlicensed therapists. Nat Med. https://doi.org/10.1038/d41591-019-00009-6
20. BBC (2020) The witches: backlash over film's portrayal of limb impairments. https://www.bbc.co.uk/news/entertainment-arts-54799930. Accessed 1 Nov 2021
21. Behrendt M (2017) Reflections on moral challenges posed by a therapeutic childlike sexbot. In: International conference on love and sex with robots. Springer, Cham, pp 96–113
22. Baai.ac.cn (2019) Beijing AI principles. https://www.baai.ac.cn/news/beijing-ai-principles-en.html. Accessed 10 Sept 2021

23. Beck J (2013) Married to a doll: Why one man advocates synthetic love. The Atlantic 6
24. Bendel O (2015) Surgical, therapeutic, nursing and sex robots in machine and information ethics. In: Machine medical ethics. Springer, Cham, pp 17–32
25. Bentham J (1791) Panopticon: or, The inspection-house. Containing the idea of a new principle of construction applicable to any sort of establishment, in which persons of any description are to be kept under inspection, etc. Thomas Byrne
26. Berlyand Y, Raja AS, Dorner SC, Prabhakar AM, Sonis JD, Gottumukkala RV, Succi MD, Yun BJ (2018) How artificial intelligence could transform emergency department operations. Am J Emerg Med 36(8):1515–1517
27. Bhatnagar G (2020) Physician burnout. Lancet 395(10221):333
28. Bilsland E, van Vliet L, Williams K, Feltham J, Carrasco MP, Fotoran WL, Cubillos EF, Wunderlich G, Grøtli M, Hollfelder F, Jackson V (2018) Plasmodium dihydrofolate reductase is a second enzyme target for the antimalarial action of triclosan. Sci Rep 8(1):1–8
29. Bogue R (2019) Exoskeletons—a review of industrial applications. Ind Robot 45(5):585–590. https://doi.org/10.1108/IR-05-2018-0109
30. Bradwell HL, Edwards KJ, Winnington R, Thill S, Jones RB (2019) Companion robots for older people: importance of user-centred design demonstrated through observations and focus groups comparing preferences of older people and roboticists in South West England. BMJ Open 9(9):e032468
31. Buchanan BG, Feigenbaum EA, Lederberg J (1968) Heuristic DENDRAL—a program for generating explanatory hypotheses in organic chemistry
32. Buchanan BG, Smith DH, White WC, Gritter RJ, Feigenbaum EA, Lederberg J, Djerassi C (1976) Applications of artificial intelligence for chemical inference. 22. Automatic rule formation in mass spectrometry by means of the meta-DENDRAL program. J Am Chem Soc 98(20):6168–6178
33. Buiten MC (2019) Towards intelligent regulation of artificial intelligence. Eur J Risk Regulat 10(1):41–59
34. Buolamwini J, Gebru T (2018) Gender shades: Intersectional accuracy disparities in commercial gender classification. In: Conference on fairness, accountability and transparency. PMLR, pp 77–91
35. Byrne L, Bottomley J, Turk A (2016) British medical association survey of GPs in England. British Medical Association, London
36. Cao B, Zheng L, Zhang C, Yu PS, Piscitello A, Zulueta J, Ajilore O, Ryan K, Leow AD (2017) Deepmood: modeling mobile phone typing dynamics for mood detection. In: Proceedings of the 23rd ACM SIGKDD international conference on knowledge discovery and data mining, pp 747–755
37. Capacity (2020) Iredell-Statesville shools. https://capacity.com/customer/iredell-statesville-schools/. Accessed 16 Aug 2021
38. Castelvecchi D (2016) Can we open the black box of AI? Nat News 538(7623):20
39. Cellan-Jones R (2020) Uber's self-driving operator charged over fatal crash. BBC News. https://www.bbc.co.uk/news/technology-54175359. Accessed 7 Sept 2021
40. Chen J, Druhl E, Ramesh BP, Houston TK, Brandt CA, Zulman DM, Vimalananda VG, Malkani S, Yu H (2018) A natural language processing system that links medical terms in electronic health record notes to lay definitions: system development using physician reviews. J Med Internet Res 20(1):e26
41. Choi E, Bahadori MT, Schuetz A (2015) Doctor AI: predicting clinical events via recurrent neural networks. arXiv 2015
42. Choi E, Schuetz A, Stewart WF, Sun J (2017) Using recurrent neural network models for early detection of heart failure onset. J Am Med Inform Assoc 24(2):361–370
43. Cleanwaterai.com (2019) Clean Water AI. https://cleanwaterai.com/. Accessed 15 Aug 2021
44. CodeBaby (2021) Home—CodeBaby. https://codebaby.com/. Accessed 26 Oct 2021
45. Cole S (2018) The house unanimously passed a bill to make child sex robots illegal. Vice.com. https://www.vice.com/en/article/vbqjx4/a-new-bill-is-trying-to-make-child-sex-robots-illegal. Accessed 15 Oct 2021

46. Corcoran CM, Cecchi GA (2020) Using language processing and speech analysis for the identification of psychosis and other disorders. Biol Psychiat: Cogn Neurosci Neuroimag 5(8):770–779
47. Cox-George C, Bewley S (2018) I, Sex robot: the health implications of the sex robot industry
48. Crevier D (1993) AI: the tumultuous history of the search for artificial intelligence. Basic Books, Inc.
49. Criddle C (2021) DeepMind uses AI to tackle neglected deadly diseases. BBC News. https://www.bbc.co.uk/news/technology-57582183. Accessed 20 Oct 2021
50. Cuthbertson A (2020) Elon Musk claims mysterious brain chip will be able to cure depression and addiction. The Independent. https://www.independent.co.uk/life-style/gadgets-and-tech/news/elon-musk-brain-chip-neuralink-depression-addiction-a9612931.html. Accessed 30 Oct 2021
51. Danaher J, McArthu, N (eds) (2017) Robot sex: social and ethical implications. MIT Press
52. Dattani S, Ritchie H, Roser M (2021) Mental health. Our world in data
53. Daut MAM, Hassan MY, Abdullah H, Rahman HA, Abdullah MP, Hussin F (2017) Building electrical energy consumption forecasting analysis using conventional and artificial intelligence methods: a review. Renew Sustain Energy Rev 70:1108–1118
54. Davenport T, Kalakota R (2019) The potential for artificial intelligence in healthcare. Fut healthc J 6(2):94
55. Deliberato RO, Celi LA, Stone DJ (2017) Clinical note creation, binning, and artificial intelligence. JMIR Med Inform 5(3):e24
56. Dmitry B (2017) Amazon caught selling child sex robots to pedophiles. News Punch. https://newspunch.com/amazon-robots-pedophiles/. Accessed 22 Oct 2021
57. Dolopikos C, Pritchard M, Bird JJ, Faria DR (2021) Electromyography signal-based gesture recognition for human-machine interaction in real-time through model calibration. In: SAI future of information and communication conference (FICC), vol 2021
58. Doshi-Velez F, Kim B (2017) Towards a rigorous science of interpretable machine learning. arXiv preprint arXiv:1702.08608
59. DreamFace Technologies (2016) Ryan—DreamFaceTech. DreamFaceTech. http://dreamfacetech.com/ryan-2/. Accessed 31 Oct 2021
60. Du M, Liu N, Hu X (2019) Techniques for interpretable machine learning. Commun ACM 63(1):68–77
61. Duan H, Sun Z, Dong W, He K, Huang Z (2019) On clinical event prediction in patient treatment trajectory using longitudinal electronic health records. IEEE J Biomed Health Inform 24(7):2053–2063
62. El Naqa I, Haider MA, Giger ML, Ten Haken RK (2020) Artificial Intelligence: reshaping the practice of radiological sciences in the 21st century. Br J Radiol 93(1106):20190855
63. ElliQ (2018) ElliQ, the sidekick for happier aging. Intuition Robotics. https://elliq.com/. Accessed 30 Oct 2021
64. ElliQ Testimonials (2021) [video] https://www.youtube.com/watch?v=Xzl0zmVtzFA: Intuition Robotics
65. Esteban C, Staeck O, Baier S, Yang Y, Tresp V (2016) Predicting clinical events by combining static and dynamic information using recurrent neural networks. In: 2016 IEEE international conference on healthcare informatics (ICHI). IEEE, pp 93–101
66. European Parliament (2017) European Parliament resolution of 16 February 2017 with recommendations to the Commission on Civil Law Rules on Robotics (2015/2103-INL)
67. Eylem O, De Wit L, Van Straten A, Steubl L, Melissourgaki Z, Danışman GT, De Vries R, Kerkhof AJ, Bhui K, Cuijpers P (2020) Stigma for common mental disorders in racial minorities and majorities a systematic review and meta-analysis. BMC Pub Health 20:1–20
68. Facchin F, Barbara G, Cigoli V (2017) Sex robots: the irreplaceable value of humanity. BMJ: British Medical Journal (Online) 358
69. Facebook (2018) Facebook. Facebook.com. https://www.facebook.com/policy.php?ref=pf. Accessed 27 Oct 2021

70. Farokhzad MR, Ebrahimi L (2016) A novel adaptive neuro fuzzy inference system for the diagnosis of liver disease. Int J Acad Res Comput Eng 1(1):61–66
71. Feigenbaum E, Buchanan B (1994) DENDRAL and META-DENDRAL: roots of knowledge systems and expert system applications. Artif Intell 59(1–2):233–240
72. Feil-Seifer D, Mataric MJ (2005) Defining socially assistive robotics. In: 9th international conference on rehabilitation robotics. ICORR 2005. IEEE, pp 465–468
73. Fiske A, Henningsen P, Buyx A (2019) Your robot therapist will see you now: ethical implications of embodied artificial intelligence in psychiatry, psychology, and psychotherapy. J Med Internet Res 21(5):e13216
74. Fitzpatrick KK, Darcy A, Vierhile M (2017) Delivering cognitive behavior therapy to young adults with symptoms of depression and anxiety using a fully automated conversational agent (Woebot): a randomized controlled trial. JMIR Mental Health 4(2):e7785
75. Fleming N (2018) How artificial intelligence is changing drug discovery. Nature 557(7706):S55–S55
76. Fournier-Tombs E (2021) The United Nations needs to start regulating the 'Wild West' of artificial intelligence. The Conversation. https://theconversation.com/the-united-nations-needs-to-start-regulating-the-wild-west-of-artificial-intelligence-161257. Accessed 1 Sept 2021
77. Fox A (2021) The (possible) future of cyborg healthcare: depictions of disability in cyberpunk 2077. Sci Cult 1–8
78. Frank L, Nyholm S (2017) Robot sex and consent: Is consent to sex between a robot and a human conceivable, possible, and desirable? Artif Intell Law 25(3):305–323
79. Fraser KC, Meltzer JA, Rudzicz F (2016) Linguistic features identify Alzheimer's disease in narrative speech. J Alzheimers Dis 49(2):407–422
80. Freeman K, Dinnes J, Chuchu N, Takwoingi Y, Bayliss SE, Matin RN, Jain A, Walter FM, Williams HC, Deeks JJ (2020) Algorithm based smartphone apps to assess risk of skin cancer in adults: systematic review of diagnostic accuracy studies. BMJ 368
81. Fumo D (2017) Why is everyone talking about artificial intelligence? [Blog] towardsdatascience. https://towardsdatascience.com/why-is-everyone-talking-about-ai-73bab31bf9c1. Accessed 4 Oct 2021
82. Gage G (2015) How to control someone else's arm with your brain. TED Talks
83. Galič M, Timan T, Koops BJ (2017) Bentham, Deleuze and beyond: an overview of surveillance theories from the panopticon to participation. Philos Technol 30(1):9–37
84. Gan R, Liang J, Ahmad BI, Godsill S (2020) Modeling intent and destination prediction within a Bayesian framework: predictive touch as a usecase. Data-Centric Eng 1
85. Gaube S, Suresh H, Raue M, Merritt A, Berkowitz SJ, Lermer E, Coughlin JF, Guttag JV, Colak E, Ghassemi M (2021) Do as AI say: susceptibility in deployment of clinical decision-aids. NPJ Digit Med 4(1):1–8
86. Geis JR, Brady AP, Wu CC, Spencer J, Ranschaert E, Jaremko JL, Langer SG, Kitts AB, Birch J, Shields WF, van den Hoven van Genderen R (2019) Ethics of artificial intelligence in radiology: summary of the joint European and North American multisociety statement. Can Assoc Radiol J 70(4):329–334
87. Gellert GA, Ramirez R, Webster SL (2015) The rise of the medical scribe industry: implications for the advancement of electronic health records. JAMA 313(13):1315–1316
88. Gideon J, Schatten HT, McInnis MG, Provost EM (2019) Emotion recognition from natural phone conversations in individuals with and without recent suicidal ideation. In: Interspeech
89. González-González CS, Gil-Iranzo RM, Paderewsky P (2019) Sex with robots: analyzing the gender and ethics approaches in design. In: Proceedings of the XX international conference on human computer interaction, pp 1–8
90. González-González CS, Gil-Iranzo RM, Paderewski-Rodríguez P (2021) Human–robot interaction and sexbots: a systematic literature review. Sensors 21(1):216
91. Graham S, Depp C, Lee EE, Nebeker C, Tu X, Kim HC, Jeste DV (2019) Artificial intelligence for mental health and mental illnesses: an overview. Curr Psychiatry Rep 21(11):1–18
92. Green RD, MacDorman KF, Ho CC, Vasudevan S (2008) Sensitivity to the proportions of faces that vary in human likeness. Comput Hum Behav 24(5):2456–2474

93. Griffis JC, Allendorfer JB, Szaflarski JP (2016) Voxel-based Gaussian naïve Bayes classification of ischemic stroke lesions in individual T1-weighted MRI scans. J Neurosci Methods 257:97–108
94. Gulliver A, Griffiths KM, Christensen H (2010) Perceived barriers and facilitators to mental health help-seeking in young people: a systematic review. BMC Psychiat 10(1):1–9
95. Hadfield H (2021) Social care facing 'unprecedented crisis' over staff shortages, say officials. Sky News. https://news.sky.com/story/social-care-facing-unprecedented-crisis-over-staff-shortages-say-officials-12395264. Accessed 16 Oct 2021
96. Halevy A, Norvig P, Pereira F (2009) The unreasonable effectiveness of data. IEEE Intell Syst 24(2):8–12
97. Halpern J (2003) What is clinical empathy? J Gen Intern Med 18(8):670–674
98. Hassali MA, Alrasheedy AA, Ab Razak BA, Al-Tamimi SK, Saleem F, Haq NU, Aljadhey H (2014) Assessment of general public satisfaction with public healthcare services in Kedah, Malaysia. Austral Med J 7(1):35
99. Heali AI (2013) Heali AI. https://heali.ai/. Accessed 14 Oct 2021
100. Heary C, Hennessy E, Swords L, Corrigan P (2017) Stigma towards mental health problems during childhood and adolescence: theory, research and intervention approaches. J Child Fam Stud 26(11):2949–2959
101. Heaven WD (2021) Hundreds of AI tools have been built to catch covid. None of them helped. MIT Technology Review. https://www.technologyreview.com/2021/07/30/1030329/machine-learning-ai-failed-covid-hospital-diagnosis-pandemic. Accessed 22 Oct 2021
102. Hirsch EM (2007) The role of empathy in medicine: a medical student's perspective. AMA J Ethics 9(6):423–427
103. Hong K (2019) The complicated truth about China's social credit system. Wired UK. https://www.wired.co.uk/article/china-social-credit-system-explained. Accessed 16 Sept 2021
104. Hussein S (2017) The English social care workforce: the vexed question of low wages and stress. In: The vexed question of low wages and stress, pp 74–87
105. Hutson M (2018) AI researchers allege that machine learning is alchemy. Science 360(6388):861
106. IDC (2021) IDC Forecasts Companies to Spend Almost $342 Billion on AI Solutions in 2021. IDC: The premier global market intelligence company. https://www.idc.com/getdoc.jsp?containerId=prUS48127321&utm_campaign=The%20Batch&utm_medium=email&_hsmi=157374105&_hsenc=p2ANqtz-9c4N0DkhhYIyl0CDasc2XgHHcQ2ZXvvPITZ13Xfg2KpHQWiOQh-luSPxkRhQOHFPQ0rZJSbh3bvwwOxP11exsctUnqSg&utm_content=157368283. Accessed 3 Oct 2021
107. Imo UO (2017) Burnout and psychiatric morbidity among doctors in the UK: a systematic literature review of prevalence and associated factors. BJPsych Bull 41(4):197–204
108. IndustryARC (2020) Haptics Technology—Forecast(2021–2026). https://www.industryarc.com/Report/15411/haptics-technology-market.html#:~:text=The%20global%20haptic%20technology%20market,the%20year%202017%20to%202022. Accessed 5 Mar 2021
109. Interview with Realdoll founder and CEO Matt McMullen at CES 2016 (2016) [video] https://www.youtube.com/watch?v=j68yDhUDCQs&ab_channel=Engadget: Engadget
110. Iqbal MZ, Campbell A (2020) The emerging need for touchless interaction technologies. Interactions 27(4):51–52
111. Iroju OG, Olaleke JO (2015) A systematic review of natural language processing in healthcare. Int J Inform Technol Comput Sci 7(8):44–50
112. Isaak J, Hanna MJ (2018) User data privacy: Facebook, Cambridge Analytica, and privacy protection. Computer 51(8):56–59
113. Jiang F, Jiang Y, Zhi H, Dong Y, Li H, Ma S, Wang Y, Dong Q, Shen H, Wang Y (2017) Artificial intelligence in healthcare: past, present and future. Stroke Vasc Neurol 2(4)
114. Jiang Y, Edwards AV, Newstead GM (2021) Artificial intelligence applied to breast MRI for improved diagnosis. Radiology 298(1):38–46
115. Jones N (2018) How to stop data centres from gobbling up the world's electricity. Nature 561(7722):163–167

116. Jumper J, Evans R, Pritzel A, Green T, Figurnov M, Ronneberger O, Tunyasuvunakool K, Bates R, Žídek A, Potapenko A, Bridgland A (2021) Highly accurate protein structure prediction with AlphaFold. Nature 596(7873):583–589

117. Jumper J, Tunyasuvunakool K, Kohli P, Hassabis D, Team A (2020) Computational predictions of protein structures associated with COVID-19. DeepMind website

118. Kashdan R (2020) Six ways urban spaces may change because of coronavirus

119. Kaur S, Singla J, Nkenyereye L, Jha S, Prashar D, Joshi GP, El-Sappagh S, Islam MS, Islam SR (2020) Medical diagnostic systems using artificial intelligence (AI) algorithms: principles and perspectives. IEEE Access 8:228049–228069

120. Keleş A, Keleş A, Yavuz U (2011) Expert system based on neuro-fuzzy rules for diagnosis breast cancer. Expert Syst Appl 38(5):5719–5726

121. Kendall G, Bai R, Błazewicz J, De Causmaecker P, Gendreau M, John R, Li J, McCollum B, Pesch E, Qu R, Sabar N (2016) Good laboratory practice for optimization research. J Oper Res Soc 67(4):676–689

122. Khan J (2021) A.I.'s Wild West moment is ending. Fortune. https://fortune.com/2021/04/27/the-sun-is-setting-on-a-i-s-wild-west/. Accessed 1 Sept 2021

123. Khan SM, Liu X, Nath S, Korot E, Faes L, Wagner SK, Keane PA, Sebire NJ, Burton MJ, Denniston AK (2021) A global review of publicly available datasets for ophthalmological imaging: barriers to access, usability, and generalisability. Lancet Digit Health 3(1):e51–e66

124. Khalil L (2020) Digital authoritarianism, China and COVID

125. King RD, Rowland J, Aubrey W, Liakata M, Markham M, Soldatova LN, Whelan KE, Clare A, Young M, Sparkes A, Oliver SG (2009) The robot scientist Adam. Computer 42(8):46–54

126. Klann JG, Szolovits P (2009) An intelligent listening framework for capturing encounter notes from a doctor-patient dialog. BMC Med Inform Decis Mak 9(1):1–10

127. Kleeman J (2020) Sex robots and vegan meat: adventures at the frontier of birth, food, sex, and death. Pegasus Books

128. Kraepelin E (1921) Manic depressive insanity and paranoia. J Nerv Ment Dis 53(4):350

129. Kretzschmar K, Tyroll H, Pavarini G, Manzini A, Singh I, NeurOx Young People's Advisory Group (2019) Can your phone be your therapist? Young people's ethical perspectives on the use of fully automated conversational agents (chatbots) in mental health support. Biomed Inform Insights 11:1178222619829083

130. Krizhevsky A, Sutskever I, Hinton GE (2012) Imagenet classification with deep convolutional neural networks. Adv Neural Inf Process Syst 25:1097–1105

131. Kun AL, Shaer O, Sadun R, Boyle LN, Lee JD (2020) The future of work and play: from automated vehicles to working from home. New Future of Work

132. Langlotz CP (2019.)Will artificial intelligence replace radiologists?

133. Larrazabal AJ, Nieto N, Peterson V, Milone DH, Ferrante E (2020) Gender imbalance in medical imaging datasets produces biased classifiers for computer-aided diagnosis. Proc Natl Acad Sci 117(23):12592–12594

134. Lee H, Lee EJ, Ham S, Lee HB, Lee JS, Kwon SU, Kim JS, Kim N, Kang DW (2020) Machine learning approach to identify stroke within 4.5 hours. Stroke 51(3):860–866

135. Leibowitz D (2020) AI now diagnoses disease better than your doctor, study finds

136. Lien B (2017) Using AI for food contamination. Medium. https://medium.com/data-science-everyday/using-ai-for-food-contamination-c2e5b47f59e3. Accessed 21 Aug 2021

137. Lighthill J (1973) Artificial intelligence: a paper symposium. Science Research Council, London

138. Lindsay RK, Buchanan BG, Feigenbaum EA, Lederberg J (1993) DENDRAL: a case study of the first expert system for scientific hypothesis formation. Artif Intell 61(2):209–261

139. Liu B, Sundar SS (2018) Should machines express sympathy and empathy? Experiments with a health advice chatbot. Cyberpsychol Behav Soc Netw 21(10):625–636

140. Liu X, Faes L, Kale AU, Wagner SK, Fu DJ, Bruynseels A, Mahendiran T, Moraes G, Shamdas M, Kern C, Ledsam JR (2019) A comparison of deep learning performance against healthcare professionals in detecting diseases from medical imaging: a systematic review and meta-analysis. Lancet Digit Health 1(6):e271–e297

141. Loggins Clay S, Griffin M, Averhart W (2018) Black/White disparities in pregnant women in the United States: an examination of risk factors associated with Black/White racial identity. Health Soc Care Commun 26(5):654–663
142. Low DM, Bentley KH, Ghosh SS (2020) Automated assessment of psychiatric disorders using speech: a systematic review. Laryngosc Invest Otolaryngol 5(1):96–116
143. Lowe D (2018) AI designs organic syntheses
144. Lucas GM, Gratch J, King A, Morency LP (2014) It's only a computer: Virtual humans increase willingness to disclose. Comput Hum Behav 37:94–100
145. Luckin R, Holmes W, Griffiths M, Forcier LB (2016) Intelligence unleashed: an argument for AI in education
146. Lundervold AS, Lundervold A (2019) An overview of deep learning in medical imaging focusing on MRI. Z Med Phys 29(2):102–127
147. Mackenzie R (2018) Sexbots: customizing them to suit us versus an ethical duty to created sentient beings to minimize suffering. Robotics 7(4):70
148. Mahapatra S (2018) Why deep learning over traditional machine learning. Towards Data Science
149. Mahmood M, Mzurikwao D, Kim YS, Lee Y, Mishra S, Herbert R, Duarte A, Ang CS, Yeo WH (2019) Fully portable and wireless universal brain–machine interfaces enabled by flexible scalp electronics and deep learning algorithm. Nat Mach Intell 1(9):412–422
150. Marshall L, Bibby J, Abbs I (2020) Emerging evidence on COVID-19's impact on mental health and health inequalities. from The Health Foundation website
151. Mayes C (2020) White medicine, white ethics: on the historical formation of racism in Australian healthcare. J Austr Stud 44(3):287–302
152. McCarthy J, Minsky ML, Rochester N, Shannon CE (2006) A proposal for the dartmouth summer research project on artificial intelligence, august 31, 1955. AI Mag 27(4):12–12
153. McClelland RT (2017) Confronting emerging new technology
154. McDonald CL, Westcott-McCoy S, Weaver MR, Haagsma J, Kartin D (2020) Global prevalence of traumatic non-fatal limb amputation. Prosthetics and orthotics international, p 0309364620972258
155. McKenzie K, Bhui K (2007) Institutional racism in mental health care
156. Megahed NA, Ghoneim EM (2020) Antivirus-built environment: Lessons learned from Covid-19 pandemic. Sustain Cities Soc 61:102350
157. Metro (2018) Poo found on every McDonald's touchscreen tested. https://metro.co.uk/2018/11/28/poo-found-on-every-mcdonalds-touchscreen-tested-8178486/. Accessed 24 Sept 2021
158. Metz C (2016) The year that deep learning took over the Internet. Wired. December 26, 2016
159. Miller RA (1994) Medical diagnostic decision support systems—past, present, and future: a threaded bibliography and brief commentary. J Am Med Inform Assoc 1(1):8–27
160. Miller AI (2019) The artist in the machine: the world of AI-powered creativity. MIT Press
161. Milne-Ives M, Lam C, De Cock C, Van Velthoven MH, Meinert E (2020) Mobile apps for health behavior change in physical activity, diet, drug and alcohol use, and mental health: Systematic review. JMIR Mhealth Uhealth 8(3):e17046
162. Mistry P (2019) Artificial intelligence in primary care
163. Moine I (2018) For the elderly who are lonely, robots offer companionship. Wall Street J
164. Monker's Garkel (2019) Monker's Garkel, the world. Aigin.io. https://aigin.io/. Accessed 10 Oct 2021
165. Moore, G.E., 1965. Cramming more components onto integrated circuits.
166. Morrell DC, Evans ME, Morris RW, Roland MO (1986) The "five minute" consultation: effect of time constraint on clinical content and patient satisfaction. Br Med J (Clin Res Ed) 292(6524):870–873
167. Mozur P (2019) One month, 500,000 face scans: How China is using AI to profile a minority. The New York Times, p 14
168. Murdoch WJ, Singh C, Kumbier K, Abbasi-Asl R, Yu B (2019) Definitions, methods, and applications in interpretable machine learning. Proc Natl Acad Sci 116(44):22071–22080

169. Neri E, Coppola F, Miele V, Bibbolino C, Grassi R (2020) Artificial intelligence: Who is responsible for the diagnosis?
170. Neuralink (2020) Science. Neuralink. https://neuralink.com/science/. Accessed 1 Nov 2021
171. Ng JH, Luk BH (2019) Patient satisfaction: concept analysis in the healthcare context. Patient Educ Couns 102(4):790–796
172. NHS (2018) MRI scan. nhs.uk. https://www.nhs.uk/conditions/mri-scan/. Accessed 16 Oct 2021
173. Nittas V, Mütsch M, Ehrler F, Puhan MA (2018) Electronic patient-generated health data to facilitate prevention and health promotion: a scoping review protocol. BMJ Open 8(8):e021245
174. Obermeyer Z, Powers B, Vogeli C, Mullainathan S (2019) Dissecting racial bias in an algorithm used to manage the health of populations. Science 366(6464):447–453
175. OECD (2021) OECD Health Statistics 2021—OECD. https://www.oecd.org/els/health-systems/health-data.htm. Accessed 16 Aug 2021
176. OECD (2021) Life expectancy at birth (indicator). https://data.oecd.org/healthstat/life-expectancy-at-birth.htm. Accessed 16 Aug 2021
177. Oelschlaeger M (1979) The myth of the technological fix. Southwestern J Philos 10(1):43–53
178. Ogden J, Bavalia K, Bull M, Frankum S, Goldie C, Gosslau M, Jones A, Kumar S, Vasant K (2004) "I want more time with my doctor": a quantitative study of time and the consultation. Fam Pract 21(5):479–483
179. Oliver D (2019) David Oliver: Does doctors' admin take up too much time? BMJ 367
180. ONS (2021) Population estimates for the UK, England and Wales, Scotland and Northern Ireland—Office for National Statistics. Ons.gov.uk. https://www.ons.gov.uk/peoplepopulationandcommunity/populationandmigration/populationestimates/bulletins/annualmidyearpopulationestimates/mid2020#age-structure-of-the-uk-population. Accessed 30 Oct 2021
181. Qlarity Imaging|Diagnostic AI for Breast Imaging (2019) Qlarity Imaging|Diagnostic AI for breast imaging. https://www.qlarityimaging.com/. Accessed 25 Oct 2021
182. Panagioti M, Geraghty K, Johnson J, Zhou A, Panagopoulou E, Chew-Graham C, Peters D, Hodkinson A, Riley R, Esmail A (2018) Association between physician burnout and patient safety, professionalism, and patient satisfaction: a systematic review and meta-analysis. JAMA Intern Med 178(10):1317–1331
183. Pande V (2018) How to democratize healthcare: AI gives everyone the very best doctor. Forbes. https://www.forbes.com/sites/valleyvoices/2018/05/23/how-to-democratize-healthcare/?sh=1ec5627b2198. Accessed 29 Oct 2021
184. Patel V, Flisher AJ, Hetrick S, McGorry P (2007) Mental health of young people: a global public-health challenge. Lancet 369(9569):1302–1313
185. Pawar U, O'Shea D, Rea S, O'Reilly R (2020) Explainable AI in healthcare. In: 2020 international conference on cyber situational awareness, data analytics and assessment (CyberSA). IEEE, pp 1–2
186. Pesapane F, Codari M, Sardanelli F (2018) Artificial intelligence in medical imaging: threat or opportunity? Radiologists again at the forefront of innovation in medicine. Eur Radiol Exp 2(1):1–10
187. Pimentel D, Cooperstein S, Randell H, Filiberto D, Sorrentino S, Kaye B, Nicklin C, Yagi J, Brian J, O'Hern J, Habas A (2007) Ecology of increasing diseases: population growth and environmental degradation. Hum Ecol 35(6):653–668
188. Plant Jammer (2020) Plant Jammer uses AI recipe technology to make grocery discounting smarter. Plantjammer.com. https://www.plantjammer.com/blog/ai-recipe-tech-discounting-smarter. Accessed 10 Oct 2021
189. Raghupathi W, Raghupathi V (2014) Big data analytics in healthcare: promise and potential. Health Inform Sci Syst 2(1):1–10
190. Rajabi M, Sadeghizadeh H, Mola-Amini Z, Ahmadyrad N (2019) Hybrid adaptive neuro-fuzzy inference system for diagnosing the liver disorders. arXiv preprint arXiv:1910.12952
191. Realbotix (2018) Realbotix. Realbotix.com. https://realbotix.com/. Accessed 29 Oct 2021

192. RealDoll (2018) "RealDoll—the World's finest love doll" Testimonials. https://www.realdoll. com/testimonials/. Accessed 30 Oct 2021

193. Real Doll X (2018) RealDoll X|Robot Sex Dolls|Silicone Dolls Adults|Love Dolls Sex. RealDoll. https://www.realdoll.com/realdoll-x/. Accessed 30 Oct 2021

194. Regalado A (2020) Elon Musk's Neuralink is neuroscience theater

195. Rehme AK, Volz LJ, Feis DL, Bomilcar-Focke I, Liebig T, Eickhoff SB, Fink GR, Grefkes C (2015) Identifying neuroimaging markers of motor disability in acute stroke by machine learning techniques. Cereb Cortex 25(9):3046–3056

196. Richardson SA (1971) Handicap, appearance and stigma. Soc Sci Med (1967), 5(6):621–628

197. Roberts H, Cowls J, Morley J, Taddeo M, Wang V, Floridi L (2021) The Chinese approach to artificial intelligence: an analysis of policy, ethics, and regulation. AI & Soc 36(1):59–77

198. Rolnick D, Donti PL, Kaack LH, Kochanski K, Lacoste A, Sankaran K, Ross AS, Milojevic-Dupont N, Jaques N, Waldman-Brown A, Luccioni A (2019) Tackling climate change with machine learning. arXiv preprint arXiv:1906.05433

199. Rudin C, Radin J (2019) Why are we using black box models in AI when we don't need to? A lesson from an explainable AI competition. Harv Data Sci Rev 1(2)

200. Rutkin A (2016) Could sex robots and virtual reality treat paedophilia. New Sci 2

201. Šabanović S, Bennett CC, Chang WL, Huber L (2013) PARO robot affects diverse interaction modalities in group sensory therapy for older adults with dementia. In: 2013 IEEE 13th international conference on rehabilitation robotics (ICORR). IEEE, pp 1–6

202. Sadeghi D, Shoeibi A, Ghassemi N, Moridian P, Khadem A, Alizadehsani R, Teshnehlab M, Gorriz JM, Nahavandi S (2021) An overview on artificial intelligence techniques for diagnosis of schizophrenia based on magnetic resonance imaging modalities: methods, challenges, and future works. arXiv preprint arXiv:2103.03081

203. Satinsky E, Fuhr DC, Woodward A, Sondorp E, Roberts B (2019) Mental health care utilisation and access among refugees and asylum seekers in Europe: a systematic review. Health Policy 123(9):851–863

204. Savage N (2021) Tapping into the drug discovery potential of AI. Biopharma Deal

205. Schork NJ (2019) Artificial intelligence and personalized medicine. In: Precision medicine in cancer therapy. Springer, Cham, pp 265–283

206. Schwartz HA, Eichstaedt J, Kern M, Park G, Sap M, Stillwell D, Kosinski M, Ungar L (2014) Towards assessing changes in degree of depression through Facebook. In: Proceedings of the workshop on computational linguistics and clinical psychology: from linguistic signal to clinical reality, pp 118–125

207. Scully JR (2020) The COVID-19 pandemic, Part 1: Can antimicrobial copper-based alloys help suppress infectious transmission of viruses originating from human contact with high-touch surfaces?

208. Segal E, Elinav E (2017) The personalized diet: The pioneering program to lose weight and prevent disease. Hachette, UK

209. Segler MH, Preuss M, Waller MP (2018) Planning chemical syntheses with deep neural networks and symbolic AI. Nature 555(7698):604–610

210. Shanafelt TD, Dyrbye LN, Sinsky C, Hasan O, Satele D, Sloan J, West CP (2016) Relationship between clerical burden and characteristics of the electronic environment with physician burnout and professional satisfaction. In: Mayo clinic proceedings, vol 91, no 7. Elsevier, pp 836–848

211. Shew A (2020) Ableism, technoableism, and future AI. IEEE Technol Soc Mag 39(1):40–85

212. Short demonstration of the LANA system (2020) [Video] Directed by R. Lander. https:// vimeo.com/481611406

213. Shortliffe EH, Davis R, Axline SG, Buchanan BG, Green CC, Cohen SN (1975) Computer-based consultations in clinical therapeutics: explanation and rule acquisition capabilities of the MYCIN system. Comput Biomed Res 8(4):303–320

214. SkinVision (2021) SkinVision|Skin Cancer Melanoma Detection App|SkinVision. SkinVision. https://www.skinvision.com/. Accessed 27 Oct 2021

215. Srivastava P, Singh N (2020) Automatized medical chatbot (medibot). In: 2020 international conference on power electronics & IoT applications in renewable energy and its control (PARC). IEEE, pp 351–354
216. Stevenson D, Farmer P (2017) Thriving at work: The Stevenson/Farmer review of mental health and employers. Department for Work and Pensions and Department of Health, London
217. Stringhini S, Carmeli C, Jokela M, Avendaño M, Muennig P, Guida F, Ricceri F, d'Errico A, Barros H, Bochud M, Chadeau-Hyam M (2017) Socioeconomic status and the 25 × 25 risk factors as determinants of premature mortality: a multicohort study and meta-analysis of 1 · 7 million men and women. Lancet 389(10075):1229–1237
218. Stockmeyer J (2019) Neuralink–Are brain-Computer Interfaces leading us into a technological utopia
219. Strubell E, Ganesh A, McCallum A (2019) Energy and policy considerations for deep learning in NLP. arXiv preprint arXiv:1906.02243
220. Susskind RE, Susskind D (2015) The future of the professions: How technology will transform the work of human experts. Oxford University Press, USA
221. Tasnim M, Stroulia E (2019) Detecting depression from voice. In: Canadian conference on artificial intelligence. Springer, Cham, pp 472–478
222. Taylor GM (2010) The physicians of Jundishapur. University of California, Irvine. Sasanika, pp 1–15
223. The Insight Partners (2017) Haptic touchscreen market development report 2017–2025. https://www.theinsightpartners.com/reports/haptic-touchscreen-market. Accessed 5 Mar 2021
224. Tibken S (2018) Questions to Mark Zuckerberg show many senators don't get Facebook. Accessed https://www.cnet.com/news/some-senators-in-congress-capitol-hill-just-dont-get-facebook-and-mark-zuckerberg/
225. Thase ME, Wright JH, Eells TD, Barrett MS, Wisniewski SR, Balasubramani GK, McCrone P, Brown GK (2018) Improving the efficiency of psychotherapy for depression: computer-assisted versus standard CBT. Am J Psychiat 175(3):242–250
226. The Alan Turing Institute (2019) Transforming medicine through AI-enabled healthcare. The Alan Turing Institute. https://www.turing.ac.uk/research/impact-stories/transforming-medicine-through-ai-enabled-healthcare. Accessed 5 Oct 2021
227. The World Bank (2020) Population, total|Data. Data.worldbank.org. https://data.worldbank.org/indicator/SP.POP.TOTL?end=2020&start=1960&view=chart. Accessed 18 Oct 2021
228. Topol EJ (2019) High-performance medicine: the convergence of human and artificial intelligence. Nat Med 25(1):44–56
229. Topol EJ (2019) Deep medicine: how artificial intelligence can make healthcare human again. Hachette, UK
230. Turing AM (1950) Computing machinery and intelligence. Mind 59(236):433–460
231. UK Gov (2018) Prevention is better than cure: our vision to help you live well for longer. Department of Health and Social Care
232. University of Cambridge (2009) Robot scientist becomes first machine to discover new scientific knowledge. University of Cambridge. https://www.cam.ac.uk/research/news/robot-scientist-becomes-first-machine-to-discover-new-scientific-knowledge. Accessed 30 Oct 2021
233. Vélez-Guerrero MA, Callejas-Cuervo M, Mazzoleni S (2021) Artificial intelligence-based wearable robotic exoskeletons for upper limb rehabilitation: a review. Sensors 21(6):2146
234. Villar JR, González S, Sedano J, Chira C, Trejo-Gabriel-Galan JM (2015) Improving human activity recognition and its application in early stroke diagnosis. Int J Neural Syst 25(4):1450036
235. Vincent DR, Deepa N, Elavarasan D, Srinivasan K, Chauhdary SH, Iwendi C (2019) Sensors driven AI-based agriculture recommendation model for assessing land suitability. Sensors 19(17):3667
236. Vincent J (2016) Twitter taught Microsoft's AI chatbot to be a racist asshole in less than a day. The Verge, p 24

237. Vu PP, Vaskov AK, Irwin ZT, Henning PT, Lueders DR, Laidlaw AT, Davis AJ, Nu CS, Gates DH, Gillespie RB, Kemp SW (2020) A regenerative peripheral nerve interface allows real-time control of an artificial hand in upper limb amputees. Sci Transl Med 12(533)
238. Wallach E (2018) An interview with Jo Aggarwal, co-inventor of Wysa. The Politic
239. Walsh F (2020) AI 'outperforms' doctors diagnosing breast cancer. BBC News. https://www.bbc.co.uk/news/health-50857759. Accessed 17 Oct 2021
240. Wang M (2020) China: Fighting COVID-19 with automated tyranny. Human Rights Watch. https://www.hrw.org/news/2020/04/01/chinafighting-covid-19-automated-tyranny
241. Wang Q, Egelandsdal B, Amdam GV, Almli VL, Oostindjer M (2016) Diet and physical activity apps: perceived effectiveness by app users. JMIR Mhealth Uhealth 4(2):e5114
242. Wang Y, Wang Q, Shi S, He X, Tang Z, Zhao K, Chu X (2020) Benchmarking the performance and energy efficiency of AI accelerators for AI training. In: 2020 20th IEEE/ACM international symposium on cluster, cloud and internet computing (CCGRID). IEEE, pp 744–751
243. Watkins J (2018) South Korea's mental health problem–that Koreans don't admit. OZY. Accessed https://www.ozy.com/acumen/south-koreas-mentalhealth-problem-that-koreans-dont-admit/83629
244. Weis JM, Levy PC (2014) Copy, paste, and cloned notes in electronic health records. Chest 145(3):632–638
245. Weizenbaum J (1966) ELIZA—a computer program for the study of natural language communication between man and machine. Commun ACM 9(1):36–45
246. West JS, Kayser L, Overton P, Saltmarsh R (1991) Student perceptions that inhibit the initiation of counseling. The School Counselor 39(2):77–83
247. West M, Kraut R, Ei Chew H (2019) I'd blush if I could: closing gender divides in digital skills through education
248. White C (2017) An overview of lifestyles and wider characteristics linked to Healthy Life Expectancy in England, June 2017
249. Williams K, Bilsland E, Sparkes A, Aubrey W, Young M, Soldatova LN, De Grave K, Ramon J, De Clare M, Sirawaraporn W, Oliver SG (2015) Cheaper faster drug development validated by the repositioning of drugs against neglected tropical diseases. J R Soc Interf 12(104):20141289
250. Willis M, Jarrahi MH (2019) Automating documentation: a critical perspective into the role of artificial intelligence in clinical documentation. In: International conference on information. Springer, Cham, pp 200–209
251. Wirtz BW, Weyerer JC, Sturm BJ (2020) The dark sides of artificial intelligence: an integrated AI governance framework for public administration. Int J Pub Adm 43(9):818–829
252. Woebot Health (2020) Relational Agent for Mental Health|Woebot Health. Woebot Health. https://woebothealth.com/. Accessed 14 Oct 2021
253. Woolhandler S, Himmelstein DU (2014) Administrative work consumes one-sixth of US physicians' working hours and lowers their career satisfaction. Int J Health Serv 44(4):635–642
254. World Health Organization (2018) 9 out of 10 people worldwide breathe polluted air, but more countries are taking action. Who.int. https://www.who.int/news/item/02-05-2018-9-out-of-10-people-worldwide-breathe-polluted-air-but-more-countries-are-taking-action. Accessed 18 Aug 2021
255. World Health Organization (2019) Mental health. Who.int. https://www.who.int/health-topics/mental-health#tab=tab_2. Accessed 26 Oct 2021
256. World Health Organization (2020) Naming the coronavirus disease (COVID-19) and the virus that causes it
257. Wysa (2021) Wysa—Everyday mental health. https://www.wysa.io. Accessed 7 Oct 2021
258. Xiao VX, Xiao B (2018) China's social credit system seeks to assign citizens scores, engineer social behaviour. The ABC, p 2
259. Yang Y, Murgia M (2019) How China cornered the facial recognition surveillance market. Los Angeles Times, p 9
260. Yuan S (2020) How China is using AI and big data to fight the coronavirus. Al Jazeera, p 1

261. Zhang X, Smith N, Webb A (2008) Medical imaging. In: Biomedical information technology. Academic Press, pp 3–27
262. Zhang P, Liang Y (2018) China's National Health Guiding Principles: a perspective worthy of healthcare reform. Primary Health Care Res Dev 19(1):99–104
263. Zhou L, Gao J, Li D, Shum HY (2020) The design and implementation of xiaoice, an empathetic social chatbot. Comput Linguist 46(1):53–93
264. Zinn W (1993) The empathic physician. Arch Intern Med 153(3):306–312

Process Mining in Healthcare: Challenges and Promising Directions

Roberto Gatta, Stefania Orini, and Mauro Vallati

Abstract Process mining for healthcare is the discipline that focuses on mining, analysing, and enhancing real-world healthcare processes. In this chapter, we provide a compelling overview of the research field, and we take the occasion to highlight current challenges and promising research directions.

1 Introduction

Process Mining (PM) is a discipline born in 2011 from the domain of Business Process Management (BPM), officially established by the creation of a dedicated Manifesto [1]. The wider field of BPM is devoted to representing the way (in terms of processes) institutions produce their goods or services, and to measuring performance by considering efficacy, efficiency, abnormal situations, or compliance between the expectations and what happens in the real world. Historically, to analyse processes, the starting point in BPM was a general idea of the process and then the effort focused on trying to understand why, where, (and what) something went wrong in a specific case or what could be improved for saving resources, time, and money. However, the increasing stream of data made available by informative sys-

R. Gatta · S. Orini
Dipartimento di Scienze Cliniche e Sperimentali, Università degli Studi di Brescia, Brescia, Italy
e-mail: roberto.gatta@unibs.it

R. Gatta
Department of Oncology, Lausanne University Hospital, Lausanne, Switzerland

S. Orini
Alzheimer's Unit - Memory Clinic, IRCCS Istituto Centro San Giovanni di Dio Fatebenefratelli, Brescia, Italy

M. Vallati (✉)
University of Huddersfield, Huddersfield, UK
e-mail: m.vallati@hud.ac.uk

tems, in particular in the last decade, paved the way for new approaches in process analysis. For this reason, in 2011 a group of researchers wrote the above-mentioned Manifesto to introduce the concept of Process Mining, where the basic idea is to exploit Artificial Intelligence (AI) techniques to mine processes directly from raw data, without any a-priori knowledge of the existing institutional processes. This approach is promising because by its data-driven nature it is not affected by any psychological bias typical of the human point of view, that is required in traditional BPM as the starting point of the analysis. A process built from scratches only by considering raw data has a higher probability of accurately representing the real-world counterpart, rather than a process that is written by hand from a domain expert, on the basis of her understanding of the process itself. To encompass all the aspects related to the discovery and maintenance of processes, the field of PM can be described by considering its three sub-disciplines:

- (i) Process Discovery (PD), aimed at mining process(es) from data. This is usually performed by exploiting Artificial Intelligence (specifically, machine learning) approaches and a range of representation languages (e.g. Finite-state machines, Petri Nets, ..).
- (ii) Conformance Checking (CC), where a given process and a given set of data are matched to measure if the data can flow through the process or if the process is representative of the provided data.
- (iii) Process Enhancement (PE), where a given process can be enriched or made more representative by the use of an additional set of data.

Conformance checking and process enhancement are also considered by traditional BPM, the main difference lays in the fact that in process mining the starting point is always an automatically mined process coupled with a strong emphasis on automatic AI-based techniques. Among the broad range of application fields for PM, healthcare stands out for the challenges that it poses and for the potential beneficial impact on society that the use of PM techniques can bring. The growing worldwide global spending [17], the heterogeneous level of computerisation among different units within the same hospitals, the abundance of still largely manual activity concerning the resource management (e.g., booking strategies, human resources), and the need for guidelines and protocols and on the other hand, the lack of tools to measure the compliance, are only some of the many facets that suggest a fruitful application of PM in healthcare. Further, there is an additional pivotal point that characterises healthcare in an almost unique fashion: the patient and the biological system. The patient is not a piece of good that should be treated with a sequence of tasks or activities: a patient has a psychological and a physiological dimension which can let her be compliant with a strategic approach or not; she can change her mind during treatment and/or the situation, in terms of caregiving or money, and this can require a radical replan of the strategy. Similarly, adverse events can often happen with or without a clear reason, and the same applies to responses to administered treatments. Further, many decisions are made under uncertainty, by humans, and this can easily lead to suboptimal results, unconventional treatment paths, waste, or even mistakes. To draw a parallel, the scenario in healthcare is like a sort of game, where for each action we have to consider a possible response that should address our next move. This greatly increases the complexity of the possible processes' paths, much more than in a manufacturing industry where the possible responses to manufacturing processes are less variegated and more predictable. Due to the characteristics of the healthcare domain, the PM community redefined the way PM should operate in healthcare, with the definition of a dedicated discipline called Process Mining for Healthcare (PM4H) [43]. Many initiatives such as MOOCs and Alliances[1] have sprung up to share experience, knowledge, methods, tools, and results among the centres working in this area of expertise.

Notably, the intrinsic complexity of the healthcare domain makes it an ideal ground to exploit AT techniques—thus highlighting the potential for PM4H to borrow existing tools and approaches. AI tools are already available in the daily clinical practice in the form of Decision Support Systems, to assist physicians in making decisions about care, balancing costs and expected benefits and risks [46]. For other applications, AI is probably going to play the role of Decision Maker: in tasks such as scheduling, for example, it has shown to have promising performance, limiting the need of human intervention to manage exceptions or minimal changes [18, 24, 25].

In this paper, we present a general overview of the PM4H discipline showing how PD, CC, and PE can be applied in healthcare (in either clinical practice or in management), and then how they have been concretely applied in many clinical domains. Based on that analysis, we then present challenges and perspectives concerning PM4H, such as the integration with electronic health records, process-oriented multicentric clinical study, privacy, and data ownership.

2   Process Mining for Healthcare

This section is devoted to presenting the characteristic of process mining for healthcare by describing how process discovery, conformance checking, and process enhancement have been implemented and specialised for the healthcare domain – taking into account both clinical and management perspectives. Figure 1 provides a graphical overview of the field in terms of input, output, and overall tasks of the three considered aspects.

2.1   Process Discovery in Healthcare

Process discovery (PD) is probably the most innovative contribution of PM, and of course PM4H, on the scene of BPM. The basic idea begins with the concept of Event

---

[1] e.g., https://www.processmining4healthcare.org/ and https://pods4h.com/alliance/.

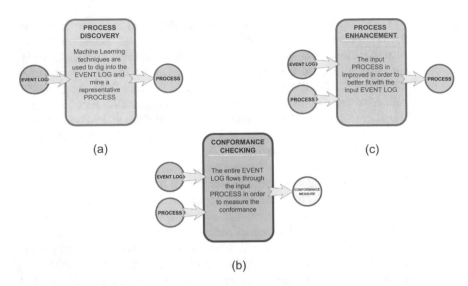

Fig. 1 **a** Process Discovery–a Machine Learning algorithm mine from a given Event Log a model of the real-world process; **b** Conformance Checking–an Event Log and a process model are compared in terms of compliance, to answer questions such as: how many patients properly flow through the given process? How is the process representative of the given Event Log? **c** Process Enhancement–an input Process model is improved by making it more compliant with a given Event Log

Log, composed of traces, which represent the input data format for PM analysis. Let us consider, for example, some events that occurred in the patient's pathway; we can define each event as a triple $<id, date, event>$ where:

- *id* is the Patient Identifier,
- *event* is the event that happened to the patient (e.g., a visit, a disease progression, a drug administration),
- *date* is the date when the considered event happened.

A sequence of *n* triples is called *trace* and can represent the entire set of Events concerning a given patient at different time points. A set of traces, regarding different patients, is called Event Log.

Pragmatically, we could imagine an Event Log as a big excel file with a single line for each Event and with three columns: Patient ID, Event, and Date. Some additional columns can be added, to provide additional attributes (e.g., the values of the LAB exams), but the most basic idea of Event Log can be thought limited to the aforementioned three columns.

The Event Log, which can be obtained for example from an electronic health record [3] or a research database, represents the minimal input for a PD algorithm. The PD system analyses the Event Log and is expected to automatically learn, by leveraging on AI techniques, the regularities in the sequence of events in the traces, which event statistically anticipates another event, if an event debars another event and, in general, the dynamics behind sequences of events. Once fully analysed, this knowledge allows the PD algorithm to build a model of a process which accurately mimics the institutional (hospital, Department, care unit, ..) organisational process on the basis of the given Event Log.

The most representative algorithm to mine a process from an Event Log is the Alpha Algorithm [2]: it allows to learn a process in the form of Petri Nets. Similarly, [54] presented a heuristic approach to generate a dependency graph. Subsequently, a range of tools was created, also leveraging on well-known approaches such as Markov Models [21].

Let us now visualise how a mined process can be represented. We consider an Event Log representing the flows of the radiotherapy palliative treatments from the prescription to the delivery that includes a cohort of 410 treatment plans. Figure 2 shows the corresponding process mined and represented by the well-known Care-FlowMiner [15]. Figure 3 shows instead the result of using a first order Markov Model. Finally, Fig. 4 shows the result of using DISCO, a commercial software for Process Mining [29], on the considered Event Log.

Examples of applications of PD in healthcare can be found in [31], where the clinical pathways of 1,050 patients affected by sepsis, leading to 15,214 events, have been analysed and mined. In [12], 460, 000 events of 30,000 patients treated in an emergency room have been analysed and the mined process has been used to test against performance indicators. In [6], the authors analysed transport pathways discovered across the time-critical phase of pre-hospital care for patients involved in road traffic crashes, on 42,603 patients and 366,754 events. PD can also be used on smaller cohorts, for example the process related to 790 patients who underwent

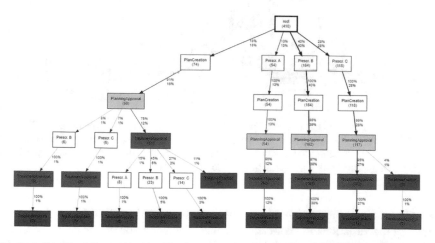

Fig. 2 A CareFlowMiner mined healthcare process. Starting from *root* it shows how the traces are built splitting the path on the different branches of the tree. Each node indicates the step (event) and the number of patients from the Event Log that navigated that node. On the edges, the percentage of patient moving to the following node with respect to the number of patients of the *root* node or of the father node

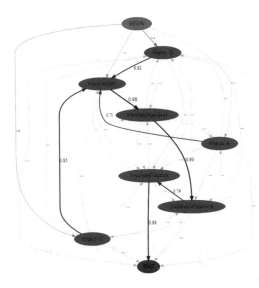

Fig. 3 A First Order Markov Process Model. Starting from *BEGIN* to *END* it plots the graph with the probability to move from a node to another one. Sometimes it is also called Direct Following Diagram and despite the simplicity it is widely used and considered communicative, in particular from physicians

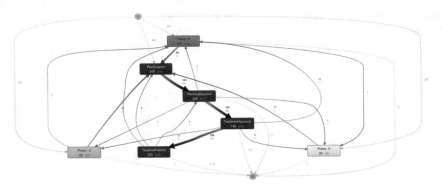

Fig. 4 A process discovered with the Fuzzy Miner [28] algorithm, as implemented in DISCO. It is a Direct Following Diagram where the edges are implemented on fuzzy rules derived from the considered traces. Thresholds are commonly used to limit the so-called *Spaghetti Effects* (the abundance of arcs that makes the graph impossible to be read)

palliative radiation therapy has been successfully mined [51]. In [38], the authors explored the variations in endometrial cancer pathways for 949 patients, from GP referral to first treatment. Finally, [53] has investigated how 184 patients affected by melanoma were treated with drugs therapies (such as immunotherapy, chemotherapy, target therapy) merging PD techniques with the most common statistical tools for survival analysis.

PD can be used for both clinical and management issues. In clinics, PD can reveal unwished or unexpected paths, can show the median and range of time the Institution, in general, requires to move the patients from a state to another state (e.g., from diagnosis to therapy) or the number of patients passing through some states representing critical areas such as treatment toxicities of nosocomial infections. From the point of view of the management, PD can reveal the bottlenecks in the institutional processes, indicating which areas of the Institution should be enforced to reduce the global from admission to dismission or waiting for queue in services (e.g., Laboratory or Radiology). In addition, a mined process can also be used to estimate how the Institution can react to hypothetical future scenarios: simulating a possible cohort of patients or clinical cases as input, the mined process can be used to estimate the effect in the different nodes and test how they can face the stress in terms of capacity. Last but not least, such mined processes can be fruitfully used to test some possible changes in the institution to reallocate the available resources, cut expenses and optimise the spending.

2.2 Conformance Checking in Healthcare

Conformance checking (CC) was initially thought to play an ancillary role, concerning PD, but in Healthcare it opens to some extremely interesting applications. The main objective of CC is to assess if a single event log, or a cohort of event logs, match with a given process model. Generally speaking, it is easy to notice two main uses of CC:

- to evaluate the goodness of a mined process; the input EL works a testing set that can reveal if the process some connections are missing or if the weight, the percentages in the edges reflect the statistics of the incoming distribution.
- to assess, given a process, the quality of the provided EL. Do some patients flow through unwished paths? Does the EL have too many patients passing through a node representing a high toxicity?

The second scenario is of particular interest because it provides a useful tool to check if a given clinical guideline (a medical process for treating a medical condition) [19] is respected in the institution, by the analysis of the data produced in the daily clinical practice (formatted as an EL). This research field was previously called Computer Interpretable Clinical Guidelines (CIGS) and was recognised to be strategic in healthcare since the 1980s [48]. However, the diffusion of CIGS was quite limited and PM4H represents a new opportunity to explore this application field, as documented in [22]. Figure 5 shows a visual representation of how PM4H techniques can be exploited for CC, by providing an analysis of a single trace with regards to a given mined process.

In literature, CC is widely adopted both in association with PD or alone. In [41] the authors measured the adherence of the patient's clinical pathways with the regional

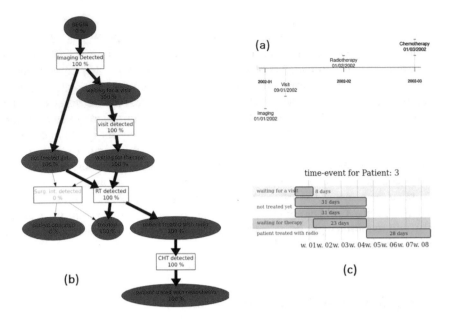

Fig. 5 A conformance checking analysis performed with PWL [41]: **a** a trace for a patient treated for rectal cancer, **b** the workflow. In each node there is the amount of patients, of the entire cohort, passing through that node. **c** how the trace in (**a**) was processed in (**b**): here we can observe how long the nodes had been activated before the end

Clinical Guidelines, for patients treated with Radiation Therapy for rectal cancer. In [34] the authors applied CC to case studies of pathways for alcohol-related illness, giant-cell arteritis, and functional neurological symptoms, and [27] measured the CG adherence for diagnostic and therapeutic events for patients with a diagnosis of stage I–III colon cancer. More in general a review [52] showed how CC was applied in 14 of 71 considered studies and a more specific review in oncology [36] counts papers using CC to measure the compliance with regards to clinical guidelines.

2.3 Process Enhancement in Healthcare

Process enhancement (PE) represents an interesting application field of PM4H and, at the same time, the most unexplored. As described in the previous sections, both PD and CC can provide tools for analysing processes, but they do not provide suggestions to improve the modelled institutional process. They can reveal bottlenecks, unwished connections or latencies but only in terms of warnings and signals that need to be interpreted by humans. PE acts differently, as it is aiming at directly enhancing a process. In particular, given as input an EL and a process, the idea of PE is to improve the provided process by making it able to (better or fully) comply with the input EL. Nowadays, in the healthcare domain PE is mostly performed manually, by humans, based on the results of PD and CC. However, it is easy to envisage a strongly AI-empowered PE, and some hints towards this direction can be found in some well-known neighbouring research fields.

In management, for example, the need to allocate the limited available resources (rooms, modalities, physicians, nurses, technicians, etc.) is one of the hardest challenges to cope with. In many care units, such as imaging departments [24], emergency rooms [30], outpatient clinics [47], endocrine unit [26], nuclear medicine [55], and operating rooms [42] the importance of having approaches to foresee the needs and consequently better allocate available resources is a well known issue. However, most of the aforementioned approaches commonly are focused on a few specific steps and do not consider the whole chain as a process. In this case, a triple composed by a process, an EL, and a set of constraints, rules, and resources for each node can potentially be used, by a PE technique, to simulate the behaviour of different possible processes, measure the expected performance, and propose the best process that should be put in place, in the real world. This can open a new perspective in developing decision support systems, specifically able to propose improvements able to save money, optimise resource allocation or put in place processes able to face stressful situations.

From the clinical point of view, a major application of PE concerns clinical guidelines. Crossing a given CG with a set of traces can easily build a confusion matrix representing the cases compliant with the CG (yes/no) and a dichotomic representation of the clinical outcome (good/bad). Under the assumption that the best CG is expected to have the best accuracy (i.e., the highest percentage of the compliant cases should have the highest percentage of successful endpoint) a PE algorithm might try to autonomously modify the CG (e.g., changing a suggested time in a transition or inserting/deleting a connection) building a new CG* and test the performance of the suggested CG*. In this way, iteratively, PE could propose a CG expected to better differentiate which traces are expected to have good or bad prognosis; in other words to better say which are the most promising pathways that should be pursued. This approach could be of interest in trying to apply a generic CG in a specific hospital, where the local availability of resources, skills, etc. makes the given CG suboptimal with the specific context.

3 Challenges and Promising Directions

Having provided an overview of the PM4H field, we are now in the position to highlight the most significant challenges that need to be addressed to allow a fruitful exploitation of PM4H in the daily practice, and the promising directions where the field can expand.

3.1   Data and Data Sources

A ubiquitous challenge for any computer science-related application to the health-care domain regards data and data sources [4]. The complexity and peculiarity of healthcare data is well-documented [14, 44], and can be summarised in three main aspects: (i) the proper interpretation requires specific considerations and the active involvement of domain experts; (ii) data sources are often heterogeneous (e.g., clinical data, images, biometric measures, etc.) and stored into informative systems not designed to support a process-oriented export (e.g., RIS, PACS, HIS, etc..), and (iii) there is a lack of a common standard to represent and transfer data. In fact, there exists a large number of standards (e.g.: SNOMED, ICD, LOINC, etc..) for data representation, and each provider is usually bound to a specific standard—or can even introduce a new one. There is the need for a standardisation of data and data sources in the medical domain, to foster the exploitation of the immense amount of knowledge that is stored in medical databases. Further, there is also the need for standardising how data is processed and manipulated [56].

In addition to the issues listed above, there is a human factor that can impact the quality of stored data. This is because users, and institutes, have different habits and common practices to complete fields where free text is required (e.g. low toxicities levels are often not compiled, co-morbidities can be interpreted differently, etc.). Issues related to data quality are well known, see e.g., [37, 39, 49], and some methodological frameworks or software tools are being made available to mitigate the specific issue [7]. Considering the PM4H field, there are some approaches proposed to support systematic event log assessment as, for example, DaQAPO [33] in R (Data Quality Assessment for process-oriented data).

3.2   Scheduling and Planning

Global spending on health is growing worldwide [17], and it is expected to grow in the near future. To maximise the use of available resources, there is a growing interest in exploiting AI approaches for scheduling treatments and optimising the way in which processes and operations are planned. General application of PM in the business management context [9, 11, 13] showed the promising role of the synergy between PM and AI in supporting resource allocation optimisation, by analysing existing processes and their actual implementation.

In the healthcare domain, this field is still in its infancy, but some effort has been devoted to designing AI-based approaches for managing Emergency Rooms [8, 40] or for supporting Radiology treatments [25]. The recent successes from the application of PM to business management suggest that there is significant scope and potential to exploit PM and AI synergies also in healthcare however, difficulties in replicating results (due the high heterogeneity of commercial solutions), different information systems lifecycle, high variability of demand, and the many different ways in which services and activities are organised in different departments make this challenge particularly hard to address.

3.3 Patients' Privacy and Multicentric Clinical Studies

The growing availability of therapies, diagnostic tools, methods, and biomarkers is increasing the heterogeneity of the patient's clinical pathways, and supporting a shift from generalised to personalised medicine. In this scenario, among all data-driven approaches also PM analysis requires a growing< number of traces, which can rarely be collected within a single hospital or research centre. For this reason, the use of multicentric clinical studies is expected to become necessary also for process-oriented analysis and this poses a new challenge to the discipline. Patient anonymisation and data encryption are recognised to be weak approaches to ensure the patients' privacy: in many cases, it can still be possible to identify a specific patient or group of patients. For this reason, methods such as distributed learning (DL) are gaining traction. DL can ensure the patient's privacy by design because no data is expected to leave the hospital: the only shared data are aggregated data which cannot reveal any useful information about specific patients. Methods to perform statistical analysis in a DL environment are quite common and well-documented [10, 16] and mostly regards ML algorithms based on convex optimisation problems.

PM still has to be framed in the DL scenario and for the moment only an explorative adaptation of the Alpha Algorithm was proposed for the distributed paradigm [23]. Currently, most of the corpus of algorithms in PD, CC, and PE still need to be adapted to be run safely in a multi-centric distributed ecosystem. However, because the topic is recognised to be crucial, a number of classical methods are being investigated for the PM scenario, such as Data swapping, Noise addition, Suppression, Generalisation, Micro-aggregation, etc. [50].

3.4 Explainability and Understandability

In a recent publication, the Alliance of Process Oriented Data Science for Healthcare identified some *Recommendations for enhancing the usability and understandability of process mining in healthcare* [45]. The authors identified the understandability of the process models, and the way they are extracted from data, as a significant barrier to the exploitation of PM in healthcare. In fact, the problem of understandability is common in medicine: physicians need to fully trust and understand a system they have to use, due to the implications on patients' health. This element is slowing down the deployment of AI-based decision support systems in healthcare, for instance [35]. In Radiomics, for example, a discipline aimed at building decision support systems by means of image analysis, the most widespread modelling tool is still the Logistic Regressor [20], due to its easy to understand nature and interpretability.

Another barrier to the use of PM4H techniques, but also AI in general, is the explainability of the provided suggestion, particularly for CC and PE. Explainability entails the possibility of a physician or a human expert to request explanations for a given suggestion or outcome [5, 32]. In other words, explainability supports an interaction between the user and the system, aimed at building trust and ensuring a correct interpretation of the results.

Understandability and explainability are of course strongly coupled, but they provide a different perspective with regards to the problem of allowing a physician to understand and trust a given system. The PM4H field should focus on approaches that can support both understandability and explainability to ensure their safe and fruitful use in daily practice.

4 Conclusion

In this chapter, we provided an overview of the process mining for healthcare field, and characterised its main sub-disciplines, namely process discovery, conformance checking, and process enhancement. We then presented challenges that need to be addressed in order to support the exploitation of PM4H, and in some cases of AI in general, and promising research directions for the field. In particular, the identified challenges and promising directions are related to data and data sources, scheduling and planning, privacy and multicentric studies, and explainability and understandability.

References

1. van der Aalst W, Adriansyah A, de Medeiros AKA, Arcieri F, Baier T, Blickle T, Bose JC, van den Brand P, Brandtjen R, Buijs J, Burattin A, Carmona J, Castellanos M, Claes J, Cook J, Costantini N, Curbera F, Damiani E, de Leoni M, Delias P, van Dongen BF, Dumas M, Dustdar S, Fahland D, Ferreira DR, Gaaloul W, van Geffen F, Goel S, Günther C, Guzzo A, Harmon P, ter Hofstede A, Hoogland J, Ingvaldsen JE, Kato K, Kuhn R, Kumar A, La Rosa M, Maggi F, Malerba D, Mans RS, Manuel A, McCreesh M, Mello P, Mendling J, Montali M, Motahari-Nezhad HR, zur Muehlen M, Munoz-Gama J, Pontieri L, Ribeiro J, Rozinat A, Seguel Pérez H, Seguel Pérez R, Sepúlveda M, Sinur J, Soffer P, Song M, Sperduti A, Stilo G, Stoel C, Swenson K, Talamo M, Tan W, Turner C, Vanthienen J, Varvaressos G, Verbeek E, Verdonk M, Vigo R, Wang J, Weber B, Weidlich M, Weijters T, Wen L, Westergaard M, Wynn M (2012) Process mining manifesto. In: Business process management workshops. Springer, Berlin, Heidelberg, pp 169–194
2. van der Aalst W, Weijters T, Maruster L (2004) Workflow mining: discovering process models from event logs. IEEE Trans Knowl Data Eng 16(9):1128–1142
3. Achampong EK (2013) Electronic health record (ehr) and cloud security: the current issues. Int J Cloud Comput Serv Sci 2(6):417
4. Altman R (2017) Artificial intelligence (ai) systems for interpreting complex medical datasets. Clin Pharmacol Ther 101(5):585–586

5. Amann J, Blasimme A, Vayena E, Frey D, Madai VI (2020) Explainability for artificial intelligence in healthcare: a multidisciplinary perspective. BMC Med Inform Decis Mak 20(1):310
6. Andrews R, Wynn MT, Vallmuur K, Ter Hofstede AH, Bosley E (2020) A comparative process mining analysis of road trauma patient pathways. Int J Environ Res Public Health 17(10):3426
7. Andrews R, Wynn MT, Vallmuur K, Ter Hofstede AHM, Bosley E, Elcock M, Rashford S (2019) Leveraging data quality to better prepare for process mining: an approach illustrated through analysing road trauma pre-hospital retrieval and transport processes in Queensland. Int J Environ Res Public Health 16(7)
8. Antunes BBP, Manresa A, Bastos LSL, Marchesi JF, Hamacher S (2019) A solution framework based on process mining, optimization, and discrete-event simulation to improve queue performance in an emergency department. In: Di Francescomarino C, Dijkman R, Zdun U (eds) Business process management workshops. Springer International Publishing, Cham, pp 583–594
9. Arias M, Rojas E, Munoz-Gama J, Sepulveda M (2015) A framework for recommending resource allocation based on process mining
10. Boyd S, Parikh N, Chu E (2011) Distributed optimization and statistical learning via the alternating direction method of multipliers. Now Publishers Inc
11. Cabanillas C (2016) Process- and resource-aware information systems. In: 2016 IEEE 20th international enterprise distributed object computing conference (EDOC), pp 1–10
12. Cho M, Song M, Park J, Yeom SR, Wang IJ, Choi BK (2020) Process mining-supported emergency room process performance indicators. Int J Environ Res Public Health 17(17):6290
13. Choueiri AC, Santos EAP (2021) Multi-product scheduling through process mining: bridging optimization and machine process intelligence. J Intell Manuf 32(6):1649–1667
14. Cios KJ, Moore GW (2002) Uniqueness of medical data mining. Artif Intell Med 26(1–2):1–24
15. Dagliati A, Tibollo V, Cogni G, Chiovato L, Bellazzi R, Sacchi L (2018) Careflow mining techniques to explore type 2 diabetes evolution. J Diabetes Sci Technol 12(2):251–259
16. Damiani A, Vallati M, Gatta R, Dinapoli N, Jochems A, Deist T, van Soest J, Dekker A, Valentini V (2015) Distributed learning to protect privacy in multi-centric clinical studies. In: Conference on artificial intelligence in medicine in Europe. Springer, pp 65–75
17. Dieleman JL, Templin T, Sadat N, Reidy P, Chapin A, Foreman K, Haakenstad A, Evans T, Murray CJ, Kurowski C (2016) National spending on health by source for 184 countries between 2013 and 2040. Lancet 387(10037):2521–2535
18. Dodaro C, Galatà G, Grioni A, Maratea M, Mochi M, Porro I (2021) An asp-based solution to the chemotherapy treatment scheduling problem. Theory Pract Log Program 21(6):835–851
19. Feder G, Eccles M, Grol R, Griffiths C, Grimshaw J (1999) Using clinical guidelines. Br Med J 318(7185):728–730
20. Gatta R, Depeursinge A, Ratib O, Michielin O, Leimgruber A (2020) Integrating radiomics into holomics for personalised oncology: from algorithms to bedside. Eur Radiol Exp 4(1):11
21. Gatta R, Lenkowicz J, Vallati M, Rojas E, Damiani A, Sacchi L, De Bari B, Dagliati A, Fernandez-Llatas C, Montesi M, Marchetti A, Castellano M, Valentini V (2017) pMineR: an innovative R library for performing process mining in medicine. In: Artificial intelligence in medicine. Springer International Publishing, Cham, pp 351–355
22. Gatta R, Vallati M, Fernandez-Llatas C, Martinez-Millana A, Orini S, Sacchi L, Lenkowicz J, Marcos M, Munoz-Gama J, Cuendet MA et al (2020) What role can process mining play in recurrent clinical guidelines issues? a position paper. Int J Environ Res Public Health 17(18):6616
23. Gatta R, Vallati M, Lenkowicz J, Masciocchi C, Cellini F, Boldrini L, Llatas CF, Valentini V, Damiani A (2019) On the feasibility of distributed process mining in healthcare. In: International conference on computational science. Springer, pp 445–452
24. Gatta R, Vallati M, Mazzini N, Kitchin D, Bonisoli A, Gerevini AE, Valentini V (2015) On the efficient allocation of diagnostic activities in modern imaging departments. In: Portuguese conference on artificial intelligence. Springer, pp 103–109
25. Gatta R, Vallati M, Pirola I, Lenkowicz J, Tagliaferri L, Cappelli C, Castellano M (2020) An empirical analysis of predictors for workload estimation in healthcare. In: Proceedings of

computational science-ICCS-20th international conference. Lecture notes in computer science, vol 12137. Springer, pp 304–311

26. Gatta R, Vallati M, Pirola I, Lenkowicz J, Tagliaferri L, Cappelli C, Castellano M (2020) An empirical analysis of predictors for workload estimation in healthcare. In: International conference on computational science. Springer, pp 304–311

27. Geleijnse G, Aklecha H, Vroling M, Verhoeven R, van Erning FN, Vissers PA, Buijs JC, Verbeek XA (2018) Using process mining to evaluate colon cancer guideline adherence with cancer registry data: a case study. In: AMIA

28. Günther C, van der Aalst W (2007) Fuzzy mining-adaptive process simplification based on multi-perspective metrics. Lecture notes in computer science. Springer, pp 328–343

29. Günther CW, Rozinat A (2012) Disco: discover your processes. BPM (Demos) 940:40–44

30. Harzi M, Condotta JF, Nouaouri I, Krichen S (2017) Scheduling patients in emergency department by considering material resources. Proc Comput Sci 112:713–722

31. Hendricks RM (2019) Process mining of incoming patients with sepsis. Online J Public health Inf 11(2)

32. Holzinger A, Biemann C, Pattichis CS, Kell DB (2017) What do we need to build explainable ai systems for the medical domain? arXiv:1712.09923

33. Janssenswillen G, Depaire B, Swennen M, Jans M, Vanhoof K (2019) bupaR: enabling reproducible business process analysis. Knowl Based Syst 163:927–930

34. Johnson OA, Dhafari TB, Kurniati A, Fox F, Rojas E (2018) The clearpath method for care pathway process mining and simulation. In: International conference on business process management. Springer, pp 239–250

35. Kundu S (2021) AI in medicine must be explainable. Nat Med 27(8):1328

36. Kurniati AP, Johnson O, Hogg D, Hall G (2016) Process mining in oncology: a literature review. In: 2016 6th international conference on information communication and management (ICICM). IEEE, pp 291–297

37. Kurniati AP, Rojas E, Hogg D, Hall G, Johnson OA (2019) The assessment of data quality issues for process mining in healthcare using Medical Information Mart for Intensive Care III, a freely available e-health record database. Health Inf J 25(4):1878–1893

38. Kurniati AP, Rojas E, Zucker K, Hall G, Hogg D, Johnson O (2021) Process mining to explore variations in endometrial cancer pathways from gp referral to first treatment. Stud Health Technol Inf 281:769–773

39. Lanzola G, Parimbelli E, Micieli G, Cavallini A, Quaglini S (2014) Data quality and completeness in a web stroke registry as the basis for data and process mining. J Healthc Eng 5(2):163–184

40. Lee YH, Rismanchian F (2018) Optimizing hospital facility layout planning through process mining of clinical pathways. Ann Opti Theory Pract 1(1):1–9

41. Lenkowicz J, Gatta R, Masciocchi C, Casà C, Cellini F, Damiani A, Dinapoli N, Valentini V (2018) Assessing the conformity to clinical guidelines in oncology: an example for the multidisciplinary management of locally advanced colorectal cancer treatment. Manag Decis

42. Lin YK, Li MY (2021) Solving operating room scheduling problem using artificial bee colony algorithm. In: Healthcare, vol 9. Multidisciplinary Digital Publishing Institute, p 152

43. Mans R, van der Aalst WMP, Vanwersch RJB (2015) Process mining in healthcare-evaluating and exploiting operational healthcare processes. Springer Briefs in Business Process Management. Springer

44. Martin N (2020) Data quality in process mining. Springer, pp 53–79

45. Martin N, De Weerdt J, Fernández-Llatas C, Gal A, Gatta R, Ibáñez G, Johnson O, Mannhardt F, Marco-Ruiz L, Mertens S, Munoz-Gama J, Seoane F, Vanthienen J, Wynn MT, Boilève DB, Bergs J, Joosten-Melis M, Schretlen S, Van Acker B (2020) Recommendations for enhancing the usability and understandability of process mining in healthcare. Artif Intell Med 109:101962

46. Moreira MWL, Rodrigues JJPC, Korotaev V, Al-Muhtadi J, Kumar N (2019) A comprehensive review on smart decision support systems for health care. IEEE Syst J 13(3):3536–3545

47. Munavalli JR, Rao SV, Srinivasan A, van Merode GG (2020) Integral patient scheduling in outpatient clinics under demand uncertainty to minimize patient waiting times. Health Inf J 26(1):435–448

48. Peleg M (2013) Computer-interpretable clinical guidelines: a methodological review. J Biomed Inform 46(4):744–763
49. Perimal-Lewis L, Teubner D, Hakendorf P, Horwood C (2016) Application of process mining to assess the data quality of routinely collected time-based performance data sourced from electronic health records by validating process conformance. Health Inf J 22(4):1017–1029
50. Pika A, Wynn MT, Budiono S, Ter Hofstede AH, van der Aalst WM, Reijers HA (2020) Privacy-preserving process mining in healthcare. Int J Environ Res Public Health 17(5):1612
51. Placidi L, Boldrini L, Lenkowicz J, Manfrida S, Gatta R, Damiani A, Chiesa S, Ciellini F, Valentini V (2021) Process mining to optimize palliative patient flow in a high-volume radiotherapy department. Techn Innov Patient Support Radiat Oncol 17:32–39
52. Rojas E, Munoz-Gama J, Sepúlveda M, Capurro D (2016) Process mining in healthcare: A literature review. J Biomed Inform 61:224–236
53. Tavazzi E, Gerard CL, Michielin O, Wicky A, Gatta R, Cuendet MA (2021) A process mining approach to statistical analysis: application to a real-world advanced melanoma dataset. In: Process mining workshops: ICPM 2020 international workshops, Padua, Italy, October 5–8, 2020, Revised Selected Papers, vol 406. Springer Nature, p 291
54. Weijters A, van Der Aalst WM, De Medeiros AA (2006) Process mining with the heuristics miner-algorithm. Technische Universiteit Eindhoven, Technical Report WP, vol 166, pp 1–34
55. Xiao Q, Luo L, Zhao SZ, Ran XB, Feng YB (2018) Online appointment scheduling for a nuclear medicine department in a Chinese hospital. Comput Math Methods Med 2018
56. Yang Y, Li R, Xiang Y, Lin D, Yan A, Chen W, Li Z, Lai W, Wu X, Wan C, Bai W, Huang X, Li Q, Deng W, Liu X, Lin Y, Yan P, Lin H (2021) Standardization of collection, storage, annotation, and management of data related to medical artificial intelligence. Intell Med

Computational Intelligence in Drug Discovery for Non-small Cell Lung Cancer

Enum S. Bilal, Mufti Mahmud, and Graham Ball

Abstract Lung cancer is a widespread disease with an incredibly high mortality rate. Hence, identifying drug targets and molecules that drive the disease state is essential. This can be done by identifying drug target pathways for specific genes related to the disease, e.g. the Kirsten rat sarcoma viral oncogene (KRAS). Machine Learning (ML) and Deep Learning (DL) techniques have been used to analyse the pathways. Still, research within this field is scarce, particularly research using sequential data such as The Cancer Genome Atlas (TCGA) and Gene Expression Omnibus (GEO). For this work, open-source ML software, WEKA, has been used to deploy ML and DL methods for the Non-Small Cell Lung Cancer. This focused specifically on the KRAS pathway and utilised TCGA and GEO datasets. The experimentations revealed that the applied methods achieved lower RMSE values for the GEO dataset. Also, networks were derived for both datasets to facilitate the identification of new drug targets.

E. S. Bilal
Nottingham Trent University, Clifton Lane, Nottingham NG11 8NS, UK
e-mail: enumbilal@outlook.com

M. Mahmud (✉)
Department of Computer Science, Nottingham Trent University, Clifton Lane, Nottingham NG11 8NS, UK

Computing and Informatics Research Centre, Nottingham Trent University, Clifton Lane, Nottingham NG11 8NS, UK

Medical Technologies Innovation Facility, Nottingham Trent University, Clifton Lane, Nottingham NG11 8NS, UK
e-mail: muftimahmud@gmail.com; mufti.mahmud@ntu.ac.uk

G. Ball
Medical Technology Research Centre, Anglia Ruskin University, Chelmsford CM1 1SQ, UK
e-mail: graham.ball@aru.ac.uk

IntelligentOMICS, Pennyfoot Street, Nottingham NG1 1GF, UK

T. Chen et al. (eds.), *Artificial Intelligence in Healthcare*, Brain Informatics and Health, https://doi.org/10.1007/978-981-19-5272-2_3

Keywords Machine learning · Deep learning · Lung cancer data · Drug pathway · Network inference

1 Introduction

Cancer is a disease in which abnormal growth of cells takes place within the body [20]. It is an incredibly prevalent disease that contributes to 10 million deaths annually. Due to lung cancer accumulating high volumes of cases consistently, it is recognised as one of the most common forms of cancer. In 2020 alone, lung cancer contributed to 11.4% of cases [57]. Approximately 13% of all lung cancers are Small Cell Lung Cancer (SCLC), and 84% are Non-Small Cell Lung Cancer (NSCLC). Research suggests that tobacco smoking, certain viruses (e.g., HPV), and materials classed as carcinogens (e.g., asbestos) can cause lung cancer, as it promotes the abnormality of cells [21].

Due to cancer's significant impact globally, many professionals have aimed to cure cancer but have been relatively unsuccessful. Although there is no definitive cure for cancer, there are treatments that have the potential to eliminate cancer, although in most cases, these act as a short term resolution. Such treatments include surgery, chemotherapy, stem cell transplant and more. Seeing as cancer is caused as a result of genetic/genomic alterations (such as mutations, small insertions or deletions of the genetic code and alternative splicing (a process in which elements are separated and joined together in a different order to the original)), targeted therapy is a common treatment for cancer. Targeted therapy intercepts the alterations the cancer cells undergo that enable them to grow and develop [30]. This process depends on identifying pathways that contribute to genetic/genomic alterations. e.g. EGFR, KRAS, MET, LKBI, BRAF etc.) and using these to target drugs [24].

KRAS mutations have been of interest within the past couple of decades, as a seminal work by Pao et al. identified its contribution to lung cancer [50]. KRAS is one of the most frequently mutated oncogenes (abnormally expressed genes) in NSCLC. KRAS mutations occur in approximately 30% of lung adenocarcinomas and 5% of squamous cell carcinomas. As it is incredibly predominant and easy to identify, it is a suitable candidate as a therapeutic target [59]. As well as this, KRAS could potentially outperform other pathways such as EGFR and ALK. The pathway for KRAS is shown in Fig. 1 and was adapted from KEGG. KEGG pathways represent the pathway maps based on the interactions amongst the molecules. The KRAS pathway was identified as the part of the 'signal transduction' pathway. Signal transduction represents the binding of extracellular signalling molecules to corresponding receptors located on the exterior of the cell [35]. Signal transduction of mutant genes (e.g. mutant KRAS) has the potential to infiltrate the cell and cause it to become cancerous, hence why the KRAS pathway is of interest.

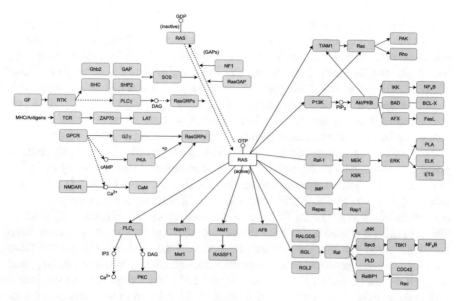

Fig. 1 KEGG KRAS Pathway for Homo Sapiens. Interactions between genes of relevance are presented here. The solid lines represent a molecular interaction or relation, and the dashed line represents an indirect link or unknown reaction. The rounded rectangle refers to other maps. This image was adapted from the KEGG pathway KRAS pathway for homo sapiens [6]

1.1 In Silico Methods of Drug Discovery

A key component of cancer research is the identification of drug targets and molecules that promote the disease state, and this research can potentially lead to a cure being found. Currently, several methods are employed to aid the identification; for example, network inference involves a network being derived from gene expression data for interaction analysis. Despite these methods being deployed, it can be challenging to determine the genes or interactions that have the most significance. In silico methods can resolve these issues. However, its potential hasn't been recognised fully in treating cancer. In silico refers to an experiment conducted on a computer, which has contributed massively to the pharmaceutical industry. For instance, in silico ligand-based methods that involve pharmacophore matching and 3D shape matching have been successful [19]. Another more prevalent method and one that has been recognised by other sectors aside from the pharmaceutical field is ML (Machine Learning). This essentially utilises algorithms to improve its accuracy in predicting results. Machine learning has been used to identify drug targets, despite it being relatively new within the biological field.

The ability to analyse biological data is incredibly important, contributing to progression within the medicinal field. However, there is a slight limitation as biological data can be complex and difficult to process. Thankfully, there has been a significant amount of development within this field due to machine learning and deep learning being deployed. Research conducted by Mahmud et al. studied the applications of Deep Learning and Reinforcement Learning for biological data. Within this work, vast examples of how Deep Learning (DL) and Reinforced Learning (RL) have been used for omics, bioimaging, medical imaging, and (brain/body)-Machine Interfaces are included and their performance. The work also highlights issues such as how existing theoretical foundations of DL need to be improved [42]. Based on the outcomes, it can be assumed that DL performs well and has contributed to higher accuracies being derived. Hence, proving its significance within this sector.

In terms of applications of ML and DL techniques pertaining to the wider range of problem domain, successful outcomes have been reported from anomaly detection [11, 12, 25–27, 38], disease detection [17, 23, 31, 37, 41–43, 52, 53] and smart data analytics [10, 16, 28, 32, 33, 48, 54, 55, 61]. With regards to research in lung cancer via in silico methods, Wang et al. focused on the classification of NSCLC. This research was based on CT images and looked to compare a state-of-the-art deep learning method (convolutional neural networks (CNN)) and four traditional machine learning methods (random forests, support vector machines, adaptive boosting, and artificial neural network). Overall, it was concluded that there was no significant difference between the two types of methods [60]. Ahmed et al. developed a data mining model and then supervised machine learning algorithms for the classification of NSCLC in lung cancer. The classifiers and machine learning methods used were support vector machines, k-nearest neighbour, and decision trees. However, these had an issue of producing a large number of false negatives [8].

Biological data can be divided into three types: images, signals and sequences. Regarding the data discussed previously, they all fall within the images category meaning there are still two other types of data not yet discussed. Another work by Mahmud et al. identified the three types of biological data and how different DL architectures can be applied. For example, TCGA and GEO datasets were identified as a part of sequence data. In addition to this, it also identifies examples of the data, one of which includes the signal transduction pathway study, which was mentioned previously [41]. Hence, the biological sequence data is of significance with regard to this work. This work shows the progression from the previous work by Mahmud et al., as more research has been conducted since the time the previous work was written. The types of biological data have been defined more within this work than in the last one shows how each type of data has its significance. And therefore, more of a focus should be on all data types instead of one in particular, which is generally CT scans. Therefore CT scans shouldn't be considered the primary source of data for lung cancer research, such as the work done by Wang et al. and Ahmed et al.. Research by Bawa et al. was based on sequential biological data, as it focused on reanalysing an existing NSCLC GEO dataset to identify significant genes. This is different from the previous lung cancer research, as it doesn't rely on CT images as a data source. From this research, Bawa, Özkan and Erol were able to determine 10 genes of significance by using only three types of machine learning methods [14]. GEO datasets generally occur within the format 'expression profiling'; this essentially refers to the stage of the sequence at a certain point [45, 63].

However, with TCGA data, which was another dataset mentioned in the 2021 work by Mahmud et al., there are varying types of data available and hence why there is limited research into the different types of data. Research by Dai et al. used the read counts and FPKM (Fragments Per Kilobase of transcript per Million mapped reads) data to determine the genes related to KRAS. Most of the genes identified here were recognised as candidates for further biological experiments [22]. This work shows that FPKM has potential, despite there being limited research. With regards to machine learning with TCGA data specifically, there has been a success with identifying target genes within research by Way et al. This research identified a certain gene that was dismissed by clinical trials as it wasn't considered effective [62]. This research emphasises the importance of using methods other than clinical trials to carry out lung cancer research. In addition to this, it also shows the importance of machine learning, as the work by Dai et al. was only able to suggest genes for further experimentation. In comparison, the research by Way et al. was able to identify a specific gene that has much more potential then the various genes from the other piece of work.

As well as this, deep learning is also beneficial with sequential datasets. Research by Patil et al. has identified the potential of deep learning to classify and predict mutations relevant to KRAS that occur within lung cancer with TCGA data. They were able to compare the accuracy values and show the significance of deep learning. However, it was identified that there was a slight issue with the deep learning identifying all of the targetable mutations [51]. This could be improved by ensuring an effective type of deep learning is selected. Mahmud et al. discussed open-source deep learning methods. One of these was dl4j, and it specified quite a few pros with minimal cons. Hence, the dl4j will be used within this work.

This work seeks to explore further the uses of machine learning methods and deep learning to mine molecular data to identify drug targets and molecules. Intelligent OMICS focus primarily on Machine Learning and AI for in silico biological discovery, specifically regarding the KRAS pathways. The aim will be to use machine learning and deep learning techniques to study NSCLC (Non-small Cell Lung Cancer) data to target the KRAS pathway. From here, networks of selected genes will be derived to determine trends of the gene interactions. The objectives of the work involve acquiring the lung cancer dataset from Public Data Repositories. The datasets selected will be sequential data: TCGA and GEO. It will also involve the implementation of various machine learning algorithms and then tuning the hyperparameters. The objective will also involve implementing deep learning via a dl4j package and then tuning the hyperparameters. In addition to this, the objectives require the network of the selected genes to be derived and to analyse its ability to identify drug targets (e.g. KRAS) and molecules that drive the disease state. And lastly, testing is required to ensure the system is robust.

In contrast, to former research conducted regarding this particular field, there will be more of a focus on RNA-seq data via FPKM. This data will be accumulated from TCGA and exclusively contain lung cancer data. Additionally, two GEO datasets will be used in addition to the TCGA to verify the methods deployed. Based on research conducted previously, the KRAS pathway will be the primary focus of this investigation. WEKA, a machine learning software, will be used to deploy both machine learning and deep learning methods.

This work will further add to research concerning in silico methods for lung cancer data. It focuses specifically on the FPKM values from the RNA-seq data instead of the traditional CT scan research. In addition to this, the work's success can determine whether WEKA is an effective tool for machine learning and deep learning. And can therefore be used as an alternative to hard-coding, machine learning, and deep learning, as hard coding can be more costly and lengthier. By using these methods, the process of identifying drug targets and molecules that drive the disease state will be simplified. This would increase the chances of success within later stages of the drug discovery process, e.g. clinical trials.

2   Methodology and Experimentation

Figure 2 demonstrates the workflow of the work. This section discusses the methods used to collect the data and organise it, ready for feature selection. After the feature selection, machine learning, network visualisation, and the deep learning methods deployed will be explained.

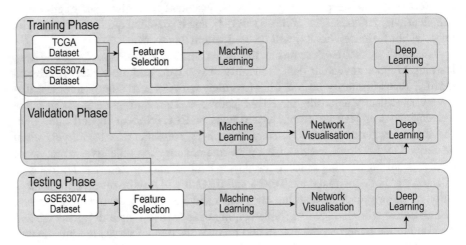

Fig. 2 Workflow Diagram of Experimentation. The process is split into training, validation and testing stages. From the two datasets, TCGA and GSE63074, the different coloured lines represent the split of the dataset. The white line represents the training data, the green line represents the validation data, and the dark blue line represents the test data. The light blue coloured boxes represent stages with results

2.1 Data Collection

Altogether two datasets, one TCGA and one GEO (GSE63074), were used to train the machine learning and deep learning. And then, one GEO dataset (GSE135304) was used to assess the quality of the machine learning and deep learning methods applied in the testing stage.

2.1.1 TCGA Dataset

The TCGA dataset was compiled from the National Cancer Institute website via the GDC (Genomic Data Commons Data) Portal [1]. The data on this website represents all types of cancers. 'Lung' cancer was selected as that was the focus of the investigation. This consisted of 11,000+ cases, making it the cancer with the largest volume of cases. After narrowing down the data selection to lung cancer, TCGA data was specifically selected to remove any other irrelevant forms of data. Primary tumours were applied as a filter to narrow down the results further, as this was the main area of interest for this work; instead of other types of data (e.g., blood samples) being included. No specific disease type was selected to ensure a variety of tumour data was being analysed.

The section of the website used was 'exploration', which enabled the user to filter the data according to the genes and mutations. The data category was filtered to transcriptomic profiling, and the experimental strategy selected was RNA-seq. The FPKM values were selected as the most appropriate file type for the research.

After this, all of the files were downloaded in a zip folder. There was an issue here, as the data needed to be extracted before continuing with the work. 7zip was used initially to mass extract the files, but it wasn't possible. Instead, a batch file was created with adapted code to extract the files in an efficient manner [7].

2.1.2 GEO Datasets

The two GEO datasets were selected from the NCBI website. The results were filtered by the term 'lung cancer'. The study type was set to expression profiling by array, so it was concordant with the data type collected for the TCGA dataset. After this, 'Homo sapiens' were selected as the organism of interest, in order to exclude any other species.

Whilst selecting datasets there were two factors considered; one of these being the acquirement of NSCLC data specifically, as the literature review mentioned identified this as the most abundant form of lung cancer. Also, the GEO dataset was required to contain a high volume of cases, so effective machine learning and deep learning could take place. The most appropriate datasets were selected: GSE63074 and GSE135304. GSE63074 was focused on patients with varying levels of NSCLC [2]. GSE135304 includes data from NSCLC with regards to cancerous nodules [3]. These were downloaded as a series matrix file.

2.2 Data Cleaning

The TCGA data were available in several separate files and were required to be in one file before opening the data in WEKA for the feature extraction. So to resolve this issue, coding was used within RStudio to compile data together by using reduce function and merge function. The code was set up so all the ENSG codes were in one column and the corresponding values for each code were in another column. The code consisted of an application function, a reduce function, and a merge function, and then the data was written to a separate file.

Following this, the ENSG codes needed to be replaced with the proper scientific terms for each code (e.g. KRAS). To resolve this issue, gene annotations that were specific to humans were downloaded from the ENSEMBL gene website [4]. Following this, there was an issue reading the gene names from the ENSG codes as the ENSG codes from the file containing the TCGA data consisted of decimal points. The Ensembl file had no decimal points. The TRUNC function was used in excel to get rid of values after the decimal points to resolve this issue. After this was done, a VLOOKUP function was used in excel to replace the ENSG codes within the file with the gene name.

The process for the GEO GSE63074 dataset didn't require any compiling of data, as it was already available in one file. With the GEO dataset, other files were available that provided more insight into the series matrix data. One of these reported the code names and their corresponding gene names. A VLOOKUP function was used here as well.

Generally, data normalisation would be carried out at this stage, but both datasets already consisted of normalised data. To prepare the data for the next stages, they needed to be filtered, so there wasn't an excess of data, as there were already high volumes of data for both the TCGA and GEO datasets. For this, the two-sample t-test was selected as shown in Eq. 1.

$$t = \frac{\bar{x}_1 - \bar{x}_2}{\sqrt{s^2(\frac{1}{n_1} + \frac{1}{n_2})}} \tag{1}$$

Here, $\bar{x}$ refers to the mean, s refers to the standard deviation, n refers to the sample size and the numbers 1 and 2 represent the two different samples.

In this instance, a t-test (as shown in Eq. 1) was applied to each dataset with two-tailed distribution and two-sample unequal variance to accommodate for the data. This was applied to each of the genes from each dataset. The data was organised, so the lowest p-value was at the top and the largest at the bottom. A cut off point was selected, and the data deemed suitable was ready for the next stage.

The data from each dataset was then transposed using a transpose function within RStudio to correctly format the data and export it to a text file. After this was done, the KRAS column was moved to the end, so it was the last column. This was done to ease the use of WEKA.

To import the data onto WEKA, the excel files needed to be saved as a csv file. So then the csv files could be loaded onto WEKA. Before feature selection, the data needed to be split into the training and the testing data. The 'RemovePercentage' filter was used in the preprocessing section from WEKA's Explorer to get the training dataset. For this work, a 60:20:20 training to validation to test ratio was used. So this was selected within the filter's settings and saved as the training set. And then, for the testing dataset, this was inverted and split into two.

2.3 Feature Selection

WEKA was used for Feature Selection; the Explorer section of WEKA was used for the attribute selection. The data sets required further filtering as there were about 100 genes present for the TCGA and GEO datasets separately; attribute selection was used to reduce the number of genes. The Wrapper method was selected as the feature selection method instead of the Filter methods or the Embedded methods because it identified the optimal genes, which is needed to reduce the time spent on machine learning. When this was carried out it didn't work initially because the algorithm set on default wasn't compatible with this particular dataset. Based upon previous research, the linear Regression was selected as the filter. After this, approximately 30 genes were narrowed down using the BestFirst Search method.

The volume of genes from the wrapper method is too large for the machine learning and deep learning. In order to resolve this, more tests need to be carried out to determine the most significant set of genes among the genes narrowed down from the wrapper method. WEKA's experimenter was the most suited candidate for this, as it enables more personalisation and detailed results being outputted.

Firstly, RStudio was then used to manipulate the data so there were csv files for each of the optimal genes from the feature selection. The main structure of the code was supplied by Graham Ball of Intelligent OMICS. Each of these files consisted of two columns: one of the selected gene and one of the gene who's pathway has been selected (KRAS in this instance).

After this was done the files were imported into the experimenter section of WEKA and a regression was carried out on the files based on the algorithm selected (e.g. Multilayer Perceptron). PCA has generally been used in this stage by other works in this stage but PCA is too linear to be used here. As the data was set using cross-validation there were 10 values for each of the 10 folds, meaning there were 100 values for each of the regression statistics. The correlation coefficient was selected to compare each of the values against each other, as shown in Eq. 2. This was done by calculating the sum of the correlation coefficients for each gene and then sorting it largest to smallest. The top 10 genes were then selected for machine learning.

$$r = \frac{\sum (x_i - \bar{x})(y_i - \bar{y})}{\sqrt{\sum (x_i - \bar{x})^2 \sum (y_i - \bar{y})^2}} \tag{2}$$

Here $\bar{x}$ and $\bar{y}$ refer to the mean, n refers to the number of data points and the numbers x and y represent the two different samples.

2.4 Application of Machine Learning

2.4.1 Training Machine Learning

There was a wide variety of Machine Learning Algorithms applied, this was to ensure a fair representation of the different types of MLMs available in WEKA: functions, lazy, meta, misc, rules and trees. Altogether, 10 Machine Learning Algorithms were applied to the TCGA and GEO data. The process of which these algorithms are run is shown in Fig. 3.

The summary statistics outputted for each of these machine learning algorithms involved the following: Correlation Coefficient, Mean Absolute Error, Root Mean Squared Error, Relative Absolute Error (%) and Root Relative Squared Error (%). Correlation coefficient is a numerical value that measures the correlation, as shown in equation 1. Mean absolute error reports the mean value of errors between instances that provide the same results, Eq. 3 shows how MAE works. Relative Mean Squared error is another numerical value that measures the differences between instances in a sample and is the root squared version of the Mean Absolute Error, this shown in Eq. 4.

$$MAE = \frac{\sum_{i=1}^{n} |y_i - x_i|}{n} \tag{3}$$

Here y refers to the prediction, x refers to the true value, n refers to the sample size.

$$RMSE = \sqrt{\frac{\sum_{i=1}^{n} (y_i - x_i)^2}{n}} \tag{4}$$

Here y_i refers to the prediction, x_i refers to the true value and n refers to the number of data points.

Relative Absolute Error is calculated by dividing the total absolute error by the total absolute error of the actual values. This is shown in Eq. 5. Root Relative Squared Error is the root squared version of the relative absolute error, as shown in Eq. 6.

$$RAE = \frac{|p_1 - a_1| + \cdot + |p_n - a_n|}{|\bar{a} - a_1| + \cdot + |\bar{a} - a_n|} \tag{5}$$

Here p refers to the predicted values, a refers to the actual values and $\bar{a}$ refers to the mean value of the actual values.

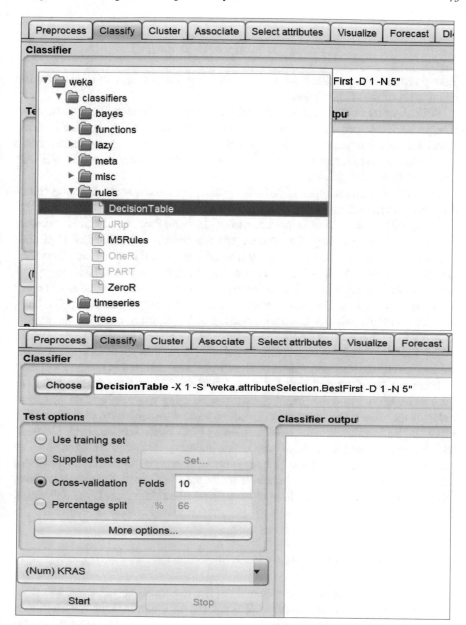

Fig. 3 Screenshots of Machine Learning in WEKA. The first screenshot shows the range of classifiers that can be selected. The second screenshot shows the cross-validation being selected and KRAS being selected as the target

$$RSE = \sqrt{\frac{|p_1 - a_1|^2 + \cdot + |p_n - a_n|^2}{|\bar{a} - a_1|^2 + \cdot + |\bar{a} - a_n|^2}} \qquad (6)$$

Here p refers to the predicted values, a refers to the actual values and $\bar{a}$ refers to the mean value of the actual values.

With all of its algorithms, WEKA enabled to user to adjust the hyperparameters if required. It also provided the user with a short summary of the machine learning algorithm, and if required how it was adapted from pre-existing algorithms. Most of the summaries of the machine learning methods below will be from the WEKA's summary mentioned previously.

Out of the different types of MLMs applied, 5 of them were from the 'functions' section from the classification and regression algorithms WEKA had to offer. The 5 algorithms were Multilayer Perceptron, Gaussian Process, Linear Regression, RBF Network and SMOreg. The Multilayer Perceptron is a classification algorithm that utilises backpropagation to classify instances in an multi-layer perceptron. The Gaussian Process in WEKA implements the typical gaussian process without hyperparameter tuning. The Linear Regression uses the linear modelling approach in order to analyse the dataset. The RBF Network involves the use of gaussian radial basis functions within a network and uses a clustering algorithm to carry out the regression. SMOreg implements a SVM for regression. These 5 algorithms were selected as the 'functions' had the largest amount of algorithms that could be applied to the dataset, and therefore a wide range of algorithms were selected to use on the data.

From the 'lazy' algorithms, IBK was selected which used k-nearest neighbor for classification. From the 'meta' algorithms, Bagging was used and this involved reducing the variance by fitting base classifiers on random subgroups of the data [49]. From the 'rules' algorithms, decision table and M5 rules were selected. Decision table involves a hierarchical table from which higher level tables are broken down by values of a pair of additional attributes to form another table [15]. M5 rules generates a decision list using separate-and-conquer for regression. From the 'trees' algorithms, Random Forest was used which involves a forest of random trees for classification and regression [5].

2.4.2 Hyperparameter Tuning

In order to further improve the values from the hyperparameter tuning was done with the validation dataset in order to decrease the error values. With the Multilayer Perceptron, there was initially some overfitting that occurred as the value for the Root Relative Squared Error was reported over 100%. In order to modify this, the learning rate was changed from 0.3 to 0.2. As for the Gaussian Process, the kernel was changed from a polykernel to normalised polykernel. For the linear regression model, the M5 attribute selection was removed. With the RBF Network the number of clusters was changed from 2 to 10. For the SMOreg, the polykernel was changed into an RBFkernel. The IBK was kept the same as changes to all elements ended up increasing the error values. As for bagging, the REPtree was kept as the classifier but the number of folds was decreased from 3 to 2. Similar to the IBK, both the decision table and M5 rules weren't changed as it lead to error values that were higher.

2.5 Network Inference

Despite the summary statistics from the machine learning being useful, they weren't able to indicate the interactions between the genes, let alone visualise them. In order to tackle this issue, Cytoscape was used to make networks that visualise the interactions the genes of interest had with other genes, as well as interactions they had with each other. The data used to form the networks were derived from the values of node weights from the Multilayer Perceptron that was run during the machine learning stage. Initially, the plan was to only analyse the interactions between KRAS and the selected genes but Cytoscape had a "STRING protein query" available, which could be used to derive another network. This was implemented as it could provide more insight into the data during the analysis stage.

2.5.1 STRING Network

First a STRING Protein network was set up with the appropriate genes. The genes selected were those formed during the feature selection. These were inputted in Cystoscope's "STRING Protein Query", and a network was set up. The majority of the genes were included within the main structure whereas the others were excluded are made smaller structures. These smaller structures were excluded. In order to highlight the selected features, the network was inputted into the software. This was able to detect the level of contribution from each of the genes. As well as this, it was able to highlight key interactions between the genes. The colour scheme was set so the strongest interaction was shown by a bright orange. KRAS inevitably had the strongest orange colour as it was the target.

2.5.2 Interactions between Selected Features

In order to form the network showing the interactions between the selected features, an appropriate network had to be formed on Excel and then imported in. This network comprised of each of the gene names, the absolute value of the sum of the nodes, the target (each of the genes were targets for every gene involved) and whether the interaction was positive or negative. After this was inputted in, the absolute value of the sum of the nodes was used to form the different widths. And the positive and negative was used to determine the type of interaction.

2.6 Application of Deep Learning

2.6.1 DL4J

Deep neural network (DNN) DNN is an artificial neural network with multi-layers
between the input and output layers. The main advantage of DNN is that it can model
complex non-linear relationships. The DNN was developed using the DL4J package
within WEKA, as shown in Fig. 4.

After adjusting the options as shown in Fig. 4, the DNN structure was determined
with the optimum values of RMSE. Figure 5 shows the layers used to form the
Deep Neural Network. The activation layer used Activation ReLu. ReLu is e a linear
function that outputs the input if its positive and outputs 0 if it is negative, so it
essentially screens the data [13]. As for the two dense layers, ActivationHardTanH
and the only difference was that the 1st dense layer had 16 outputs and the 2nd dense
layer has 4 outputs and the 3rd dense layer had 8 outputs. And lastly the output
layer had 1 output. The activation function for this was ActivationHardTanH and the
loss function was LossL1. The overall RMSE with just this structure alone is 4.2575
and 0.3318, for the TCGA and GEO datasets respectively. This is an improvement
compared to the previous value before the dense layers, which were 4.3133 and
0.3179, for the TCGA and GEO datasets respectively.

2.6.2 Hyperparameter Tuning

In order to improve the values of RMSE furthermore, hyperparameter tuning was
carried out, as shown in appendix 10. It was determined the optimum conditions for
the network configuration were the following:

- Updater–Nadam
- Bias Updater–AdaGrad
- Weight Initialisation Method–Xavier

The hyperparameter tuning was able to improve the values of both the TCGA
and GEO dataset. The TCGA dataset changed from 4.2575 to 4.0744 and the GEO
dataset change from 0.3318 to 0.3025.

2.7 KnowledgeFlow

Further investigation was conducted into easing the process that has been used up
until this point. This was investigated, as it could ensure machine learning and deep
learning could be carried out more efficiently and more easily. WEKA's Knowledge-
Flow enables the user to combine components from different parts of WEKA.

In order to set up the workflow on KnowledgeFlow, the CSV loader is inputted
and then the training and testing split occurs with the Remove Percentage filter. And

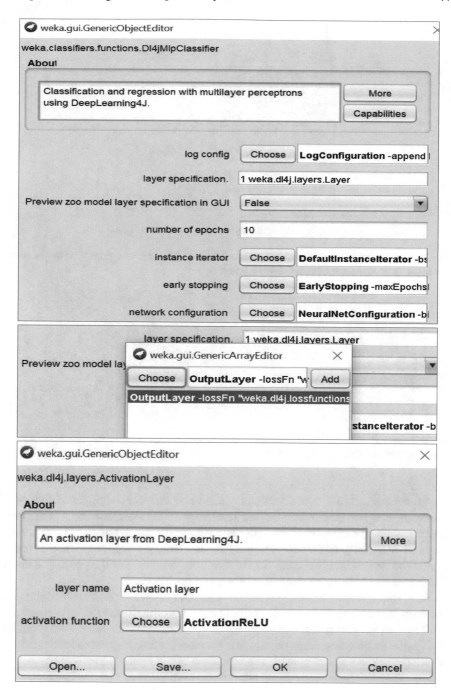

Fig. 4 Screenshots of Deep Learning in WEKA. The first screenshot shows the properties of the dl4j. The second screenshot shows the properties of the layers. The third shows the properties of a specific layer type

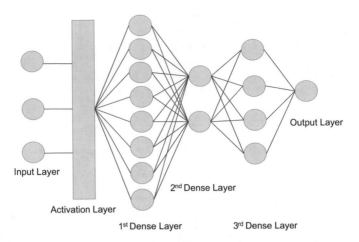

Fig. 5 Deep Neural Network layout. This network shows the input layers up until the output layer. It consists of an activation layer and 3 dense layers

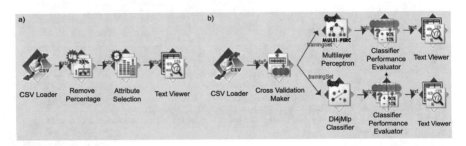

Fig. 6 KnowledgeFlow workflow. The first part of the workflow **a** shows the stages until the feature selection. The second part of the workflow **b** shows the stages after the experimenter stage

then from here, the attribute selection is added and set on the wrapper method and finally the data can be viewed from the TextViewer. This workflow could have been continued for the entirety of the process used for the work but the experimenter couldn't be added to this section as it uses features from the explorer. Hence it would have to be broken into two parts. So the first selection involves the procedure up to and including the feature selection, as shown in the Fig. 6a.

After the experimenter stage would be conducted, then the machine learning and the deep learning could be carried out. These are normally carried out separately but KnowledgeFlow enables the user to use both of these together. As shown in Fig. 6b, the multilayer perceptron, which is the machine learning method and the deep learning, are run simultaneously. The workflow in the figure below was simplified to show only one machine learning algorithm, when many can be run together.

3 Results and Discussion

3.1 Traditional Machine Learning for TCGA and GEO Data

The results of the various machine learning methods when applied to the TCGA and GEO data revealed that the different metrics indicate different methods to perform better (see Table 1). After hyperparameter tuning the results get slightly better (see Table 2), though no concrete method performed well for all metrics. One interesting point to observe here is that, the different datasets exhibit different behaviour when the same method is applied. For the TCGA dataset the Gaussian process showed the least correlation among the features with values 0.4828 and 0.4323 before and after hyperparameter tuning respectively. The SMOreg achieved minimum MAE and RAE with values 2.3417 and 64.3356 (before) and 2.3135 and 64.1945 (after) hyperparameter tuning, respectively. The Random Forest achieved the minimum RMSE (3.6097) and RRSE (67.9603) values which were not affected by the hyperparameter tuning. For the GEO dataset the Decision Table showed the least correlation with value 0.6214 which was not affected by the hyperparameter tuning. Prior to hyperparameter tuning, the Random Forest performed superior for the rest of the metrics (MAE: 0.2011, RMSE: 0.2712, RAE: 51.8023, RRSE: 56.2145) which remained unchanged for MAE, RAE and RRSE but the Bagging performed better than Random Forest in

Table 1 Summary statistics of various machine learning methods for the TCGA and GEO data

ML method	CC		MAE		RMSE		RAE (%)		RRSE (%)	
	TCGA	GEO	TCGA	GEO	TCGA	GEO	TCGA	GEO	TCGA	GEO
Multilayer perceptron	0.621	0.732	3.280	0.260	5.345	0.347	90.106	67.075	100.630	71.951
Gaussian process	0.483	0.770	3.592	0.236	4.771	0.307	98.689	60.846	89.824	63.571
Linear regression	0.717	0.780	2.435	0.231	3.703	0.301	66.895	59.587	69.721	62.335
RBF network	0.522	0.662	2.909	0.279	4.529	0.361	79.925	71.823	85.270	74.725
SMOreg	0.720	0.777	2.342	0.233	3.764	0.303	64.336	59.892	70.861	62.852
IBK	0.559	0.781	3.053	0.229	4.729	0.317	83.885	58.962	89.039	65.782
Bagging	0.659	0.802	2.609	0.220	4.132	0.289	71.672	56.659	77.796	59.853
Decision table	0.571	0.621	2.993	0.285	4.373	0.383	82.235	73.442	82.328	79.449
M5 rules	0.689	0.784	2.473	0.232	3.854	0.299	67.937	59.681	72.566	61.979
Random forest	0.738	0.828	2.404	0.201	3.610	0.271	66.052	51.802	67.960	56.215

Legend— ML Method: Machine Learning Method, cc: Correlation Coefficient, MAE: Mean Absolute Error, RMSE: Root Mean Squared Error, RAE: Relative Absolute Error, RRSE: Root Relative Squared Error

Table 2 Summary statistics of the hyperparameter tuned machine learning methods for the TCGA and GEO data

ML method (TCGA)	CC		MAE		RMSE		RAE (%)		RRSE (%)	
	TCGA	GEO	TCGA	GEO	TCGA	GEO	TCGA	GEO	TCGA	GEO
Multilayer perceptron	0.641	0.725	3.205	0.249	4.725	0.335	90.149	67.025	88.025	71.903
Gaussian process	0.432	0.759	3.557	0.225	4.745	0.300	98.629	60.592	89.527	63.525
Linear regression	0.717	0.776	2.424	0.239	3.693	0.295	66.839	59.425	69.586	62.314
RBF network	0.502	0.645	2.803	0.292	4.563	0.348	79.794	71.783	85.159	74.649
SMOreg	0.691	0.756	2.314	0.202	3.737	0.302	64.195	59.743	70.529	62.249
IBK	0.559	0.781	3.053	0.229	4.729	0.317	83.885	58.962	89.039	65.782
Bagging	0.654	0.801	2.593	0.214	4.023	0.264	71.248	56.644	77.115	59.240
Decision table	0.571	0.621	2.993	0.285	4.373	0.383	82.235	73.442	82.328	79.449
M5 rules	0.689	0.784	2.473	0.232	3.854	0.299	67.937	59.681	72.566	61.979
Random forest	0.738	0.828	2.404	0.201	3.610	0.271	66.052	51.802	67.960	56.215

Legend— ML Method: Machine Learning Method, cc: Correlation Coefficient, MAE: Mean Absolute Error, RMSE: Root Mean Squared Error, RAE: Relative Absolute Error, RRSE: Root Relative Squared Error

RMSE after the hyperparameter tuning (0.2639). One trend that appears evident is that the models perform better in terms of error values in GEO data in comparison to TCGA data.

For the machine learning methods, the RMSE values of the testing were computed based on previous research. The training and the testing RMSE values were added into a table 5 but the difference between TCGA and GEO datasets was more apparent. The Table 3 included the RMSE values for the training with TCGA and GEO datasets and the testing for TCGA and GEO datasets for two variants (GSE63074 and GSE135304), where the last one is the new dataset.

When comparing the tests with each other, the TCGA and the GEO relevant data were kept separate. This was due to the TCGA reporting significantly higher values of RMSE, and GEO reporting less, hence meaning it would be difficult to interpret the GEO data. As shown in Fig. 7, the RMSE of the TCGA training reported higher than the TCGA testing. This is due to the testing dataset being much smaller so than the training dataset, so there is more room for error. Figure 8 shows the comparison

Table 3 RMSE values of machine learning methods during training and testing

ML method	Training		Test		
	TCGA	GEO	TCGA	GEO	
				GSE63074	GSE135304
Multilayer perceptron	4.72	0.33	5.32	0.42	0.22
Gaussian process	4.75	0.30	5.29	0.49	0.22
Linear regression model	3.69	0.29	4.70	0.42	0.21
RBF network	4.56	0.35	5.95	0.52	0.26
SMOreg	3.74	0.30	4.29	0.49	0.20
IBK	4.73	0.32	5.73	0.48	0.21
Bagging	4.02	0.26	5.52	0.47	0.15
Decision table	4.37	0.38	5.37	0.53	0.22
M5 rules	3.85	0.30	4.55	0.42	0.20
Random forest	3.61	0.27	4.30	0.42	0.19

between the RMSE values of the GEO Training, Testing and New dataset. The RMSE of the GEO training reported higher than the GEO testing. This is due to the testing dataset being much smaller so than the training dataset, so there is more room for error. On the other hand, however, the new dataset has much lower RMSE values compared to the training and testing. This is because the new dataset had less error in comparison to the former dataset, due to hyperparameterisation of the machine learning. This shows that the hyperparameterisation of machine learning was very efficient.

3.1.1 Discussion of Machine Learning Methods Deployed

Machine learning within WEKA to study TCGA and GEO lung cancer data has been incredibly useful. The vast range of machine learning methods available meant that several machine learning algorithms could be analysed, as opposed to alternative methods that would be much more time consuming. Despite this, the values reported as a result of the regression analysis were quite high. This was more prevalent in the TCGA data, and this was most likely due to the TCGA data being a lot more complex prior to the feature selection and data cleaning. As well as this, the hyperparameter tuning appeared to be successful as the values of RMSE decreased after this process was done.

In order to determine the machine learning methods with the most potential, one specific numerical value would need to be used to compare the algorithms to each

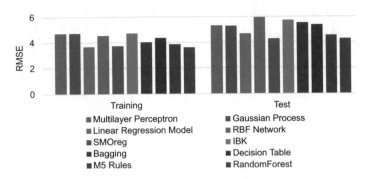

Fig. 7 Comparison of TCGA Training and Testing RMSE values. This graph represents the TCGA datasets, these are split into two, training and testing. For each of these the machine learning methods used are deployed

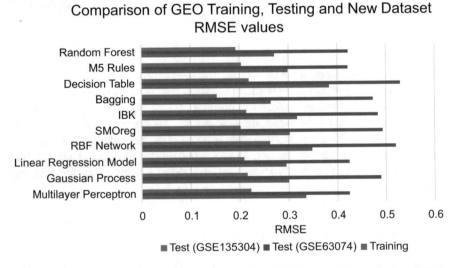

Fig. 8 Comparison of GEO Training, Testing and New GEO dataset. This graph represents the RMSE values of GEO datasets, and is divided by the machine learning algorithm. The different colours denotes the different datasets

other. There were 5 values recorded: Correlation Coefficient, Mean Absolute Error, Root Mean Squared Error, Relative Absolute Error (%) and Root Relative Squared Error (%). Out of these values, the most common and most effective are MAE and RMSE. MAE scales the error linearly whereas RMSE doesn't. In addition, RMSE accounts for larger weights having larger error values, so it penalises large errors. MAE uses absolute value, which isn't considered ideal in terms of mathematical calculations [18]. Despite this, MAE is more robust with regards to outliers [56]. Overall, RMSE is more beneficial as a value to compare the values against each other.

Overall, the highest RMSE was reported to be Multilayer Perceptron for the TCGA data and Decision Table for the GEO data. Ideally, for the RMSE the values have to be as low as possible. The three lowest values of RMSE for the TCGA dataset from smallest to largest is: Random Forest, Linear Regression and SMOreg. The three lowest values of RMSE for the GEO dataset from smallest to largest is: Random Forest, Bagging and M5 Rules.

Multilayer Perceptron is a relatively popular machine learning algorithm and is still prevalent within recent research. Within the work, it performed poorly for the TCGA dataset compared to the machine learning algorithms. Initially, the learning rate was set at default, at 0.3. But as the value of the RSE exceeded 100%, the learning rate was changed to 0.2 in order to prevent the overfitting from occurring. Research conducted by Mirzakhani studied the use of multilayer perceptron on lung tumor data. This research was different compared to that done within the work because the data used by Mirzakhani was CT scans, which is similar to most research done within this field. This work identified MLPs as being effective as it had an accuracy of 98.31% [44]. The difference with this is that the learning rate used here was significantly lower than the one used in this work. It would be interesting to further study the effects of the learning rate for the multilayer perceptron to see if results like that in the work are obtainable. The decision table also performed poorly but for the GEO dataset. Within research it has been identified as a sophisticated tool and how they had the potential to be developed. [39] The vast majority of the works are from a considerably long time ago, hence meaning there have been no advancements. This is most likely due to developments being unsuccessful and hence why it is justifiable for the decision table to perform the worst. As for the best performing algorithms, it is to be noted that the random forest considered the best for both the TCGA and the GEO datasets. This is evidenced by literature research as well that is relevant to the work. A work by Feng et al. conducted research into signaling pathways for cancers, it was noted that random forests are useful for this particular field, especially for KRAS and EGFR pathways [29]. This particular work consisted of many MLMs that are incredibly prevalent within in this particular field, hence it is incredibly valid and it can be presumed that random forest is one of the best candidates for machine learning. In addition to this, by Bawa et al. identified that Random Forests were able to identify strong gene candidates efficiently for NSCLC, which is concordant with the aims and objectives of this work. This particular work focused on three main machine learning methods, one of which being random forest. As well as this, it identified the combination of random forest and another MLM, SVM were incredibly powerful [14]. The SMOReg, that was identified as one of the best performing machine learning algorithms for TCGA, is based on SVM and is used for regression. For future research, it would be interesting to see the overlapping genes identified between the random forest and the SMOreg and how useful the genes identified can be for NSCLC research. In contrast to the research into Random Forest, there are some works that indicate there are potentially better methods than random forest. One such work mentions how Cox machine learning algorithms perform better than random forests [64]. This particular algorithm isn't available on WEKA and hence highlighting the limitations of using WEKA.

3.2   Network Interactions

3.2.1   Protein Network Interaction Visualisation from TCGA and GEO Data

Cytoscape was used to visualise the interactions between the genes that were selected. There were two types of networks made. One of which being the STRING network. The STRING network was derived from the STRING database which consisted of well-known protein-protein interactions. After the proteins were imported onto the system, there were some that weren't present on the 'main' network. These external genes were excluded. From here, the genes of interest (gathered from the feature selection stage) were imported here to signify the interactions between the nodes. For the TCGA data, there were 5 genes that were highlighted in the main structure in Fig. 9: KRAS, AMMERC1L, BRAP, ADIPOR2 and IPO8. For the GEO data, there were 3 genes that were highlighted in the main structure in Fig. 10: KRAS, STRRAP and PPP2R2A.

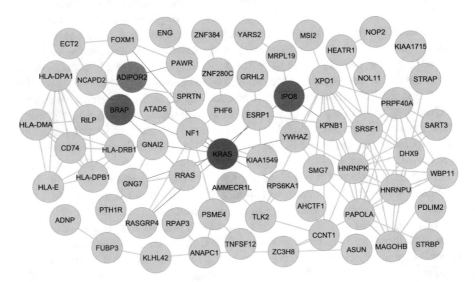

Fig. 9 STRING Protein Network for the TCGA data. This network presents all of the genes within the main network. The colours are used to signify the genes of interest identified from the feature selection, with green being the weakest interaction and dark orange being the strongest interaction

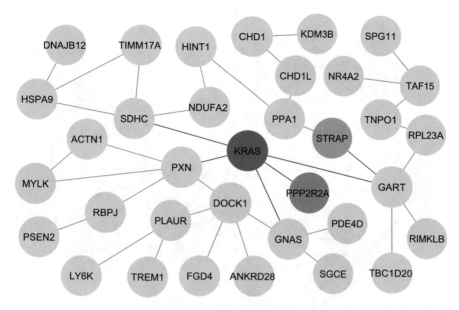

Fig. 10 STRING Protein Network for the GEO data. This network presents all of the genes within the main network. The colours are used to signify the genes of interest identified from the feature selection, with green being the weakest interaction and dark orange being the strongest interaction

3.2.2 Interactions Between KRAS and Other Significant Genes from TCGA and GEO Data

The other network made was based on the interactions the genes of interest had with each other. This involved both positive and negative interactions. For the TCGA inter-actions (as shown in Fig. 11), the most negative interaction was recorded between MFSD9 and AEBP2 as the target. Neither of these were included within the main structure of STRING network. On the other hand the most positive interaction recorded between the TCGA interactions were C2CD5 and IPO8 as the target. IPO8 was identified within the STRING network but there was no interactions between it and C2CD5. As for the GEO data (as shown in Fig. 12), the most negative inter-action recorded between YARS2 and MTSS1L as the target. Neither of these were included within the main structure of STRING network. On the other hand the most positive interaction recorded between the GEO interactions were CENPT and KRAS as the target. KRAS was identified within the STRING network but there was no interactions between it and CENPT. In addition to this, there were many other new interactions identified.

After conducting a search on works that contain the interactions between C2CD5 and IPO8, and CENPT and KRAS, there were none found. It was anticipated the TCGA with the FPKM files and the unique GEO dataset would contain gene inter-

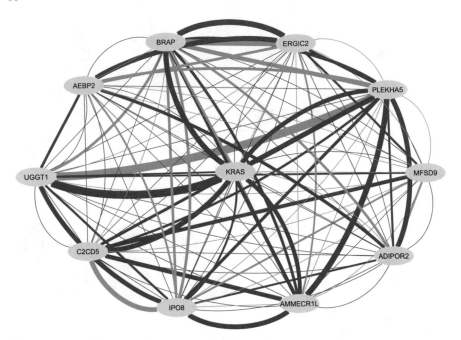

Fig. 11 STRING Feature Interactions for the TCGA data. This network presents all of the interactions between the selected genes. The colours are used to signify the type of interaction, with green is a negative interaction and blue is a positive interaction. The weight signifies the strength of the interaction

actions that were rare but not completely unidentified. The ability to identify gene interactions is incredibly important by the work Nastiuk et al. identified [47].

There has been previous work carried out to indicate that gene interactions identified by in silico methods have been effective using network interactions, and hence supports the fact that successful gene interactions have been identified previously. One of which being that during a research into mTOR inhibitors affecting the RAF/MEK/ERK pathway, there were 10 identified drug candidates based on network interferences. At the time of the research, three of these were undergoing clinical testing. This proves that network interference models are useful in predicting gene interactions that have potential, and also expanding the identification of useful gene interactions [36]. As well as this, there has been work done by Luo et al. that identified the novel interactions between a gene and three drug candidates, and these were experimentally verified and proved to be successful at preventing anti-inflammatory disease [40]. There have been many cases like the ones mentioned previously which shows that gene interactions that have been identified by other methods may not be useful as in silico methods.

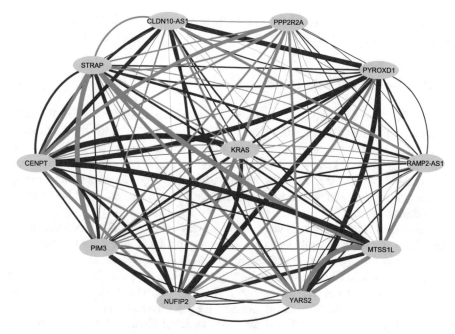

Fig. 12 STRING Feature Interactions for the GEO data. This network presents all of the interactions between the selected genes. The colours are used to signify the type of interaction, with green is a negative interaction and blue is a positive interaction. The weight signifies the strength of the interaction

Table 4 RMSE values of deep learning during the training and testing stages

	Training		Testing		
	TCGA	GEO	TCGA	GEO (GSE63074)	GEO (GSE135304)
RMSE values	4.0744	0.3025	4.1893	0.3827	0.2393

3.3 Performance with Deep Learning

3.3.1 RMSE Values Across Training and Testing stages with DL4J Package

As for the deep learning, only one value was computed for each of the training and testing of the TCGA and GEO datasets. The data is within Table 4, which showed similar results to the machine learning. The TCGA RMSE values are much higher and the testing value is higher than the training value as there is a smaller set of values. The GEO data shows the same results aswell between the training and the testing (GSE63074) but as the GSE135304 is a new dataset with more values compared to the other test, it has a much lower RMSE.

The Table 4 included the RMSE values for the following: TCGA Training, GEO Training. TCGA Testing, GEO Test (GSE63074) and GEO Test (GSE135304).

3.3.2   Discussion of Deep Learning

The results from the deep learning were moderately successful as the final results yielded as RSME value of 4.0744 for the TCGA and 0.3025 for the GEO data, after the hyperparameter tuning was done. In comparison to the RMSE values of the machine learning data these were relatively similar. The deep learning implemented was more successful than 6 of the machine learning algorithms. As for the deep learning of the GEO dataset, it was more successful than 6 of the machine learning algorithms as well.

With regards to research, it was noted by Wang et al. that deep learning might sometimes not work as well as machine learning methods, which could potentially justify the results [41]. However, in contrast to this, Moreno et al. have recently published a work in which deep learning models performed better than their machine learning counterparts in terms of accuracy [46]. In addition to this, another work by Tabares-Soto et al., identified the accuracy of the machine learning method they used (logistic regression) as 90.6% and the Convolutional Neural Network as 94.43% [58]. There is more research that confirms deep learning is meant to yield better accuracies however, this data is based on CT images in which a CNN is used. For this particular research FPKM values were used in order to determine drug targets and the molecules that drive the disease state. As mentioned previously there is a lack of research regarding the data aside from CT images within NSCLC. Research done by Ahn et al. used TCGA and GEO data but included normal human data as well as cancer data. Interestingly, they utilised a certain structure involves multiple layers within their DNN, which is generally considered detrimental to the accuracy values. The DNN structure was comprised of with six hidden layers with 500, 500, 200, 300, 200, and 100 nodes; it also used ReLu as the activation function which was similar to the research conducted in this work [9]. There is no currently no research conducted on the deep learning of numerical NSCLC datasets (e.g., FPKM) along the KRAS pathway, let alone with WEKA's deep learning dl4j being used.

3.3.3   KnowledgeFlow

Lastly, KnowledgeFlow was included as a way to ease the process in which the feature selection, machine learning and deep learning were carried out. This was done so efficiently and was able to yield the same results as those gathered in the previous stages. In addition to this, it worked well with the testing stages as well. This doesn't necessarily relate with the aims and objectives and the original goal was to ensure the machine learning and the deep learning were carried out efficiently, and not whether they were easily usable. Despite the system being able to accommodate for most parts of the experiment, there was the experimenter section that wasn't possible.

In order to resolve this, the current system would need to be more sophisticated. Gnanambal et al. studied the use of KnowledgeFlow in WEKA and proposed a more complex layout, that involved several different layers being involved as opposed to the one layout process used [34]. This research was based on breast cancer data, and hence why it varies slightly. There has been no research into the use of WEKA's KnowledgeFlow in to lung cancer data.

4 Conclusion

With regards to the aims and objectives the work has been relatively successful, as it has been able to produce new drug targets and molecules that drive the disease state. The aim involved using ML and DL to analyse the lung cancer data, which was done so successfully. In addition to this, networks were derived from data acquired from one of the machine learning methods. All of the objectives were met as a diverse range of methods were produced and these were are all tested and succeeded. As well as this, further research was done into using WEKA's KnowledgeFlow to simplify the process.

As for the next steps after this work, it would be interesting to compare the research conducted to that of the same experiments but done in another e.g. python coding. As well as this, it would be interesting to study other datasets aside from TCGA and GEO and see whether the system implemented could accommodate for them. It would also be interesting to carry out the same experiments on other pathways such as EGFR in order to study its effect and see whether the effect is the same as that from other works that compared KRAS and EGFR. As well as this, another line of work could incorporating other types of lung cancer as well and not only NSCLC.

References

1. GDC. https://portal.gdc.cancer.gov/
2. GEO Accession viewer. https://www.ncbi.nlm.nih.gov/geo/query/acc.cgi?acc=GSE63074
3. GEO Accession viewer. https://www.ncbi.nlm.nih.gov/geo/query/acc.cgi?acc=GSE135304
4. Homo_sapiens-Ensembl genome browser 106. https://www.ensembl.org/Homo_sapiens/Info/Index
5. Hweka 3: Machine learning software in java. https://www.cs.waikato.ac.nz/ml/weka/
6. KEGG PATHWAY: Ras signaling pathway-Homo sapiens (human). https://www.genome.jp/pathway/hsa04014+N00103
7. How do I extract all archives in the subdirectories of this folder? (Mar 2015). https://serverfault.com/q/8092
8. Ahmed SRA, Al Barazanchi I, Mhana A, Abdulshaheed HR (2019) Lung cancer classification using data mining and supervised learning algorithms on multi-dimensional data set. Period Eng Nat Sci 7(2):438–447
9. Ahn T, Goo T, Lee CH, Kim S, Han K, Park S, Park T (2018) Deep learning-based identification of cancer or normal tissue using gene expression data. In: 2018 IEEE international conference on bioinformatics and biomedicine (BIBM). IEEE, pp 1748–1752

10. Al Banna MH et al (2021) Attention-based bi-directional long-short term memory network for earthquake prediction. IEEE Access 9:56589–56603
11. Al Nahian MJ, Ghosh T et al (2020) Towards artificial intelligence driven emotion aware fall monitoring framework suitable for elderly people with neurological disorder. In: Proceedings brain information, pp 275–286
12. Al Nahian MJ et al (2021) Towards an accelerometer-based elderly fall detection system using cross-disciplinary time series features. IEEE Access 9:39413–31
13. Apicella A, Donnarumma F, Isgrò F, Prevete R (2021) A survey on modern trainable activation functions. Neural Netw 138:14–32
14. Bawa TA, Özkan Y, Erol ÇS (2021) Reanalysis of non-small-cell lung cancer microarray gene expression data. In: Multidisciplinary digital publishing institute proceedings, vol 74, p 22
15. Becker BG (1998) Visualizing decision table classifiers. In: Proceedings IEEE symposium on information visualization (Cat. No. 98TB100258), pp 102–105
16. Biswas M, Tania MH, Kaiser MS et al (2021) Accu3rate: a mobile health application rating scale based on user reviews. PloS one 16(12):e0258050
17. Biswas M et al (2021) An xai based autism detection: the context behind the detection. In: Proceedings brain information, pp 448–459
18. Chai T, Draxler RR (2014) Root mean square error (rmse) or mean absolute error (mae)?-arguments against avoiding rmse in the literature. Geosci Model Dev 7(3):1247–1250
19. Chikhale H, Nerkar A (2020) Review on in-silico techniques an approach to drug discovery. Curr Tre Phar Pharma Chem 2(1):24–32
20. Cooper GM, Hausman RE, Hausman RE (2007) The cell: a molecular approach, vol 4. ASM Press Washington, DC, USA
21. Cruz CSD, Tanoue LT, Matthay RA (2011) Lung cancer: epidemiology, etiology, and prevention. Clin Chest Med 32(4):605–644
22. Dai D, Shi R, Han S, Jin H, Wang X (2020) Weighted gene coexpression network analysis identifies hub genes related to kras mutant lung adenocarcinoma. Medicine 99(32)
23. Deepa B et al (2022) Pattern descriptors orientation and map firefly algorithm based brain pathology classification using hybridized machine learning algorithm. IEEE Access 10:3848–3863
24. El-Telbany A, Ma PC (2012) Cancer genes in lung cancer: racial disparities: are there any? Genes Cancer 3(7–8):467–480
25. Fabietti M, Mahmud M, Lotfi A (2021) Anomaly detection in invasively recorded neuronal signals using deep neural network: effect of sampling frequency. In: Proceedings AII, pp 79–91
26. Fabietti M, Mahmud M, Lotfi A (2022) Channel-independent recreation of artefactual signals in chronically recorded local field potentials using machine learning. Brain Inform 9(1):1–17
27. Fabietti M et al (2020) Artifact detection in chronically recorded local field potentials using long-short term memory neural network. In: Proceedings AICT 2020, pp 1–6
28. Faria TH et al (2021) Smart city technologies for next generation healthcare. In: Data-driven mining, learning & analytics for secured smart cities, pp 253–274
29. Feng J, Zhang H, Li F (2021) Investigating the relevance of major signaling pathways in cancer survival using a biologically meaningful deep learning model. BMC Bioinform 22(1):1–13
30. Gerber DE (2008) Targeted therapies: a new generation of cancer treatments. Am Fam Phys 77(3):311–319
31. Ghosh T et al (2021) Artificial intelligence and internet of things in screening and management of autism spectrum disorder. Sustain Cities Soc 74:103189
32. Ghosh T et al (2021) An attention-based mood controlling framework for social media users. In: Proceedings brain information, pp 245–256
33. Ghosh T et al (2021) A hybrid deep learning model to predict the impact of covid-19 on mental health form social media big data. Preprints 2021(2021060654)
34. Gnanambal DS, Thangaraj DM, Meenatchi DV, Gayathri DVG (2018) An effective framework for breast cancer diagnosis using weka knowledge flow environment. In: 2018 IADS International conference on computing, communications & data engineering (CCODE)
35. Krauss G (2006) Biochemistry of signal transduction and regulation. Wiley

36. Krentel F, Singer F, Rosano-Gonzalez ML, Gibb EA, Liu Y, Davicioni E, Keller N, Stekhoven DJ, Kruithof-de Julio M, Seiler R (2021) A showcase study on personalized in silico drug response prediction based on the genetic landscape of muscle invasive bladder cancer. Sci Rep 11(1):1–14

37. Kumar I et al (2022) Dense tissue pattern characterization using deep neural network. Cogn Comput 1–24. [ePub ahead of print]

38. Lalotra GS, Kumar V, Bhatt A, Chen T, Mahmud M (2022) iReTADS: an intelligent real-time anomaly detection system for cloud communications using temporal data summarization and neural network. Secur Commun Netw 2022:9149164

39. Lu H, Liu H (2000) Decision tables: Scalable classification exploring rdbms capabilities. In: Proceedings of the 26th international conference on very large data bases, VLDB'00, p 373

40. Luo Y, Zhao X, Zhou J, Yang J, Zhang Y, Kuang W, Peng J, Chen L, Zeng J (2017) A network integration approach for drug-target interaction prediction and computational drug repositioning from heterogeneous information. Nat Commun 8(1):1–13

41. Mahmud M, Kaiser MS, McGinnity TM, Hussain A (2021) Deep learning in mining biological data. Cogn Comput 13(1):1–33

42. Mahmud M et al (2018) Applications of deep learning and reinforcement learning to biological data. IEEE Trans Neural Netw Learn Syst 29(6):2063–2079

43. Mammoottil MJ, Kulangara LJ, Cherian AS, Mohandas P, Hasikin K, Mahmud M (2022) Detection of breast cancer from five-view thermal images using convolutional neural networks. J Healthc Eng 2022:4295221

44. Mirzakhani F (2017) Detection of lung cancer using multilayer perceptron neural network. Med Technol J 1(4):109–109

45. Monti M (2012) Gene expression profiling: methods and protocols. Eur J Histochem 56(3), br12–br12

46. Moreno S, Bonfante M, Zurek E, Cherezov D, Goldgof D, Hall L, Schabath M (2021) A radiogenomics ensemble to predict egfr and kras mutations in nsclc. Tomography 7(2):154–168

47. Nastiuk KL, Krolewski JJ (2016) Opportunities and challenges in combination gene cancer therapy. Adv Drug Deliv Rev 98:35–40

48. Nawar A, Toma NT, Al Mamun S et al (2021) Cross-content recommendation between movie and book using machine learning. In: Proceedings AICT, pp 1–6

49. Panov P, Džeroski S (2007) Combining bagging and random subspaces to create better ensembles. In: International symposium on intelligent data analysis, pp 118–129

50. Pao W, Wang TY, Riely GJ, Miller VA, Pan Q, Ladanyi M, Zakowski MF, Heelan RT, Kris MG, Varmus HE (2005) Kras mutations and primary resistance of lung adenocarcinomas to gefitinib or erlotinib. PLoS Med 2(1):e17

51. Patil PD, Hobbs B, Pennell NA (2019) The promise and challenges of deep learning models for automated histopathologic classification and mutation prediction in lung cancer. J Thorac Dis 11(2):369

52. Paul A et al (2022) Inverted bell-curve-based ensemble of deep learning models for detection of covid-19 from chest x-rays. Neural Comput Appl 1–15

53. Prakash N et al (2021) Deep transfer learning covid-19 detection and infection localization with superpixel based segmentation. Sustain Cities Soc 75:103252

54. Satu M et al (2020) Towards improved detection of cognitive performance using bidirectional multilayer long-short term memory neural network. In: Proceedings brain information, pp 297–306

55. Satu MS et al (2021) Tclustvid: a novel machine learning classification model to investigate topics and sentiment in covid-19 tweets. Knowl-Based Syst 226:107126

56. Shcherbakov MV, Brebels A, Shcherbakova NL, Tyukov AP, Janovsky TA, Kamaev VA et al (2013) A survey of forecast error measures. World Appl Sci J 24(24):171–176

57. Sung H, Ferlay J, Siegel RL, Laversanne M, Soerjomataram I, Jemal A, Bray F (2021) Global cancer statistics 2020: Globocan estimates of incidence and mortality worldwide for 36 cancers in 185 countries. CA Cancer J Clin 71(3):209–249

58. Tabares-Soto R, Orozco-Arias S, Romero-Cano V, Bucheli VS, Rodríguez-Sotelo JL, Jiménez-Varón CF (2020) A comparative study of machine learning and deep learning algorithms to classify cancer types based on microarray gene expression data. Peer J Comput Sci 6:e270

59. Tomasini P, Walia P, Labbe C, Jao K, Leighl NB (2016) Targeting the kras pathway in non-small cell lung cancer. Oncologist 21(12):1450–1460

60. Wang H, Zhou Z, Li Y, Chen Z, Lu P, Wang W, Liu W, Yu L (2017) Comparison of machine learning methods for classifying mediastinal lymph node metastasis of non-small cell lung cancer from 18f-fdg pet/ct images. EJNMMI Res 7(1):1–11

61. Watkins J, Fabietti M, Mahmud M (2020) Sense: a student performance quantifier using sentiment analysis. In: Proceedings IJCNN, pp 1–6

62. Way GP, Sanchez-Vega F, La K, Armenia J, Chatila WK, Luna A, Sander C, Cherniack AD, Mina M, Ciriello G et al (2018) Machine learning detects pan-cancer ras pathway activation in the cancer genome atlas. Cell Rep 23(1):172–180

63. Zhang J, Hu H, Xu S, Jiang H, Zhu J, Qin E, He Z, Chen E (2020) The functional effects of key driver kras mutations on gene expression in lung cancer. Front Genet 11:17

64. Zhu W, Xie L, Han J, Guo X (2020) The application of deep learning in cancer prognosis prediction. Cancers 12(3):603

AI for Brain Disorders

The Emerging Role of AI in Dementia Research and Healthcare

Janice M. Ranson⊙, Magda Bucholc⊙, Donald Lyall, Danielle Newby⊙,
Laura Winchester⊙, Neil Oxtoby⊙, Michele Veldsman⊙,
Timothy Rittman⊙, Sarah Marzi⊙, Nathan Skene⊙, Ahmad Al Khleifat⊙,
Isabelle Foote⊙, Vasiliki Orgeta⊙, Andrey Kormilitzin⊙,
and David J. Llewellyn

1 Introduction to Dementia Research and Healthcare

Dementia is caused by an acquired, sustained decline in brain function, leading to difficulty with everyday activities. With multiple aetiologies, clinical presentation varies, typically including problems with memory, cognition, and communication [1]. Dementia research aims to identify risk factors, disease mechanisms and treatments. However, progress has been limited. Many cases remain undiagnosed, and there is currently no cure.

David J. Llewellyn—On behalf of the Deep Dementia Phenotyping (DEMON) Network.

J. M. Ranson
College of Medicine and Health, University of Exeter, Exeter, UK

M. Bucholc
Cognitive Analytics Research Lab, School of Computing, Engineering and Intelligent Systems, Ulster University, Derry, UK

D. Lyall
Institute of Health and Wellbeing, University of Glasgow, Glasgow, UK

D. Newby
Department of Psychiatry, Warneford Hospital, University of Oxford, Oxford, UK

L. Winchester · A. Kormilitzin
Department of Psychiatry, University of Oxford, Oxford, UK

N. Oxtoby
University College, London, UK

M. Veldsman
Wellcome Centre for Integrative Neuroimaging, University of Oxford, Oxford, UK

Department of Experimental Psychology, University of Oxford, Oxford, UK

T. Rittman
Department of Clinical Neurosciences, University of Cambridge, Cambridge, UK

There is an increasing availability of rich, multimodal data from experimental models, population-based cohorts, clinical trials, and electronic health records. This chapter covers 5 key areas where AI has the potential to achieve impact; genetics and omics, experimental medicine, drug discovery and trials optimisation, imaging, and prevention.

2 Genetics

Genomic data-generating methods are proliferating rapidly, spurred on by the falling costs of DNA sequencing and microfluidic technologies enabling single cell genomics. A major advance is the emergence of well-powered genome-wide association (GWAS) studies [2]. Statistical methods such as LDSC [3] and MAGMA [4] have enabled the full genomic signal to be considered by accounting for confounding from linkage disequilibrium. However, we do not know what effect most genetic variants have, how they relate to cellular changes, or how genetic factors interact with modifiable risks.

2.1 How Do We Determine the Biological Effect of Genetic Variants?

GWAS results tell us which variants are associated with disease. While these are commonly discussed as single nucleotide variants (SNPs) we don't necessarily know

S. Marzi
UK Dementia Research Institute, Imperial College, London, UK

Department of Brain Sciences, Imperial College, London, UK

N. Skene
Faculty of Medicine, Department of Brain Sciences, Imperial College, London, UK

A. Al Khleifat
Basic and Clinical Neuroscience, King's College London, London, UK

I. Foote
Unit for Psychological Medicine, Wolfson Institute of Population Health, Barts and The London School of Medicine and Dentistry, Queen Marry University of London, London, UK

Preventive Neurology Unit, Wolfson Institute of Population Health, Barts and The London School of Medicine and Dentistry, Queen Marry University of London, London, UK

V. Orgeta
Division of Psychiatry, University College London, London, UK

D. J. Llewellyn (✉)
College of Medicine and Health, Alan Turing Institute, University of Exeter, Exeter, UK
e-mail: David.Llewellyn@exeter.ac.uk

the actual base pair in the genome responsible for increased risk, as alleles found at nearby genetic variants are correlated. This is known as linkage disequilibrium. Statistical techniques can determine which genetic variant in a region is likely to be causal, by considering conditional probabilities and functional (e.g. epigenetic) annotations [5]. Supervised learning is a useful adjunct to statistical fine mapping: the genomic features associated with known expression- Quantitative Trait Loci (QTL) can be used to train a classifier, whose output from new variants could then be used to set the priors for statistical fine mapping [6]. Identifying the causal variant does not tell us what those variants do though; machine learning (ML) models [7] have therefore been developed to predict genomic features such as transcription factor binding [8], RNA–protein binding [9], RNA splicing [10], and 3D genome structure [11]. These models use cutting-edge techniques, such as attentional networks, to enable predictions of variant effects to be made over long distances (e.g. 100,000 bp) [8].

2.2 How Do We Get from Genetic Epidemiology and -Omics to Practical Applications?

GWAS investigate the association of dementia with genetic variants across the genome, and individual associations often have modest effect sizes. Successful early stage drug trials have substantial corroboration in independent GWAS, and targets with genetic evidence of disease association are almost twice as likely to succeed across multiple phases [12]. Similarly, GWAS provide an opportunity to identify existing drugs which could be repurposed on the basis of shared targets [13] to improve drug trial efficiency.

Many people are interested in their genetic risk for dementia [14]. However, translating data into usable information benefitting public health is a major challenge. Polygenic scores are single values reflecting an individual's cumulative genetic risk. Common complex traits and disorders primarily have polygenic, high-frequency but low-penetrance architectures. These scores have utility in predicting lifetime risk of dementia, but major challenges include how they can be used reliably at the individual level, across ethnicities, and at different stages of lifecourse [15, 16].

Key areas in which AI and ML can help include meta-analyses of GWAS and RNA-Seq data, development of polygenic scores for dementia subtypes, and combining -omics data to enhance our understanding of functional implications of identified genetic associations. The next step is to integrate these promising approaches for real-world impact.

3   Experimental Medicine

Animal [17] and cellular [18] models provide vital evidence of mechanism to better understand disease hypotheses and causal pathways. These results can give rise to new drug targets, and discovery of biomarkers to allow identification of dementia-related diseases in their preclinical form. Experimental models for dementia include mice with specific genetic mutations or knock-ins, patient-derived induced pluripotent stem cell (iPSC) cultures [19], and human tissues [20]. Complex multi-cellular and multi-species models include organoids of the human brain [21], multi-species models of the blood–brain barrier [22] and chimeric mouse models, containing live human cells [23]. All these models capture different aspects of disease biology, and allow varying extents of control over genetic and environmental experimental intervention.

Intelligent experimental medicine is a relatively new field encapsulating some of the most promising opportunities for innovation using AI in dementia research. Data-driven approaches can tackle integrative analyses across multiple studies and heterogeneous model systems. Advanced informatics methodologies are able to detect results that might be missed by a direct analysis. By integrating data modalities within a single cohort, we can make stronger inferences of underlying changes and specific patterns. Using ML and AI, we can find new associations that may be obscured by data noise to make new disease inferences. To progress the field of experimental medicine for dementia, we need to address three key questions.

3.1   What Makes a Good Experimental Model?

We need measurable criteria to determine suitability and representativeness of experimental models. Which aspects of disease biology can be captured by various model systems? For example, given that iPSC-derived cell cultures or organoids show gene regulatory ageing markers of very early development, do they represent suitable models of neurodegenerative disease processes in the context of old age? Or could ageing signatures even be simulated experimentally or computationally in these in vitro systems?

3.2   How Can We Make Best Use of Multimodal Data?

Robust studies should control for experimental factors and batch effects that can have an impact on the measured phenotype, by harmonising, randomising across experimental conditions and including appropriate covariates in analyses. This is challenging for small, single modality studies, with limited statistical power and reliability. Development of analytic methods and tools that can span across modalities and leverage these links, is a rapidly evolving and promising field. Connecting brain activity with gene expression patterns for example, could give new insights into gene regulation in the context of functional activation of neurons. In the same way, atlases across phenotypes and omics, carefully collected on matched samples are set to provide novel insights into disease biology [24].

3.3 How Can We Translate Insights from Experimental Models to Human Disease Biology?

Clinical trials for drugs developed using animal models are generally unsuccessful [25]. We need strong quantitative approaches for cross-model translation. ML approaches can be leveraged to translate gene-regulatory networks and the response to experimental perturbation across species. By reviewing existing approaches [26] and those used in other fields, we can address these kinds of translational challenges. Armed with prior biological knowledge and large-scale reference datasets for baseline and perturbed conditions, development of novel translation algorithms is possible.

4 Drug Discovery and Trials Optimisation

Despite a concerted and sustained international effort in developing disease-modifying therapies for dementia, progress has been poor. Some treatments can produce short-term symptomatic relief, but the disease continues unabated. Of the plethora of experimental drugs tested in hundreds of trials, only one disease-modifying therapy, Aducanumab, has been approved by the US Food and Drug Administration [27].

Clinical trials aim to recruit at-risk individuals who may benefit from a drug. The ideal scenario is a large, population-representative sample of individuals at the same stage of disease progression or with the same risk of disease [28]. In reality, sample sizes are limited, and assessment of disease severity and risk is not straightforward; these diseases are heterogeneous and lack well-defined disease progression [29, 30]. Recent efforts to improve recruitment for clinical trials include use of biomarker data [31], especially in the pre-symptomatic phase [32, 33]. Current biomarker-based screening is quite crude, for example values are typically dichotomised using predefined cut points. There is much room for improvement [29, 34].

Identification of suitable candidates for clinical trials is a challenge well-suited to advanced data science methods. Multimodal data from large cohort and population studies can be used to characterise and quantify disease severity [35] and subtype [36] even in the absence of a well-defined disease progression axis [37]. Such approaches promise the precision that has been thwarting clinical trials to date. Applications of AI and related methods for computational drug discovery include unsupervised learning to discover unseen patterns [38], and meta models for understanding disease mechanisms [39].

While data from large observational studies is readily available, this is not the case for interventional studies, particularly clinical trial data [40]. Pharmaceutical sponsors of neurology trials often only share patient-level data following regulatory approval of an experimental drug. Opportunities for optimising clinical trials include utilising publicly available data, and improving the state of the art in precision understanding and forecasting of dementia [16]. The former lends itself to traditional data science methods (e.g., gradient boosting for feature selection or weighting) and AI (e.g., feature generation from neuroimaging data). The latter is an active area of research that will benefit from large multidisciplinary collaborative initiatives leveraging available data. Examples include the EuroPOND consortium (http://europo nd.eu) and Fraunhofer SCAI (http://www.diseaseprogressionmodels.eu/).

Another challenge is that following participants over the time which dementia typically develops is generally impractical and prohibitively expensive, particularly for dementia prevention trials. One low-cost solution is interrogation of electronic health records to identify patients who are subsequently diagnosed with dementia or experience adverse events. Relevant information is often recorded in free-text clinical notes which is problematic for conventional analytic approaches [41]. Advances in text mining and Natural Language Processing facilitate analysis of relevant information [42]. This approach can also inform future care by identifying how treatments benefit patient subgroups, and develop drug-response predictive models, thus capturing real-world effectiveness.

5   Neuroimaging

Structural neuroimaging using CT or MRI is routine in the diagnosis and management of dementia [43]. Additional neuroimaging modalities can help analyse: (1) brain activity, using functional MRI [44], electroencephalography (EEG) [45] or magnetoencephalography (MEG) [46]; (2) metabolic changes, using positron emission tomography (PET) [47]; (3) specific pathologies, using PET ligands for protein aggregation such as beta-amyloid [48] or tau [49].

Neuroimaging generates large, complex data beyond the ability of human interpretation or traditional statistical approaches, but ideally suited to AI methods for supporting clinical diagnosis, and understanding disease mechanisms. Existing datasets include ADNI [50], NACC [51], OASIS [52], and GeNFI [53].

AI methods in structural MRI outperform traditional approaches, for example using hippocampal volume for diagnostic classification [54, 55], or conversion from mild cognitive impairment to Alzheimer's disease [56]. One promising approach combined structural MRI, PET and clinical data to train a ML model that subsequently predicted conversion to Alzheimer's disease from structural MRI alone [57].

Whilst barriers remain in validation and clinical translation, we are optimistic that meaningful AI decision support tools for neuroimaging will be in clinical practice within the next decade.

The anatomical specificity of neuroimaging provides insights into disease mechanisms of neurodegeneration across the brain. The first study to apply a 'big data' approach to this challenge used multimodal MRI and PET imaging combined with plasma and CSF markers in a multifactorial generative model, to infer that vascular changes occurred earliest in Alzheimer's disease [58]. This approach using neuroimaging to infer disease progression has since been extended, most notably using the Subtype and Stage Interference (SuStAiN) model. This model has been applied to genetic frontotemporal dementia [36] investigating the complex relationship between genotype and structural brain changes, and more recently in Alzheimer's disease to identify patterns of tau accumulation [59].

The issue of interpretability remains a challenge, particularly for 'black box' deep learning methods [60]. Understanding the features used for classification is important to relate changes to anatomical brain regions, and to ensure that classification is not based on noise signals such as motion in functional imaging methods [61]. Methods to identify features within neural networks are emerging and have been successfully applied to neuroimaging data in Alzheimer's disease [62].

Whilst we are optimistic about AI in neuroimaging for dementia, some challenges remain. One key challenge is ensuring that research populations represent the real world setting. AI is notoriously sensitive to bias within the data that trains its algorithms [63], and selection bias has been highlighted in datasets of neuroimaging for dementia [64]. Future data collection must recruit strategically to address this issue. A second key challenge is the practical issue of regulatory approval. Only four AI methods have been approved for clinical use in neuroimaging for dementia in the US or EU, but most of these perform image segmentation, and none directly classify patient groups [65]. This low rate of success suggests a significant barrier at the point of translation from research to clinical practice.

6 Prevention

Epidemiological studies of recent birth cohorts demonstrate a decrease in age-specific dementia incidence [66], demonstrating the potential for dementia prevention by targeting modifiable risk factors [67, 68]. A multitude of interacting risk factors and pathologies contribute to dementia risk. The 2020 Lancet Commission on Dementia Prevention, Intervention and Care identified 12 modifiable risk factors, which could prevent up to 40% of dementia cases [67]. These are low education, hearing loss, traumatic brain injury, hypertension, high alcohol intake, obesity, smoking, depression, social isolation, physical inactivity, air pollution and diabetes. Several systematic reviews have identified additional risk factors [69]. AI and ML methods can be used to improve our understanding of commonality and causality of risk factors, in order to develop and test effective preventative interventions.

A major challenge in this field is the issue of reverse causation. Traditional statistical approaches often fail to distinguish causal risk factors from prodromal dementia symptoms. Methods such as Mendelian randomization are providing new insights into causal pathways [70], but can be inadequately powered and suffer from weak instrument and survival bias. ML methods, such as deep learning approaches, could improve the way risk variants are identified within genome-wide association studies [71], creating stronger genetic instruments to improve causal analysis.

Most dementia risk factors are moderately correlated [72]; despite this, many studies fail to consider the interactions between modifiable and non-modifiable risk factors (e.g. age and sex) or non-linear effects. This leads to overly simplistic methods that do not reflect true biological relationships. For example, mid-life hypertension increases risk for dementia, but becomes apparently 'protective' during prodromal dementia [73], suggesting the onset of dementia itself influences blood pressure. ML approaches can measure these interactions and nonlinear effects, which could uncover pathways that underpin the influence that multimorbidity has on dementia risk [72]. Approaches such as path signature-based methods [74], allow us to model complex relationships and identify the optimal duration and timing of lifestyle or drug interventions to reduce dementia risk.

Existing dementia risk prediction tools such as the Cardiovascular Risk Factors, Aging, and Incidence of Dementia (CAIDE) Dementia Risk Score, incorporate risk factors such as age, education, physical activity, vascular and cardiometabolic risk factors, to predict dementia ~20 years later [75]. However, these are based on linear models, leaving substantial scope for more advanced modelling, including extreme gradient boosting trees or neural networks.

Deep learning [76] and network-based approaches [77] are being used to identify and validate existing drugs as potential preventative interventions to reduce risk and delay dementia onset. ML approaches could help identify how and why certain drugs reduce risk [78]. The development of preventative interventions could in turn enable the use of personalised medicine by applying network meta-analytics [79] and other ML methods to recommend interventions and predict treatment response to improve patient outcomes.

Underpinning all these advances is the need for more high-quality, longitudinal and multimodal data, which currently remains unavailable from a single source. Better harmonisation of existing cohorts and multimodal datasets using AI/ML methods will also help to inform guidance set out by policymakers and professional bodies for public health management.

7 A Global Initiative for AI Applied to Dementia Research and Healthcare

The Deep Dementia Phenotyping (DEMON) Network is an international collaborative initiative launched in 2019 to support the growing interest in data science and AI applied to dementia research and healthcare. Collaborative research and knowledge transfer activities are coordinated by multidisciplinary Working Groups covering all areas of dementia research, with over 1300 members worldwide. Membership is free, and those interested in the application of AI to dementia are invited to find out more at demondementia.com.

8 Conclusions

The intimidating challenge that dementia represents reflects the sheer complexity and heterogeneity of the human brain. AI and related methods can help to embrace this complexity. Current applications are most advanced in the subfield of neuroimaging, where features can now be efficiently extracted and incorporated into powerful diagnostic and predictive models. The use of AI in genetics shows promise for identifying genomic features, although the translation of this knowledge to clinically-relevant tools remains challenging. The use of AI in drug discovery, experimental medicine and prevention is less established, though preliminary studies provide proof of principle. Our ability to make sense of this rich data with more sophisticated techniques will depend on the global research community working beyond traditional disciplinary and geographic boundaries.

References

1. Alzheimer's Association. What is Dementia? https://www.alz.org/alzheimers-dementia/what-is-dementia. Accessed 16 Feb 2019
2. Wightman DP, Jansen IE, Savage JE et al (2020) Largest GWAS (N=1,126,563) of Alzheimer's disease implicates microglia and immune cells. medRxiv 2020:2020.2011.2020.20235275
3. Finucane HK, Bulik-Sullivan B, Gusev A et al (2015) Partitioning heritability by functional annotation using genome-wide association summary statistics. Nat Genet 47:1228–1235
4. de Leeuw CA, Mooij JM, Heskes T, Posthuma D (2015) MAGMA: generalized gene-set analysis of GWAS data. PLoS Comput Biol 11:e1004219
5. Weissbrod O, Hormozdiari F, Benner C et al (2020) Functionally informed fine-mapping and polygenic localization of complex trait heritability. Nat Genet 52:1355–1363
6. Wang QS, Kelley DR, Ulirsch J et al (2021) Leveraging supervised learning for functionally informed fine-mapping of cis-eQTLs identifies an additional 20,913 putative causal eQTLs. Nat Commun 12:3394
7. Avsec Ž, Kreuzhuber R, Israeli J et al (2019) The Kipoi repository accelerates community exchange and reuse of predictive models for genomics. Nat Biotechnol 37:592–600
8. Avsec Ž, Agarwal V, Visentin D et al (2021) Effective gene expression prediction from sequence by integrating long-range interactions. bioRxiv 2021:2021.2004.2007.438649
9. Pan X, Shen H-B (2018) Predicting RNA–protein binding sites and motifs through combining local and global deep convolutional neural networks. Bioinformatics 34:3427–3436
10. Paggi JM, Bejerano G (2018) A sequence-based, deep learning model accurately predicts RNA splicing branchpoints. RNA 24:1647–1658
11. Schwessinger R, Gosden M, Downes D et al (2020) DeepC: predicting 3D genome folding using megabase-scale transfer learning. Nat Methods 17:1118–1124

12. King EA, Davis JW, Degner JF (2019) Are drug targets with genetic support twice as likely to be approved? Revised estimates of the impact of genetic support for drug mechanisms on the probability of drug approval. PLoS Genet 15:e1008489
13. Visscher PM, Wray NR, Zhang Q et al (2017) 10 years of GWAS discovery: biology, function, and translation. Am J Hum Genet 101:5–22
14. Hoell C, Wynn J, Rasmussen L et al (2020) Participant choices for return of genomic results in the eMERGE Network. Genet Med 22
15. Lewis CM, Vassos E (2020) Polygenic risk scores: from research tools to clinical instruments. Genome Med 12:44
16. Myszczynska MA, Ojamies PN, Lacoste AMB et al (2020) Applications of machine learning to diagnosis and treatment of neurodegenerative diseases. Nat Rev Neurol 16:440–456
17. Götz J, Bodea L-G, Goedert M (2018) Rodent models for Alzheimer disease. Nat Rev Neurosci 19:583–598
18. Arber C, Lovejoy C, Wray S (2017) Stem cell models of Alzheimer's disease: progress and challenges. Alzheimer's Res Therapy 9:42
19. Penney J, Ralvenius WT, Tsai LH (2020) Modeling Alzheimer's disease with iPSC-derived brain cells. Mol Psychiat 25:148–167
20. Nott A, Schlachetzki JCM, Fixsen BR, Glass CK (2021) Nuclei isolation of multiple brain cell types for omics interrogation. Nat Protoc 16:1629–1646
21. Grenier K, Kao J, Diamandis P (2020) Three-dimensional modeling of human neurodegeneration: brain organoids coming of age. Mol Psychiat 25:254–274
22. Gerhartl A, Pracser N, Vladetic A, Hendrikx S, Friedl HP, Neuhaus W (2020) The pivotal role of micro-environmental cells in a human blood-brain barrier in vitro model of cerebral ischemia: functional and transcriptomic analysis. Fluids Barriers CNS 17:19
23. Mancuso R, Van Den Daele J, Fattorelli N et al (2019) Stem-cell-derived human microglia transplanted in mouse brain to study human disease. Nat Neurosci 22:2111–2116
24. Hartl CL, Ramaswami G, Pembroke WG et al (2021) Coexpression network architecture reveals the brain-wide and multiregional basis of disease susceptibility. Nat Neurosci 24:1313–1323
25. Rhrissorrakrai K, Belcastro V, Bilal E et al (2015) Understanding the limits of animal models as predictors of human biology: lessons learned from the sbv IMPROVER species translation challenge. Bioinformatics 31:471–483
26. Brubaker DK, Lauffenburger DA (2020) Translating preclinical models to humans. Science 367:742–743
27. Walsh S, Merrick R, Milne R, Brayne C (2021) Aducanumab for Alzheimer's disease? BMJ 374:n1682
28. Sakpal TV (2010) Sample size estimation in clinical trial. Perspect Clin Res 1:67–69
29. Ryan J, Fransquet P, Wrigglesworth J, Lacaze P (2018) Phenotypic heterogeneity in dementia: a challenge for epidemiology and biomarker studies. Front Pub Health 6:181
30. Friedman LG, McKeehan N, Hara Y et al (2021) Value-generating exploratory trials in neurodegenerative dementias. Neurology 96:944–954
31. Rafii MS, Zaman S, Handen BL (2021) Integrating biomarker outcomes into clinical trials for Alzheimer's disease in down syndrome. J Prev Alzheimers Dis 8:48–51
32. Jack CR Jr, Bennett DA, Blennow K et al (2016) A/T/N: An unbiased descriptive classification scheme for Alzheimer disease biomarkers. Neurology 87:539–547
33. Weston PSJ, Nicholas JM, Henley SMD et al (2018) Accelerated long-term forgetting in presymptomatic autosomal dominant Alzheimer's disease: a cross-sectional study. Lancet Neurol 17:123–132
34. Bullain S, Doody R (2020) What works and what does not work in Alzheimer's disease? From interventions on risk factors to anti-amyloid trials. J Neurochem 155:120–136
35. Golriz Khatami S, Robinson C, Birkenbihl C, Domingo-Fernández D, Hoyt CT, Hofmann-Apitius M (2020) Challenges of integrative disease modeling in Alzheimer's disease. Front Mol Biosci 6
36. Young AL, Marinescu RV, Oxtoby NP et al (2018) Uncovering the heterogeneity and temporal complexity of neurodegenerative diseases with subtype and stage inference. Nat Commun 9:4273

37. Hascup ER, Hascup KN (2020) Toward refining Alzheimer's disease into overlapping subgroups. Alzheimers Dement (NY) 6:e12070
38. Harrer S, Shah P, Antony B, Hu J (2019) Artificial intelligence for clinical trial design. Trends Pharmacol Sci 40:577–591
39. Domingo-Fernández D, Kodamullil AT, Iyappan A et al (2017) Multimodal mechanistic signatures for neurodegenerative diseases (NeuroMMSig): a web server for mechanism enrichment. Bioinformatics 33:3679–3681
40. Brassington I (2017) The ethics of reporting all the results of clinical trials. Br Med Bull 121:19–29
41. Goodday SM, Kormilitzin A, Vaci N et al (2020) Maximizing the use of social and behavioural information from secondary care mental health electronic health records. J Biomed Inform 107:103429
42. Kormilitzin A, Vaci N, Liu Q, Nevado-Holgado A (2021) Med7: a transferable clinical natural language processing model for electronic health records. Artif Intell Med 118:102086
43. Filippi M, Agosta F, Barkhof F et al (2012) EFNS task force: the use of neuroimaging in the diagnosis of dementia. Eur J Neurol 19:1487–1501
44. Greicius MD, Srivastava G, Reiss AL, Menon V (2004) Default-mode network activity distinguishes Alzheimer's disease from healthy aging: evidence from functional MRI. Proc Natl Acad Sci USA 101:4637–4642
45. Horvath A, Szucs A, Csukly G, Sakovics A, Stefanics G, Kamondi A (2018) EEG and ERP biomarkers of Alzheimer's disease: a critical review. Front Biosci (Landmark Ed) 23:183–220
46. Babiloni C, Blinowska K, Bonanni L et al (2020) What electrophysiology tells us about Alzheimer's disease: a window into the synchronization and connectivity of brain neurons. Neurobiol Aging 85:58–73
47. Kato T, Inui Y, Nakamura A, Ito K (2016) Brain fluorodeoxyglucose (FDG) PET in dementia. Ageing Res Rev 30:73–84
48. Chételat G, Arbizu J, Barthel H et al (2020) Amyloid-PET and 18F-FDG-PET in the diagnostic investigation of Alzheimer's disease and other dementias. Lancet Neurol 19:951–962
49. Lowe VJ, Curran G, Fang P et al (2016) An autoradiographic evaluation of AV-1451 Tau PET in dementia. Acta Neuropathol Commun 4:58
50. Jack CR Jr, Bernstein MA, Fox NC et al (2008) The Alzheimer's disease neuroimaging initiative (ADNI): MRI methods. J Magn Reson Imag 27:685–691
51. Beekly DL, Ramos EM, Lee WW et al (2007) The National Alzheimer's Coordinating Center (NACC) database: the uniform data set. Alzheimer Dis Assoc Disord 21:249–258
52. Marcus DS, Wang TH, Parker J, Csernansky JG, Morris JC, Buckner RL (2007) Open access series of imaging studies (oasis): cross-sectional MRI data in young, middle aged, nondemented, and demented older adults. J Cogn Neurosci 19:1498–1507
53. Rohrer JD, Nicholas JM, Cash DM et al (2015) Presymptomatic cognitive and neuroanatomical changes in genetic frontotemporal dementia in the genetic frontotemporal dementia initiative (GENFI) study: a cross-sectional analysis. Lancet Neurol 14:253–262
54. Li F, Liu M (2019) A hybrid convolutional and recurrent neural network for hippocampus analysis in Alzheimer's disease. J Neurosci Methods 323:108–118
55. Morin A, Samper-Gonzalez J, Bertrand A et al (2020) Accuracy of MRI classification algorithms in a tertiary memory center clinical routine cohort. J Alzheimers Dis 74:1157–1166
56. Costafreda SG, Dinov ID, Tu Z et al (2011) Automated hippocampal shape analysis predicts the onset of dementia in mild cognitive impairment. Neuroimage 56:212–219
57. Giorgio J, Landau S, Jagust W, Tino P, Kourtzi Z (2020) Modelling prognostic trajectories of cognitive decline due to Alzheimer's disease. NeuroImage: Clin 26:102199
58. Iturria-Medina Y, Sotero RC, Toussaint PJ et al (2016) Early role of vascular dysregulation on late-onset Alzheimer's disease based on multifactorial data-driven analysis. Nat Commun 7:11934
59. Vogel JW, Young AL, Oxtoby NP et al (2021) Four distinct trajectories of tau deposition identified in Alzheimer's disease. Nat Med 27:871–881

60. Liu M, Li F, Yan H et al (2020) A multi-model deep convolutional neural network for automatic hippocampus segmentation and classification in Alzheimer's disease. Neuroimage 208:116459
61. Power JD, Barnes KA, Snyder AZ, Schlaggar BL, Petersen SE (2012) Spurious but systematic correlations in functional connectivity MRI networks arise from subject motion. Neuroimage 59:2142–2154
62. Qiu S, Joshi PS, Miller MI et al (2020) Development and validation of an interpretable deep learning framework for Alzheimer's disease classification. Brain 143:1920–1933
63. Parikh RB, Teeple S, Navathe AS (2019) Addressing bias in artificial intelligence in health care. JAMA 322:2377–2378
64. Mendelson AF, Zuluaga MA, Lorenzi M, Hutton BF, Ourselin S (2017) Selection bias in the reported performances of AD classification pipelines. NeuroImage: Clinical 14:400–416
65. Muehlematter UJ, Daniore P, Vokinger KN (2021) Approval of artificial intelligence and machine learning-based medical devices in the USA and Europe (2015–20): a comparative analysis. Lancet Digit Health 3:e195–e203
66. Global, regional, and national incidence, prevalence, and years lived with disability for 354 diseases and injuries for 195 countries and territories, 1990–2017: a systematic analysis for the Global Burden of Disease Study 2017 (2018) Lancet 392:1789–1858
67. Livingston G, Huntley J, Sommerlad A et al (2020) Dementia prevention, intervention, and care: 2020 report of the Lancet Commission. Lancet 396:413–446
68. Norton S, Matthews FE, Barnes DE, Yaffe K, Brayne C (2014) Potential for primary prevention of Alzheimer's disease: an analysis of population-based data. Lancet Neurol 13:788–794
69. Deckers K, van Boxtel MP, Schiepers OJ et al (2015) Target risk factors for dementia prevention: a systematic review and Delphi consensus study on the evidence from observational studies. Int J Geriatr Psychiat 30:234–246
70. Kuźma E, Hannon E, Zhou A et al (2018) Which risk factors causally influence dementia? A systematic review of mendelian randomization studies. J Alzheimers Dis 64:181–193
71. Nicholls HL, John CR, Watson DS, Munroe PB, Barnes MR, Cabrera CP (2020) Reaching the end-game for GWAS: machine learning approaches for the prioritization of complex disease loci. Front Genet 11
72. Peters R, Booth A, Rockwood K, Peters J, D'Este C, Anstey KJ (2019) Combining modifiable risk factors and risk of dementia: a systematic review and meta-analysis. BMJ Open 9:e022846
73. Sproviero W, Winchester L, Newby D et al (2021) High blood pressure and risk of dementia: a two-sample mendelian randomization study in the UK Biobank. Biol Psychiat 89:817–824
74. Moore PJ, Lyons TJ, Gallacher J (2019) for the Alzheimer's disease neuroimaging I. Using path signatures to predict a diagnosis of Alzheimer's disease. PloS One 14:e0222212
75. Kivipelto M, Ngandu T, Laatikainen T, Winblad B, Soininen H, Tuomilehto J (2006) Risk score for the prediction of dementia risk in 20 years among middle aged people: a longitudinal, population-based study. Lancet Neurol 5:735–741
76. Liu R, Wei L, Zhang P (2021) A deep learning framework for drug repurposing via emulating clinical trials on real-world patient data. Nat Mach Intell 3:68–75
77. Fang J, Zhang P, Wang Q et al (2020) Network-based translation of GWAS findings to pathobiology and drug repurposing for Alzheimer's disease. medRxiv 2020:2020.2001.2015.20017160
78. Tsuji S, Hase T, Yachie-Kinoshita A et al (2021) Artificial intelligence-based computational framework for drug-target prioritization and inference of novel repositionable drugs for Alzheimer's disease. Alzheimer's Res Therapy 13:92
79. Tomlinson A, Furukawa TA, Efthimiou O et al (2020) Personalise antidepressant treatment for unipolar depression combining individual choices, risks and big data (PETRUSHKA): rationale and protocol. Evid Based Ment Health 23:52–56

Effective Diagnosis of Parkinson's Disease Using Machine Learning Techniques

Bilash Dash, Tianhua Chen, and Richard Hill

Abstract Parkinson's disease (PD) is a progressive neurological disorder that impairs the physical abilities of human beings such as speech, gait, and complex muscle-and-nerve actions. Early diagnosis of PD is important for alleviating the symptoms and reducing the overall socio-economic burden in healthcare. However, the key to the success is cost-effective and convenient telemedicine technology to overcome the challenges around the availability of expensive diagnoses and skilled clinicians. Almost 90% of PD patients suffer from a speech disorder and hence speech signals can be used as a non-invasive and cost-effective technique for diagnosis. Recent advances in machine learning and sensor technologies facilitate automated PD diagnosis for increased prediction accuracy and the capability to handle diverse biomarkers in an effective and timely manner. In establishing an effective predictive model for PD diagnosis, this study explores several popular machine learning classifiers in combination with feature set extraction, with and without Principal Component Analysis (PCA). Evaluating performance with a PD benchmark data set, our research discovered that Deep Neural Networks and Gradient Boosting Machines achieved 1st and 2nd places with an accuracy of **94.44%** and **89.74%**, with a weighted average **f1-score of more than 93%**. It is expected that this outcome will help clinicians achieve effective differentiation of the PD group from healthy controls based on voice data.

1 Introduction

Parkinson's Disease (PD), firstly described by the British Physicians James Parkinson [1, 2], is a neurological progressive disorder that involves degeneration of the central nervous system around specific nerve cells or neurons based in a region of the brain (mid brain area) called substantia niagra [1, 3–8]. The degeneration of these neurons results in reduced production of dopamine, leading to restricted motor control, which

B. Dash · T. Chen (✉) · R. Hill
Department of Computer Science, School of Computing and Engineering,
University of Huddersfield, Huddersfield, UK
e-mail: T.Chen@hud.ac.uk

© The Author(s), under exclusive license to Springer Nature Singapore Pte Ltd. 2022
T. Chen et al. (eds.), *Artificial Intelligence in Healthcare*, Brain Informatics and Health,
https://doi.org/10.1007/978-981-19-5272-2_5

progressively gets worse. The rate of progression is so slow that the symptoms are visible only after 70–80% of neurons have died which could be too late from an individual's wellbeing perspective [3, 5–7, 9]. It is believed that a combination of age, genetic and environmental factors could be the cause behind the degeneration of neurons [1, 3, 7, 10].

The symptoms of PD can be categorised as follows: (1) **Motor** symptoms affecting the movement & co-ordinations of body parts and can be seen by others, (2) **Non-motor** symptoms, sometimes called non-visible symptoms. Non-motor symptoms are manifested through sleep disorder, affecting mental health, eyesight, memory, speech & communication and sometimes resulting in pain and fatigue [7–9, 11]. The clinician, in the absence of well-proven tests for diagnosis of Parkinson's, use the symptoms and results of several invasive and non-invasive tests such as neurological, imaging and pathological etc. which are expensive, not accurate enough and could be misleading [2, 6–8, 12].

Studies show that an estimated of more than 10 million people around the world are suffering from PD and men are 1.5 times more likely to get affected with PD than women [5]. A statistical compilation made in 2018 found around 145 K registered PD patients in the United Kingdom i.e., 1 in 350 adults which is set to rise to 1 in 5 by 2025 with 50 new patients are diagnosed every day [1, 7, 11, 13]. The life expectancy is not impacted by the onset of PD but makes the person vulnerable to severe infections and/or death [9, 13–15]. As there is no cure to the PD, hence monitoring and treatment, comprising a combination of medications, & therapies such as physiotherapy, speech & language therapy, becomes an ongoing option with a possibility of a surgical option, called Deep Brain Stimulation (DBS), which could be financially not viable for the majority of the mass. The dearth of neurological and movement disorder experts poses an added challenge for the timely diagnosis & treatment [11].

It has been established that more than 25% of PD patients are misdiagnosed (or missed diagnosis) and around 48% were diagnosed and treated for their non-existent condition due to the absence & untimely of tests to predict the onset of the disease [3, 5, 6, 16, 17]. One of the most effective & non-invasive diagnoses is done by measuring the frequency of various speech signals over a period of time for the progression of PD [2, 8, 10–13, 17–19] as the critical mass of PD subjects suffer from speech disorders.

With faster adoption of digital healthcare systems & cloud-native technologies, a plethora of digital healthcare data, real-time sensors data and research outcomes are widely available at central places for the analysis and extraction of knowledge and patterns that may facilitate the understanding, diagnosis and treatment of PD. This is accelerated with the recent advancement of machine learning (ML) techniques, an area of Artificial Intelligence that is concerned with learning automatically from the data, which has witnessed successes in numerous health and medicine areas [20–24].

A cost-effective way for diagnosis and hence the treatment could be delivered through employing computer-assisted diagnosis by analysing data from various sensors, medical & wearable devices acquired through IoT technology and then subject to ML model(s) for the timely prediction/detection of PD. A lot of research has been done on the feasibility of predicting the onset of PD through using various machine learning & neural network classifiers such as Support Vector Machine (SVM), Deep Neural Network (DNN), Convolutional Neural Network (CNN), Regression and Decision Trees integrating data from multi-modal sensors, wearing and audio devices. It was noticed that most of the contributions highlighting the automatic detection of PD were based on the continuous speech samples representing the periodicity and regularity of the voice signals [1, 2, 7–10, 13–15, 18]. Numerous reviewed research incorporating a combination of conventional ML & neural network algorithms had different performance outcomes based on the feature set & algorithm selected with DNN & SVM topping in the list [2]. Some papers used Principal Component Analysis (PCA) and Kernel Principal Component Analysis (KPCA) used as part of feature selection strategy to choose the most significant features and obtained a high degree of accuracy with low computational time [5–7]. The key emphasis of each paper was to devise an evaluative approach following different feature engineering & optimisation techniques to develop the best performing model.

In working towards establishing a case study to demonstrate the effectiveness of recent machine learning models in diagnosing PD, this paper attempted a machine learning pipeline to improve the accuracy of the prediction of PD group from the healthy controls by comparing the performance of linear, non-linear, ensemble and neural network algorithms with the original feature sets as well as the PCA based feature set. A comparative study was conducted using various statistical performance metrics of both sets to start with and then progressing in steps based on the best outcome of the previous step of the pipeline.

2 Related Works

In order to inform and guide this work, several relevant works delivered in the last five years (2016–2020) on the application of ML predicting the PD using different motor/non-motor data, predominantly speech impairment data, was reviewed at the time when this study was reviewed. Those works generally used a combination of both linear, non-linear machine learning algorithms combined with advanced feature engineering techniques and achieved different but impressive performance scores showing the effectiveness of ML in predicting PD at an early stage [2, 7, 8, 10, 13, 15, 17–19]. For instance, Agarwal et al. [8] used Extreme Learning Machine (ELM) using a single hidden layer Feed Forward Network with randomly chosen weights & biases for predicting PD on the speech data set from UCI Machine learning Repository. The **ELM** model was very fast in training & achieved better generalisation with an accuracy of 81.55%, better than SVN and Artificial Neural Network (ANN) used for comparison. From the perspective of used predictors, some research evaluated the performance of standard machine learning classifiers both on Original Feature Set and reduced feature set of different component sizes following the application of dimensionality reduction using PCA and KPCA on UCI speech data. Although, several researches [7, 15, 18] were impressive with a reduced feature set with accuracy reported between 90–97% but the best algorithm reported was different on each occasion.

In addition, the application of standard ML classifiers and Neural Network algorithms were also applied to complex data sets such as digitised handwriting data by Shamrat et al. [13] to identify movement disorder potential leading to PD, complex genetic & transcriptomic data by Su et al. [25] in early identification of PD subtypes and phonation data by Almeida et al. [26]. In a recent review article [25] that summarises 15 literatures highlighted the advanced application of ML on complex genetic & transcriptomic data set, and highlighted the significant improvement in the diagnosis of PD using ML on such complex data structure, and how that helped clinicians not just predicting the PD but also identifying risky gene expression (PD subtypes) for effective treatment and the need of further research using ML for better understanding of the pathogenesis of PD.

Alternatively, the specific application of (deep) neural network-based models for predicting the PD in some research proved more effective over standard ML classifiers [2, 27–29] on different data sets from UCI ML repository, PPMI database and wearable devices. Belić et al. [29] had done a systematic review of 48 literature on the application of ML covering conventional & neural network algorithms on body kinematics data including both upper & lower body extremities using different instrumentations for diagnosis, monitoring and assessment of PD. Those researches revealed that the data from wearable devices combined with supervised machine learning algorithms such as SVM, SVR, NB, LR, ANN, k-NN, EML, LDA, DT etc., with ANN topping the rank, can provide significant diagnostic support to the clinician in early detection of PD with an accuracy of more than 90%. This is also consistent with a recent work done by Wang et al. [28] involved a comparison of the performance of deep learning framework involving 3 different architectures, one ensemble model combining those three neural models and 11 machine learning algorithms for early detection of PD using data from Parkinson's Progression Markers Initiative (PPMI) database. The deep learning model resulted in superior performance with an accuracy of 96.45% without resorting to any feature selection techniques.

Generally, the use of machine learning to facilitate PD diagnosis typically involves applying various feature engineering techniques, followed by the employment of specific machine learning algorithms to establish a predictive model for diagnosis. The use of both motor and non-motor data sets, collected from clinical and/or wearable instruments, proved the huge potential of ML across data types helping clinicians in forecasting the onset of a terminal illness. It is evident from the above review that ML-based prediction of PD could help clinicians significantly in taking early clinical decisions for interventions of most PD subjects. It was observed that PCA based feature set (PFS) had delivered far better model performance over the original feature set (OFS). The DNN algorithm in general delivered better performance over linear and non-linear ML algorithms across all literatures reviewed for both original and reduced feature data sets. However, there are instances where k-NN and SVM modelled on dataset following application of different feature extraction/selection criteria and imputation techniques delivered better performance with an accuracy of more than 95%. Hence, it is evident from the literature review that there is no free lunch available & hence prudent to have a performance evaluation framework comprising multiple ML algorithms on PD speech impairment data combined with DR technique to identify the best performing classifier.

Work in this paper, motivated by past works mentioned above, extends the approach followed in the literatures. The ML pipeline experimented in this paper includes feature engineering & extraction using PCA to address multi-collinearity in the dataset, K-fold cross-validation to address unbalance in the UCI speech data set, evaluating the performance of multiple linear, non-linear, ensemble classifiers and Deep Neural Network (DNN) followed by model optimisation using Grid search. The extended framework helps in identifying the best classifier & demonstrate effective use of ML algorithms in predicting PD with higher performance. It is expected that this framework will motivate others to apply to data set in healthcare or in other sectors as well to identify the best performing algorithm for a given use case.

3 Experimental Pipeline and Setup

The diagram in Fig. 1 describes the methodology followed for the research using a myriad of algorithms (linear, non-linear, ensemble and neural network) in combination with the use of two feature sets, i.e., original feature set (OFS) and PCA-informed feature set (PFS). In general, the experimentation comprised several exploratory analysis and ML engineering tasks executed in sequence. The initial & exploratory data analysis provided various structural, relational and statistical insights about the data set emphasizing the need for feature engineering. The data set was stratified to overcome the imbalanced distribution of the classification label and then subject to test/train split with cross-validation. The experiment involved 6 standard ML, 3 ensemble and 1 DNN algorithms which were trained & tested with default hyper-parameters in stage 1(Baseline). The 2nd Stage (Tuning) took the 3 best models out of standard & ensemble classifiers and the DNN in stage 1. All models in stage 2 were optimised with an extensive hyper-parameter grid using Grid search. The best of the fine-tuned ML algorithms and the DNN in stage 2 were trained on the full training data set and tested with the test data set in stage 3(Finalise). Both models' performance was compared using various performance metrics such as accuracy, f1-score, specificity, ROC, Log loss and Precision-Recall graph to choose the best fitting algorithm.

The dataset used is a popular benchmark from UCI website [14], composed of a set of biomedical voice markers of 195 data points from 31 people out of which 23 are diagnosed with PD. The dataset has 24 attributes with each observation identified by the subject with the 'name' attribute and the 'status' attribute with binary values, i.e., '1' for PD afflicted and '0' for healthy subjects. The time since diagnoses ranged from 0 to 28 years and the ages of the subjects ranged from 46 to 85 years (mean 65.8, standard deviation 9.8). On an average of six phonations were recorded from each subject, ranging from one to 36 s in length. Although amplitude normalization affects

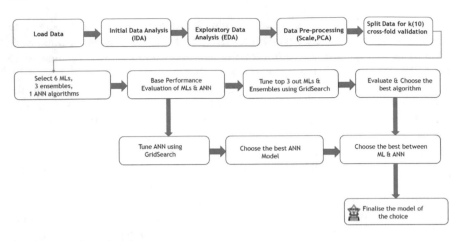

Fig. 1 Research methodology

the calibration of the samples, the study is focused on measures insensitive to changes in absolute speech pressure level. Thus, to ensure the robustness of the algorithms, all samples were digitally normalized in amplitude prior to the calculation of the measures.

As some machine learning algorithms may be affected significantly by dramatically different ranges of attributes, standardization was applied which transforms features in a dataset with mixed Gaussian and non-Gaussian distributions into a standard Gaussian distribution with a mean of 0 and standard deviation of 1.

The dimensionality reduction process in ML pipeline helps to reduce the number of dimensions in a high dimensional dataset either through features selection or feature extraction. **Principal Component Analysis (PCA),** a dimensionality reduction method, is employed to extract the best possible features of a dataset with 'd' number of vectors to reduce the dimensionality by making a set 'k' PCA feature (vector) orthogonal to each other. *Each* PCA vector is formed with higher variance i.e., the first PCA vector/component will have the largest variance followed by the second and so on. Hence, there is a need to choose the minimum number of PCA components from the orthogonal space representing the maximum number of variances of the data set [7, 10, 11, 15].

In order to establish an effective model for PD diagnosis, the following popular 10 machine learning techniques have been explored.

- **Linear Algorithms:**

  - Logistic Regression (LR) uses a logistic function to model a binary classification problem and in this research is used to classify the positive PD patients.
  - Linear Discriminant Analysis (LDA) predicts the class label by using a linear model of independent vectors (object) and estimating the probability of each class in the k-finite set and assigning the class to the vector with the highest probability.

- **Non-linear Algorithms**:

  - A Decision Tree is a non-parametric ML model that predicts the value of the target (class label) by learning the decision rules inferred from the features i.e., with a set of 'If–Then-Elses'. Each feature is represented as the node, the branch as the decision on the node and the leaf node is the outcome/class label in the tree structure and hence is the name.
  - k-Nearest Neighbour (KNN) is a supervised classification algorithm where each independent vector or the input object is assigned to the class that most commonly exists in its k-neighbours voted the object in plurality.
  - Naïve Bayes (NB) uses Bayes' theorem in which the feature vectors are assigned to a class label drawn out of k-finite values with an assumption that each feature independently contributes to the underlying class value.
  - Support Vector Machine (SVM) algorithm classifies each vector by distributing those vectors on both sides of a hyper-plane in such a manner that all vectors are kept as far from the plane as possible. Vectors close to the hyperplane are called Support Vectors.

- **Ensemble Algorithms**:

  - Random Forest (RF) utilises ensemble learning using multiple decision trees on a distinct group of data points to predict the class label for each sub-tree. The RF uses the majority of the votes from sub-trees to assign the class to the test/new data.
  - AdaBoost (AB) is an ensemble boosting algorithm and works by building a series of models starting with weaker and gradually strengthened models through learning from the previous model through assigning higher weights to misclassified & lower weights to correctly classified points by previous base algorithm resulting in the final model with better accuracy. This experiment used a Decision Tree classifier with depth = 1 as the base estimator.
  - Gradient Boosting Machine (GBM) ensembles decision tree models optimised through a loss function and gradient descent algorithm so as to minimise the gradient loss in order to deliver a better fit model.

- **Deep Neural Network (DNN)** is an extension of Artificial Neural Network (ANN), where it uses multiple dense layers of fully connected neurons to establish the relationship between the input and output layers through a differentiable Activation Function and optimised weight & bias matrix linked to hidden layers.

Despite the implementation of machine learning algorithms that come with default parameter settings, the grid search was also performed, which search over a given subset of the hyper-parameters space (search grid) of a training algorithm. Each model was then built and evaluated based on every combination of parameters (each small square) defined in the grid, with a hyper-parameter of the best machine learning model reported in the next section.

In order to generate more reliable results, cross-validation has been used to split the dataset to have less variance. The whole data set is split into k (k = 10 in this paper)

Fig. 2 Confusion matrix

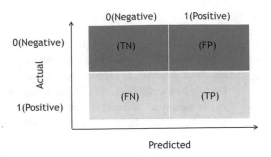

folds to inform the algorithm to cross-validate in a cyclic manner. The algorithm is trained on (k–1) folds i.e. 90% of the data with one held back fold for testing in each cycle. The process is repeated so that each fold of the dataset is given a chance to be the held back test set. The outcome of the process results in k different performance scores (E_i) which is averaged out to establish the single performance of the algorithm, which is a reliable estimate [17] (Fig. 2).

In terms of performance evaluation of the resultant models, several metrics are employed and introduced here. These include the confusion matrix, which tables the predicted score against the actual ones as shown in Table 2, where TN is True Negative that records subjects that do not have PD and correctly predicted; FN is False Negative, where a positive PD patient is predicted as non-PD case; FP is False Positive, where a non-PD patient is incorrectly predicted as positive and TP is True Positive, where a PD patient is correctly predicted as the positive.

- Accuracy of the prediction made by the model is measured as the ratio of correctly classified data with respect to total data points
  i.e.= $\frac{TP+TN}{TP+FP+TN+FN}$
- The Precision of a prediction is measured as the number of points predicted correctly positive out of the total number of positives predicted by the model i.e. $\frac{TP}{(TP+FP)}$
- The Recall is measured as the number of points predicted positive correctly out of the total number of actual positive i.e. $\frac{TP}{(TP+FN)}$

Both Precision and Recall should be as high as possible to have an effective model. The harmonic mean of precision and recall metric, called F1-score, as described below, better describes the model performance. This experimentation is a health care use case, where FP and FN play a crucial role in delivering financially efficient and clinically risk-averse service respectively and hence F1-score is considered equally important as accuracy.

$$F1-Score = \frac{2*Precision*Recall}{(Precision+Recall)}$$

Receiver Operating Characteristic (ROC) is the plot of TPR against FPR producing a curved line for various threshold values as shown in Fig. 3, where TPR is the Ratio of True positive to total positive and FPR is the ratio of False-positive to total negative. AUC is the Ares Under Curve and lies in the range of [0,1]. The value of AUC in the range [0.5,1] is considered good and hence better model should give AUC score closer to 1.

It uses the probability score computed by the model to compute loss incurred between the real and predicted label value. The log-loss is inversely proportional to the predicted probability as seen in Fig. 4, hence the log-loss has to be as minimum as possible for predicted probability to be as closer to 1. The research used as this is an important metric for both binary & multi-class classification.

The experimentation was conducted in a laptop with a dual-core Intel i7 @2.5 GHz with 8 GB RAM running Windows 10 Professional edition. The research used Spyder 5.1.0 of Anaconda distribution for the Parkinson's dataset pre-processing, EDA (Exploratory Data Analysis), model building & performance analysis using Python 3.8.8. The outputs generated, including graphs by Spyder, have been used in this research. The Spyder environment was updated with TensorFlow/Keras, Scikit-learn, Scipy, Matplotlib, Yellowbricks and Stats model packages in addition to defaults packages it is shipped with.

Fig. 3 ROC curve

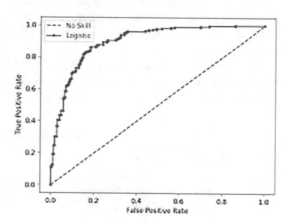

Fig. 4 Log loss working model

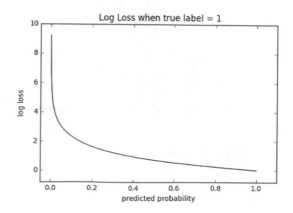

4 Experimental Results and Discussion

An EDA (Exploratory Data Analysis) was performed on the PD data set for missing data, outlier and data distribution. It turned out there does not exist any missing values, hence advanced interpolation techniques such as [30] is not required, for data imputation and the data set had a mix of Gaussian & Exponential distribution.

The following bar graph in Fig. 5 shows the distribution of class variable, 'status', 1(PD patients) and 0(Healthy subjects), which shows that value distribution is imbalanced, approximately in 1:3 ratio—this is also maintained through stratification when splitting the data into training and test sets.

Multivariate data analysis was further conducted to understand the data distribution and correlation among them, following the standardisation of original data. As shown in Fig. 6, a strong correlation among features was found using Pearson's correlation algorithm which is evident from the heat map with a correlation coefficient >= 0.9. Hence, it was critical to go for feature extraction for effective model performance and the Principal Component Analysis (PCA) was used.

The PCA analysis using the cumulative sum of variance ratio demonstrated that 96% of the variance could be explained by 8 components with 1% increase in variance for each additional component. Figure 7 shows the cumulative variance graph showing the maximum variance achieved with n = 8, which was used for this research.

The scaled PCA features and the class variable were empirically split in 80:20 to create train& test data segments for independent testing on the final model. The training set, for each ML model, was subject to K-tenfold cross-validation. The

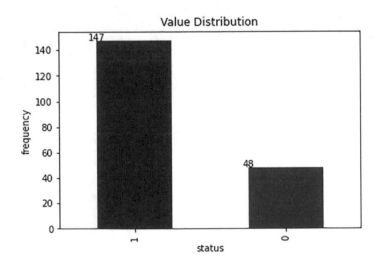

Fig. 5 Class distribution

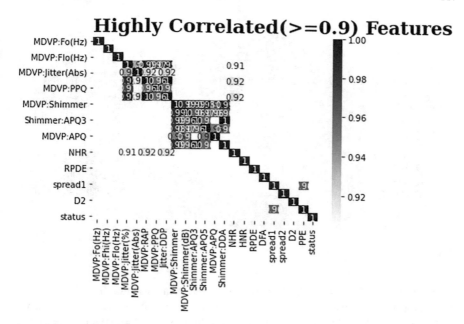

Fig. 6 Highly correlated feature heat map

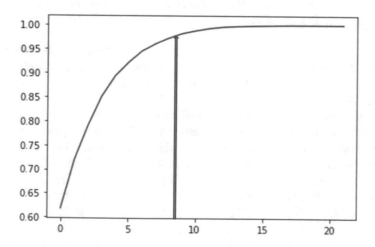

Fig. 7 PCA cumulative variance graph (n = 22)

labels were stratified between train & test data split (80:20) and within K-fold cross-validation as well for effective training of the model. The diagram in Fig. 8 describes various stages followed during the experimentation.

All 10 models were evaluated with tenfold cross-validation with default parameter settings and on both standardised (OFS) and PCA (8 component) features set (PFS) to compare the performance of models on both feature sets.

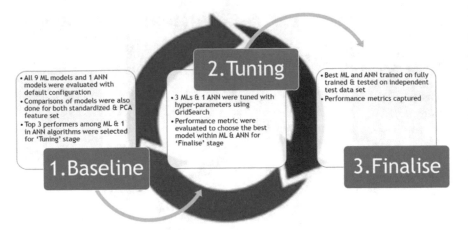

Fig. 8 Model training strategy

The above model training strategy was followed in the research for selecting algorithms for the subsequent stage based on their relative performance. It was observed that almost all algorithms fared better on PFS over OFS and an accuracy cut-off of 89% was decided to choose three ML algorithms i.e. KNN, SVM, GBM and DNN were selected for the next level of experimentation i.e. to tune further to get the best performance. Table 1 describes the mean accuracy of each algorithm for each feature set.

Table 1 above shows that PCA based feature set with drastically reduced features (by 36%) has delivered the same or better performance. The PCA-based feature set will be explored onwards for subsequent experimentation to have optimal computation complexity.

All four selected algorithms in the previous stage were subject to tuning through setting different values to key hyper-parameters. All key hyper-parameters, potentially impacting the performance, were defined in grid implementing through Python dictionary object & Grid search, a brute force technique, and evaluating the performance of the model for all combinations of hyper-parameters. This stage identifies the best model within each algorithm and validates against the independent validation data set (Not PD = 10, PD = 29 observations) held back at the time data split.

Table 2 above describes the performance of the best model within each algorithm against the independent validation data set along with the best parameter values following the grid search strategy to identify the best algorithm. The best algorithms, one each from ML and DNN, were further selected for the next stage for finalising the winner of this research. GBM and SVM have a tie in terms of model accuracy i.e., 94.87%. However, GBM has a recall for 1 as 100% with 0(zero) 'False Negative' as shown in the confusion matrix. Though SVM has a better f1-score than GBM and being a healthcare project, more emphasis would be given to the 'Recall' value of positive cases i.e. '**status**' = 1 and hence has chosen GBM over SVM–GBM and DNN models hence go to next stage i.e. '**Finalise**'.

Table 1 Model performance with OFS versus PFS

Algorithm	Standardised feature set (%)	PCA feature set (8 components) (%) ✔	Next stage selection
Logistic Regression (LR)	81	83	✖
Linear Discriminant Analysis (LDA)	86	84	✖
Decision Tree (DT)	83	86.3	✖
k-Nearest Neighbors (KNN)	89	89	✔
Gaussian Naïve Bayes (NB)	69	81	✖
Support Vector Machine (SVM),	86	86.5	✔
Random Forest (RF),	86	86	✖
AdaBoost (AB)	91	86	✖
Gradient Boosting Machine (GBM)	88	89	✔
DNN (Sequence)	87	88	✔

The GBM and the DNN models in the previous stage were fully trained on the training data set with the best parameters identified and they were now validated against the independent validation data set previously held, with the outcomes represented in Confusion Matrix as shown in Fig. 9.

The DNN has a better type-I error (False Positive) than GBM which has no consequence on health risk as more follow-up tests are done for PD confirmation but may not be financially appealing. Both models have very low (1 number) type-II error (False Negative), which is not solicited in the healthcare service but could be improved by choosing a representative sample as the data set is imbalanced as shown in Fig. 5 and/or providing some biases to the minority class.

The accuracy of DNN, as shown in Table 3, is better than GBM and with TNR 90% and hence is more effective than GBM. The accuracy should be read in conjunction with the f1-score in Fig. 10 for overall effectiveness, where the overall f1-score of DNN is higher than that of GBM and both the recall & precision of the 'Parkinson' label is better in the case of DNN.

The ROC of DNN has very high 'steepness' and hence AUC is larger than GBM is close to 1 as shown in Fig. 11 and hence is more effective.

Table 2 Optimised model performance

Algorithm	Conf. matrix	Accuracy (Baseline)	Class	Precision	Recall	F1 score	Best grid parameters
KNN	[[8 2] [1 28]]	82.3% (89.0%)	0	0.89	0.80	0.84	{'algorithm': 'ball_tree', 'n_neighbors': 4, 'p': 2, 'weights': 'distance'}
			1	0.93	0.97	0.95	
SVM	[[9 1] [1 28]]	87.8% (86.5%)	0	0.90	0.90	0.90	{'C': 10, 'gamma': 0.2, 'kernel': 'rbf'}
			1	0.97	0.97	0.97	
GBM	[[7 3] [1 28]]	89.74% (89.0%)	0	0.87	0.70	0.77	{'learning_rate': 0.3, 'max_depth': 5, 'min_samples_leaf': 2, 'min_samples_split': 3, 'n_estimators': 40, 'subsample': 1.0}
			1	0.90	0.96	0.93	
DNN	[[9 1] [1 28]]	94.44% (88.0%)	0	0.90	0.90	0.90	{'batch_size': 10, 'epochs': 750, 'optimizer': 'RMSprop'}

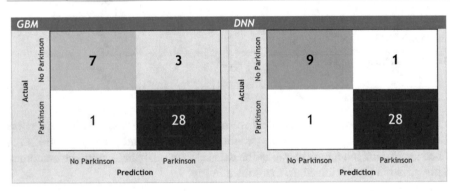

Fig. 9 Model confusion matrix comparison

Table 3 Model accuracy comparison

Algorithm	Accuracy (%)	Misclassification (%)	Specificity (%)
GBM	89.74	10.26	70.00
DNN	94.44	5.13	90.00

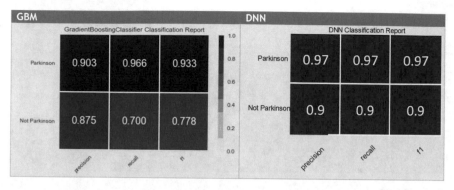

Fig. 10 Model classification report comparison

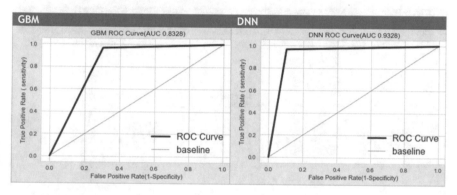

Fig. 11 Model ROC & AUC comparison

This is supported further by the area under the curve (AUC) for DNN, shown in Fig. 12, which is almost 1 and is higher than GBM signifying the strong predictability power of the algorithm. The log loss of DNN is also better than GBM as shown in Fig. 13.

Overall, this suggests the effectiveness of using a **Deep Neural Network** for diagnosing Parkinson's disease. The above conclusion is in line with the outcome of reviewed papers where DNN [2, 8], SVM [10, 13, 15] and KNN [7, 19] delivered the best result on speech signal data using different feature extraction/selection techniques. In general, KNN & SVM performed well with feature reduction technique with accuracy well above 90% but with a low number of reduced dimensions using PCA. The DNN, wherever compared with ML algorithms fared well with an accuracy above 90% using hyper-parameter tuning. However, no single paper had mentioned the use of the GBM as part of the evaluation.

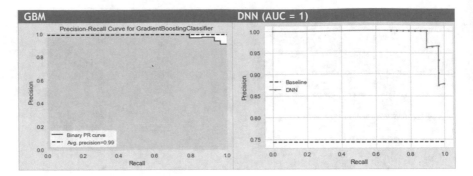

Fig. 12 Model precision-recall curves

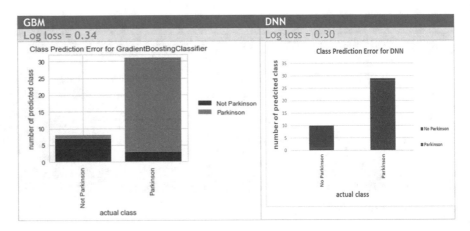

Fig. 13 Model Loss and error comparison

5 Conclusion

In this study, a gradual evaluation of ten different machine learnings was experimented including linear, non-linear, ensemble methods and one deep learning algorithm with & without PCA on the Parkinson benchmark. It turned out most algorithms delivered good **accuracies (>85%)** on reduced feature set (PCA = 8 components), which demonstrate the effectiveness of applying machine learning for PD diagnosis. In particular, the DNN produced the best accuracy as high as 94% with just eight features and with a weighted average f1-score of 0.97. Another finding was that most of the algorithms gave better results with a fewer number of features that have significantly reduced employing Principal Component Analysis, which would also result in the computational time efficiency. In future work, it would therefore be worth investigating further the advantage of different feature selection and extraction techniques, which in addition to bringing the advantage of improving model performance and reducing computational load, but also deliver significant benefits in clinical practice & cost optimisation through conducting a fewer number of tests. Another interesting future work may consider establishing the model with data collected under COVID19 that has resulted in influence over several factors such as mental wellbeing [31].

References

1. Pereira CR et al (2019) A survey on computer-assisted Parkinson's Disease diagnosis. Artif Intell Med 95:48–63
2. Haq AU et al (2018) Comparative analysis of the classification performance of machine learning classifiers and deep neural network classifier for prediction of parkinson disease. 2018 15th international computer conference on wavelet active media technology and information processing (ICCWAMTIP)
3. ParkinsonsUK (2021) Parkinson's UK. Retrieved 05/06/2021, from https://www.parkinsons.org.uk/
4. Team PSNT (2018) Parkinson's News Today, from https://parkinsonsnewstoday.com/
5. Foundation PS (2016) Parkinson's foundation. Retrieved 05/06/2021, from https://www.parkinson.org/understanding-parkinsons
6. WebMD (2021) WebMD -Parkinson's Disease Health Center. Retrieved 06/06/2021, from https://www.webmd.com/parkinsons-disease/
7. Anand A et al (2018) Evaluation of machine learning and deep learning algorithms combined with dimensionality reduction techniques for classification of Parkinson's Disease. 2018 IEEE International symposium on signal processing and information technology (ISSPIT)
8. Agarwal A et al (2016) Prediction of Parkinson's disease using speech signal with Extreme Learning Machine. 2016 international conference on electrical, electronics, and optimization techniques (ICEEOT)
9. Bind S et al (2015) A survey of machine learning based approaches for Parkinson disease prediction. Int J Comput Sci Inf Technol 6(2):1648–1655
10. Shahbakhti M et al (2013) Combination of PCA and SVM for diagnosis of Parkinson's disease. 2013 2nd international conference on advances in biomedical engineering
11. Little M et al (2008) Suitability of dysphonia measurements for telemonitoring of Parkinson's disease. Nature Proceedings
12. Lew M (2007) Overview of Parkinson's disease. Pharmacotherapy: J Human Pharmacol Drug Therapy 27(12P2):155S–160S
13. Shamrat FM et al (2019) A comparative analysis of parkinson disease prediction using machine learning approaches 1:2576–2580
14. Dua DAGC (2017) UCI machine learning repository—Parkinson's sataset. Retrieved 05/06/2021, from https://archive.ics.uci.edu/ml/datasets/Parkinsons
15. Kaninika, Tayal A (2018) Determination of Parkinson's disease utilizing Machine Learning Methods. 2018 International conference on advances in computing, communication control and networking (ICACCCN)
16. Jankovic J (2008) Parkinson's disease: clinical features and diagnosis. J Neurol Neurosurg Psychiatry 79(4):368
17. Nilashi M et al (2016) Accuracy improvement for predicting Parkinson's disease progression. Sci Rep 6(1):34181
18. Aich S et al (2018) A nonlinear decision tree based classification approach to predict the Parkinson's disease using different feature sets of voice data. 2018 20th international conference on advanced communication technology (ICACT)

19. Ozkan H (2016) A comparison of classification methods for Telediagnosis of Parkinson's Disease. Entropy 18(4):115
20. Chen T, Antoniou G, Adamou M, Tachmazidis I, Su P (2021) Automatic diag-nosis of attention deficit hyperactivity disorder using machine learning. Appl Artif Intell, 1–13, 2021
21. Su P, Chen T, Xie J, Zheng Y, Qi H, Borroni D, Zhao Y, Liu J (2020) Corneal nerve tortuosity grading via ordered weighted averaging-based feature extraction. Med Phys
22. Chen T, Keravnou-Papailiou E, Antoniou G (2021) Medical analytics for health-care intelligence—recent advances and future directions. Artif Intell Med 112:102009
23. Stirlng J, Chen T, Bucholc M (2020) Diagnosing alzheimer's disease using a self-organising fuzzy classifier. In Fuzzy logic: recent applications and developments. Springer
24. Chen T, Shang C, Su P, Keravnou-Papailiou E, Zhao Y, Antoniou G, Shen Q (2020) A decision tree-initialised neuro-fuzzy approach for clinical decision sup-port. Artif Intell Med 111:101986
25. Su C et al (2020) Mining genetic and transcriptomic data using machine learning approaches in Parkinson's disease. npj Parkinson's Disease 6(1):1–10
26. Almeida JS et al (2019) Detecting Parkinson's disease with sustained phonation and speech signals using machine learning techniques. Pattern Recogn Lett 125:55–62
27. Eskofier BM et al (2016) Recent machine learning advancements in sensor-based mobility analysis: deep learning for Parkinson's disease assessment. 2016 38th annual international conference of the IEEE engineering in medicine and biology society (EMBC), IEEE
28. Wang W et al (2020) Early detection of Parkinson's disease using deep learning and machine learning. IEEE Access 8:147635–147646
29. Belić M et al (2019) Artificial intelligence for assisting diagnostics and assessment of Parkinson's disease—a review. Clin Neurol Neurosurg 184:105442
30. Chen T, Shang C, Yang J, Li F, Shen Q (2020) A new approach for transformation-based fuzzy rule interpolation. IEEE Trans Fuzzy Syst 28(12):3330–3344
31. Chen T, Lucock M (2022) The mental health of university students during the COVID-19 pandemic: an online survey in the UK. PLoS ONE 17(1):e0262562

Brain Networks in Autism Spectrum Disorder, Epilepsy and Their Relationship: A Machine Learning Approach

Tanu Wadhera and Mufti Mahmud

Abstract The aim of the chapter is threefold: (i) to find the brain topology in ASD, (ii) to find the brain topology in epilepsy, and finally, (iii) to quantitatively find the bidirectional relationship between ASD and epilepsy. The functional brain networks are explored using a complex network approach and graph-theory-based measures. To fulfil the aims, the chapter has moved beyond the traditional comparisons (TD vs ASD or TD vs E) and included the additional comparisons such as ASD vs E, ASD vs ASD+E, and E vs ASD+E. The statistical comparisons and Machine Learning-based classifications have provided distinct and robust neural metrics to reveal brain network topologies in ASD, epilepsy, and ASD+E phenotype. The impact of age on the brain topology metrics has also been analysed and reasoned, respectively. The complex brain network methodology proved significant in finding neurological mechanisms underlying ASD. Also, it demonstrated the association of co-morbidity (epilepsy) with the disorder- and age-induced atypical behaviour in ASD.

1 Introduction

Bridging the complex relationship between ASD and epilepsy (E) phenotypes can provide robust markers to account for the mechanisms underlying ASD, epilepsy, and even for a subset of disordered individuals who demands more research at the

T. Wadhera
Indian Institute of Information Technology Una, Una, Himanchal Pradesh, India
e-mail: tanu.wadhera@iiitu.ac.in

M. Mahmud (✉)
Department of Computer Science, Nottingham Trent University, Nottingham NG11 8NS, UK
e-mail: Mufti.Mahmud@ntu.ac.uk

Computing and Informatics Research Centre, Nottingham Trent University, Nottingham NG11 8NS, UK

Medical Technologies Innovation Facility, Nottingham Trent University, Nottingham NG11 8NS, UK brain circuit level. The overlap between ASD and epilepsy is significant as screening one condition can prove beneficial for the early intervention of another domain.

EEG recordings are the best way to rule out epilepsy in ASD, and thus, EEG signals have been explored and analysed in this chapter. Among different graph-theory methods to convert brain EEG signals into complex networks, the visibility graph (VG) approach is highly preferred by researchers [14]. The VGs have the potential to quantify the synchronisation of time series (identical as well as non-identical) without any need for stimulating parameters such as threshold value and inherit non-linear attributes of time series (such as EEG) [1]. Compared to traditional methods such as Fourier Transforms, VGs do not require any preprocessing or noise removal step. In this manner, VG can never miss any critical information from the recorded signal. Thus, the studies utilise VGs as a visualising tool and feature extraction method.

The VGs convert the brain signals into temporal networks with each node as the time point, and the link/edge between two nodes is formed according to their visibility to each other, which is a criterion explained by [11]. This method validates dynamic correlations in a time series for mapping complex graphs without pre-processing. Various studies have employed the VG method to map EEG into a complex network, as explained in the literature. The information is then taken out via graph-based measures such as an average degree or modularity, clustering coefficient, or characteristic path length. For example, recently, a study used the VG algorithm and average degree metric for EEG (only C3 channel) to differentiate ASD and TD with an accuracy of 81.67% [3]. In sum, VGs have the potential to extract the information objectively and simplify the computation process while keeping the periodic, stochastic, and chaotic nature of time series intact.

Most research studies have analysed one or two neural metrics, which restricts the accurate identification of the disorder and thus hinders the detection of relevant biomarkers. The present chapter has overcome such limitations and extracted multiple graph-based complex measures to detect neural dysfunction. In Sect. 2, the EEG time series is mapped into a complex brain network, and then graph-based measures are computed to compare the brain network of ASD, E, and ASD+E conditions with the TD group.

2   Mapping Eeg Time-Series to Complex Network

The procedure to convert a time series into a VG-based network is explained in [11] and stepwise in the following section. The steps for any weighted graph- G (N, E, W) are:

STEP1: Data-point of the time series is node (N) of the network. As for the given time-series $y_1(t_k) = \{y_1(t_1), y_1(t_2), \ldots\ldots\ldots y_1(t_N)\}$,, $1 < k < N$ with $N = n_k$.

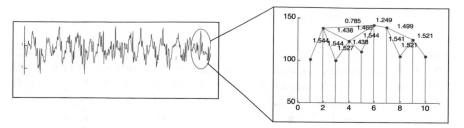

Fig. 1 Schematic representation of weighted visibility graphs

STEP2: Build all links forming edges amongst nodes using visibility criteria formulated as:

$$y(t_2) < y(t_1) + (y(t_3) - y(t_1))\frac{t_2 - t_1}{t_3 - t_1} \tag{1}$$

where $y(t_1)$, $y(t_2)$ and $y(t_3)$ represent the data-points at t_1, t_2, t_3 instants.

STEP 3: Figure out absolute weight assessment of edge to form a robust network by employing equation, explained in (2) given as:

$$w_{12} = abs\left(arctan\frac{n_2 - n_1}{t_2 - t_1}\right) \tag{2}$$

where w_{12} is the weight of the edge between n_2 and n_1 nodes. The function *arctan* detects rapid variation in time series. After following these steps, the schematic of the signal is shown in Fig. 1.

The figure reflects that the data points in the time series with the highest or lowest value are more visible in VG graphs and contribute to the degree in the graph.

3 Material and Method

3.1 Dataset

The EEG signals were acquired by experienced hospital neurophysiologists. For comparison, the standard datasets of ASD and Epilepsy described in [2] were also processed and analysed by using the proposed approach. Additionally, 50 individuals with ASD+E conditions were selected to fulfil the present chapter's objective.

3.2 Network Metrics and Analysis

A complex network based on the VG algorithm is evaluated using different network metrics from the connectivity matrix. The weighted variants were computed for all the metrics- Average weighted degree (AD^w), Global efficiency (GE^w), Weighted clustering coefficient (CC^w), Local efficiency (LE^w), characteristic path length (CPL^w), weighted modularity (Q^w), eigenvector centrality (EC^w), and small-world (SW) index. The parameters are explained as follows:

1. Average Weighted Degree: The average sum of edge weights linked with any node p in the network.

$$AD^w = \sum_{p,q \in S_g} w_{pq} \tag{3}$$

2. Weighted Global efficiency: It quantises the capacity of parallel data transferring in the brain network. It is inversely related to short path lengths in the network. For a fully connected network, $GE = 1$, whereas $GE = 0$ in the case of a completely disconnected network. Here, N represents total nodes in the network and w_{pq}^s represents the smallest weight between nodes p and q.

$$GE^w = \frac{1}{N(N-1)} \sum_{p,q \in S_g, p \neq q} \frac{1}{w_{pq}^s} \tag{4}$$

3. Weighted clustering coefficient: It computes whether any two nodes (p and q) are neighbours of any other node (say r) can be connected. It provides a cluster of nodes representing that any network with large clusters reveals higher connection density.k_p: neighbours of p; $k_p(k_p - 1)$: total links; $\max(w)$ is the maximum weight of the network that normalises CC between 0 and 1.

$$CC_p^w = \frac{1}{k_p(k_p - 1)} \sum_{q,r} \frac{(w_{pq}w_{qr}w_{pr})^{1/3}}{\max(w)} \tag{5}$$

4. Weighted Local efficiency: It measures information transfer among local subnetworks or neighbourhoods. In a given node, it is assessed via the inverse of the path length of the node.

$$LE^w = \frac{1}{2} \sum_{p,q \in S_g, p \neq q} \left(\frac{w_{pq}w_{pr}}{w_{qr}} \right)^{1/3} \frac{1}{k_p(k_p - 1)} \tag{6}$$

5. Weighted Characteristic Path Length (CPL): It gives an average of the shortest path between all node pairs in the network. It is widely referred to as the integration capacity of the network.

$$CPL^w = \frac{1}{n} \sum_{p=n} \frac{\sum_{q \in N, p \neq q} w_{pq}}{n-1} \tag{7}$$

6. Small-World Index: A high segregation and high integration simultaneously in-network is called small-world architecture. To have small-world features, the value SW > 1 should hold.

$$SW = \frac{CC^w / CC^w_{rand}}{CPL^w / CPL^w_{rand}} \tag{8}$$

7. Weighted Modularity: It computes partitioning network strength into diverse sub-networks. It has a $[-1\ 1]$ range with high values marking close connection amongst related nodes with scattering between nodes of a different community.

$$Q^w = \frac{1}{2w} \sum_p \sum_q \left(w_{pq} - \frac{w_p w_q}{2w} \right) \delta(C_p C_q) \tag{9}$$

For computing modularity, the connectivity matrix was computed at a group level by averaging all the individual connectivity matrices of subjects from ASD, ASD+E, TD, and Epilepsy groups.

8. Weighted Eigenvector Centrality: The centrality value acquired after combining the neighbour nodes' centrality values. It offers node centrality by totalling centralities of nodes in its neighbour, thus enhancing layer sensitivity in the network hierarchy.

$$C_p^w = \frac{1}{\lambda} \sum_q w_{pq} C_q \tag{10}$$

where $N(a)$ denotes neighbouring nodes, $b \in N(a)$, $A^{w\ characterises}$ weighted adjacency matrix, λ is the largest eigenvalue of A^w, and C is network centrality.

The network metrics computed in this chapter have been shown diagrammatically in Fig. 2.

To statistically examine the dataset, a repeated-measure ANOVA is designed for matrix 4 (Group: ASD, ASD+E, TD, E) $\times$ 2 (Hemisphere: Left, Right) $\times$ 19 (Electrodes) to determine brain connectivity significance across brain regions. The Hemisphere and Electrodes act as with-in subject elements and Group as a between-subject element.

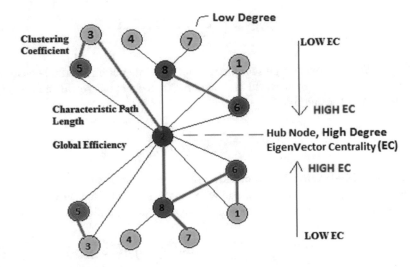

Fig. 2 Schematic of network metrics related to node properties

3.3   Classification and Performance Evaluation of Metrics

A tenfold cross-validation method is charted in constructing poised training and testing datasets. At the same time, the training dataset division is carried as 80% for training and 20% for validation purposes. The effectiveness of state-of-art classifiers is validated utilising various performance factors like sensitivity, specificity, and AUC.

4   Results

4.1   Brain Network Topology

The wired diagrams for 50 nodes in individuals with ASD, E, ASD+E, and TD are shown in Fig. 3 (i, ii, iii, iv). The connectivity is sparser in ASD+E individuals, whereas it is highly integrated into E condition individuals. The figure demonstrates the variation in the brain's topology of all the individuals.

4.2   Statistical Analysis of Network Metrics

The trivial Mauchly's investigation for AD^w(p $=$ 0.33), CC^w(p $=$ 0.12), GE^w(p $=$ 0.46), Q^w(p $=$ 0.58), and EC^w(p $=$ 0.24), confirmed sphericity hypothesis. The

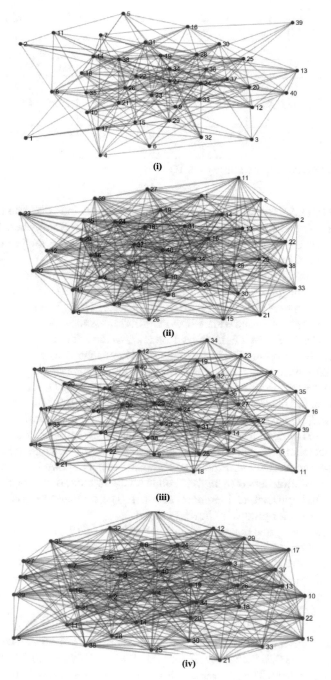

Fig. 3 Wire diagrams showing connectivity outlines in (i) ASD+E, (ii) ASD, (iii) TD, and (iv) E using 50 Nodes

Table 1 Description of 4 × 2x19 ANOVA with significant effect of group, hemisphere, and electrode on ASD, TD, E, and ASD+E participants

Interaction	d.f	F-value							
		AD^w	CC^w	GE^w	Q	EC	LE	SW	CPL
Group	1	195.64*	1.38**	2.88**	1.97*	3.01*	3.67*	5.43**	8.89**
Electrodex Group	2	136.75*	1.65*	2.06*	1.68*	3.24**	3.52*	4.56*	12.54*
Group x Hemisphere	2	175.45*	1.46*	2.45**	2.01*	3.33**	3.20*	4.81*	10.9**

(d.f.: degree of freedom; *p < 0.001;**p < 0.05)

$SW(p = 0.001)$, $LE^w(p = 0.03)$, and $CPL(p = 0.01)$ values disrupted sphericity ($p = 0.001$). The GroupxElectrode ($p < 0.05$) and GroupxHemisphere ($p < 0.05$) interactions were also found significant. No other effect and interaction were found trivial. The summary of the results is provided in Table 1.

The hemisphere influence revealed possible changes in lateralisation and electrode level for different groups, as shown by t-test data (Table 2). In ASD versus TD group, left hemisphere lateralisation is found compared to the E versus TD group. In comparing the ASD+E group with ASD, lateralisation towards the right hemisphere is observed. In ASD+E versus E, lateralisation towards the left hemisphere is observed, whereas in ASD+E versus TD, towards the right hemisphere. The lobes comparison showed ASD connectivity much higher for the frontal, and parietal lobe, and relative connectivity in the occipital lobe. In contrast, in E versus TD, more connectivity is observed in the temporal lobe and relatively among central and frontal lobes. In ASD versus E, higher connectivity is traced in frontal and comparative connectivity in temporal and parietal lobes. The ASD+E cohort described higher connectivity in temporal, occipital, and frontal regions compared to ASD, whereas ASD+E versus E has greater connectivity in frontal and comparative in temporal lobes, and ASD+E versus TD condition reflected higher connectivity in frontal and occipital, while lesser in central, parietal, and temporal sections. The evaluation of mean values of computed metrics for groups is shown in Fig. 4.

The average weighted degree is higher in E (324.34 ± 17.3) and ASD+E (298.87 ± 14.9) conditions compared to TD (278.41 ± 14.4) and ASD (283.26 ± 14) group participants. The GE^w is higher in TD (0.64 ± 0.04) followed by ASD (0.59 ± 0.03), E (0.43 ± 0.03) and ASD+E (0.35 ± 0.05) condition in decreasing order. The EC^w values are higher in TD (0.53 ± 0.04) followed by ASD (0.42 ± 0.02), ASD+E (0.38 ± 0.05) and E (0.33 ± 0.03) conditions in decreasing order. The CC^w value is higher in ASD+E (0.64 ± 0.04) followed by TD (0.57 ± 0.06), ASD (0.52 ± 0.0.2) and E (0.43 ± 0.03) group. The SW index value is higher in TD (1.56 ± 0.07), followed by ASD (1.02 ± 0.02), then ASD+E (0.95 ± 0.04) and E (0.93 ± 0.04) conditions in decreasing manner. The Q^w value is high in TD (0.55 ± 0.03) then, followed by ASD+E (0.49 ± 0.04), ASD (0.42 ± 0.02), and E(0.34 ± 0.03) in decreasing order. The LE^w is higher in TD (0.58 ± 0.03) than ASD+E (0.50 ± 0.02) and then followed

Table 2 Summary of network metrics in ASD, E, TD, ASD+E

Group			t-values							
			AD^w	CC^w	GE^w	Q^w	EC^w	LE^w	CPL^w	SW
ASD versus TD	HEMISPHERE	Left	16.45	xx	xx	−0.09	−0.08	−0.16	−0.09	−0.44
		Right	13.32	−0.08	−0.03	−0.16	−0.14	−0.12	0.11	−0.56
ASD versus E		Left	−42.56	0.05	0.14	xx	0.03	0.05	−0.27	xx
		Right	−30.72	0.09	0.10	0.08	0.06	0.11	−0.18	0.08
ASD versus ASD + E		Left	−18.32	xx	0.26	xx	0.05	−0.08	−0.20	0.08
		Right	−15.21	−0.12	0.24	−0.06	xx	−0.03	−0.27	0.05
E versus TD		Left	26.48	−0.09	−0.11	−0.13	−0.14	−0.10	xx	−0.56
		Right	34.53	−0.15	−0.20	−0.18	−0.23	−0.21	0.12	−0.69
E versus ASD+E		Left	25.64	−0.24	xx	−0.15	xx	−0.21	−0.13	xx
		Right	18.76	−0.16	xx	−0.07	−0.05	−0.16	−0.09	xx
TD versus ASD + E		Left	−16.78	xx	0.27	0.05	0.09	xx	−0.33	0.50
		Right	−12.45	0.07	0.29	0.08	0.13	0.06	−0.45	0.63
ASD versus TD	LOBES LOBES	Frontal	8.98	0.15	−0.12	0.08	0.004	0.18	0.10	−0.32
		Parietal	11.23	−0.05	0.11	−0.16	−0.08	−0.26	0.08	−0.28
		Occipital	−15.18	−0.13	xx	−0.13	−0.15	0.11	0.16	xx
ASD versus E		Frontal	11.32	xx	−0.05	0.12	0.05	0.08	0.05	0.09
		Temporal	−54.35	−0.11	0.16	xx	0.06	xx	−0.14	0.11
		Parietal	−67.54	−0.09	0.18	0.05	0.09	0.13	−0.18	0.05
ASD versus ASD + E		Frontal	−10.61	−0.12	0.21	0.11	xx	−0.12	−0.22	0.08
		Temporal	−13.76	−0.08	0.17	xx	−0.08	−0.07	−0.19	0.05

(continued)

Table 2 (continued)

Group		t-values							
		AD^w	CC^w	GE^w	Q^w	EC^w	LE^w	CPL^w	SW
E versus TD	Occipital	-12.24	-0.04	0.13	-0.09	-0.11	-0.08	xx	0.10
	Frontal	36.73	-0.11	-0.18	-0.16	-0.12	-0.21	0.17	-0.36
	Central	38.21	xx	-0.22	-0.11	-0.23	-0.12	0.14	xx
	Temporal	28.54	0.05	-0.15	-0.20	-0.13	-0.23	0.10	-0.40
E versus ASD+E	Frontal	13.61	-0.18	0.03	-0.11	-0.05	-0.22	xx	xx
	Temporal	11.42	-0.15	0.05	-0.16	xx	-0.17	-0.12	xx
TD versus ASD + E	Frontal	-14.13	0.03	0.32	0.03	0.09	xx	0.14	0.34
	Central	xx	0.09	0.11	0.12	xx	-0.05	-0.09	xx
	Parietal	-16.73	0.06	0.15	0.05	0.11	0.03	-0.18	xx
	Temporal	-9.01	0.03	0.29	xx	0.15	0.08	-0.16	0.39
	Occipital	xx	xx	0.18	xx	0.05	0.04	-0.21	0.28

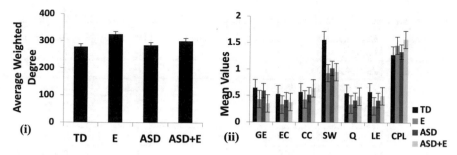

Fig. 4 Mean values of complex network metrics (i) Average weighted degree (AD^w), (ii) GE^w, EC^w, CC^w, LE^w, SW, Q^w, LE^w, and CPL^w in TD, E, ASD, and ASD+E Participants

by ASD (0.42 ± 0.03) and E(0.31 ± 0.02) in a decreasing manner. The CPL^w value is higher in ASD+E (1.57 ± 0.03) than followed by E(1.46 ± 0.02), ASD (1.34 ± 0.05) and TD (1.28 ± 0.04) in decreasing order.

4.2.1 Classifying Brain Networks

In comparing SVM and KNN classifiers, it is found that the SVM classifier outperformed the KNN classifier. The performance of the SVM classifier is summarised in Table 3. The sensitivity, specificity, accuracy, and AUC (ROC) revealed average values of important metrics for diverse classes.

The AUC (ROC) has been computed to discover the importance of individual metrics in characterising the groups. The results demonstrating the AUC (ROC) for significant network metrics are demonstrated in Fig. 5.

4.2.2 Functional Overlapping Regions in ASD and Epilepsy

The overlapping regions in ASD and epilepsy groups are computed using a paired-samples t-test on the topological metrics. The test revealed shared brain areas, which are given in Table 4, represented by an electrode number in their respective lobes. A probabilistic approach is followed to compute the overlap quantitatively. The commonality in ASD and Epilepsy is 53%; ASD and ASD+E is 47%; and epilepsy and ASD+E is 51% in AD^w, CC^w, LE^w, CPL^w, Q^w, EC^w measures (6 metrics × 19 electrodes = 114). Globally, ASD and Epilepsy intersection is 57%, ASD and ASD+E overlap is 49%, and epilepsy and ASD+E overlap is 55% for GE^w and SW metric s.

4.2.3 Variation in Complex Metrics with Age

To examine the effect of age for ASD, ASD+E, E, and TD participants, the metric-based data was calculated over two age groups (0–11 years and 11–18 years). A

Table 3 Summary of SVM classifier performance metrics for classification of different groups

Category	Classification group	Accuracy (%)	Specificity (%)	Sensitivity (%)	AUC (ROC)
Two classes	ASD versus TD	99.7	93.4	100	0.992
	ASD versus E	95.4	90.3	98.2	0.978
	ASD versus ASD+E	94.5	88.8	97.8	0.958
	E versus TD	95.4	91.5	97.2	0.964
	E versus ASD+E	96.6	97.2	96.2	0.974
	TD versus ASD+E	94.8	90.7	96.8	0.968
Three classes	ASD versus TD versus E	98.4	100	100	0.993
	ASD versus TD versus ASD+E	97.8	90.4	97.3	0.985
	ASD versus E versus ASD+E	98.1	93.5	98.8	0.990
	TD versus E versus ASD+E	97.4	100	97.6	0.963
Four classes	ASD versus TD versus E versus ASD+E	98.7	98.9	100	0.988

manifold linear-regression model is applied with network metrics as independent variables and age as well as the group as dependent variables. As illustrated in Table 5, with increasing age, the metrics AD^w, Q^w, LE^w, SW, and CC^w increases in TD, while other factors remain unaffected. In ASD individuals, the metrics CC^w, LE^w, and SW reduces whereas CPL and EC^w metrics increase with the age factor. In Epilepsy (E) group, the parameters, Q^w, GE^w, LE^w, EC^w and SW decrease whereas CPL and AD^w increase with age. In ASD+E group, Q^w, CC^w, EC^w and SW rise whereas LE^w reduce significantly with age compared to other insignificant metrics.

For TDs, the EC and CPL were indifferent to age recommending maintenance of global network association with age. In contrast to TDs, meaningful sensitivity to EC with cumulative age was initiated in ASD, E, and ASD+E groups that's a probable indicator for an uncommon global organisation. In ASD+E individuals, the age reduces LE^w and significantly increases CC^w, Q^w, EC^w and SW paralleled to additional metrics.

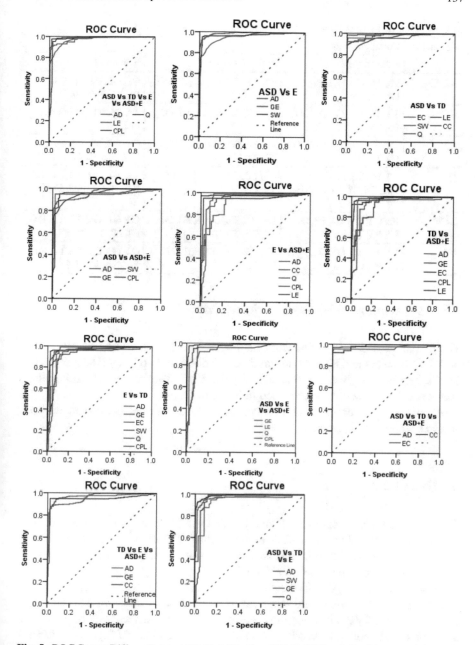

Fig. 5 ROC Curves Differentiating ASD, E, ASD+E and TD for Different Combination of Network Metrics

Table 4 Similarities of brain metrics reflecting shared brain area among different cohorts

Parameter	Commonalities		
	ASD and E	ASD and ASD+E	E and ASD+E
AD^w	F8, T6, C4, Fp2, F7, C3, O2, O1, P4	F3, T3, T5, Fz, C3, P3, P4, Cz, Fp1, F8, F4	O1, O2, P3, T6, F3, C4, P4, F4, Fp2, Pz
CC^w	T3, T5, O1, Fp1, C3, O2, P3, P5, Fp2, F3, Fz	Fp1, FP2, F8, C3, T6, O2, P4	T3, P3, P4, F8, F3, O1, Fp1
CPL^w	T3, Fp1, Fp2, F7, F3, O1, O2, P4, T6	F8, F4, O1, O2, P4, C4, T6, T3, T4	O1, O2, T3, P4, Fp1, Fp2, F4, F8, Pz
Q^w	C3, Fz, T3, F8, P3, O1, Fp1, T4, T6, O2, F7, F4, Fp2	O1, P3, T6, Fp2, C3, T5, T3, C4	T3, T4, Fp1, F3, Cz, C3, P3, P4, O2, Fp2, Fz, Pz
EC^w	Fz, C3, C4, O1, P3, O2, F4, F8, T3, T4	O1, T6, Fp1, Fp2, F8, F4, P4, C3, T3, T4	C3, O1, O2, T3, T5, Fp1, F4, F8, T6, P4, P3
SW	P3, T3, T6, O1, O2, Fp2, F4, F3, C4, F8	T3, T5, T4, O2, Fp1, P3, P4, F8	O1, O2, P3, T3, T4, Fp1, Fp2, F4, F8, F7, P4

4.3 Assessment With Standardized Data

The recommended complex network method is also run on two standardised data of ASD (Dataset I and II) and one standardised dataset of epilepsy (Dataset III; [2]. Similar features are given in SVM and KNN classifiers. The features where classifiers performed better are only summarised in Table 6.

A contrast of present chapter outcomes with the current automated network analysis technique is briefed in Table 7.

5 Discussion

The functional neural topology, its changes and overlapping with complex network metrics are identified between ASD, epilepsy, and ASD+E group via statistical and ML-based methods. The brain is a complex network via weighted VG approaches & complex graph measures ($AD^w, GE^w, CC^w, LE^w, CPL^w, Q^w, EC^w$, and SW index) are evaluated to show ASD+E condition with variations in ASD than epilepsy. It is found that frontal, parietal and temporal lobes generate changes in ASD+E. With the usage of the SVM classifier, the present chapter forwards a subset of metrics to discriminate one cohort from others. Combining AD^w, LE^w, CPL^w, Q^w can discriminate ASD, E, ASD+E, and TD with an accuracy 98.7%. Thus, the brain topology is a possible set to differentiate neural abnormalities and underlying processes.

Differences in network metrics revealed that the ASD+E cohort shows dissimilar metric outlines compared to TDs, the prime cause of atypicality and behavioural

Table 5 Effect of age on functional connectivity metrics in all groups

Group	CC^w	Q^w	GE^w	LE^w	CPL^w	AD^w	EC^w	SW
ASD	$\beta = -0.39$ [$-0.49, -0.3$]	xx	xx	$\beta = -0.32$ [$-0.26, -0.37$]	$\beta = 0.38$ [$0.29, 0.43$]	xx	$\beta = 0.35$ [$0.30, 0.39$]	$\beta = -0.22$ [$-0.18, -0.29$]
E	xx	$\beta = -0.35$ [$-0.24, -0.38$]	$\beta = -0.16$ [$-0.12, -0.24$]	$\beta = -0.27$ [$-0.24, -0.32$]	$\beta = 0.26$ [$0.22, 0.34$]	$\beta = 3.11$ [$2.19, 3.24$]	$\beta = -0.29$ [$-0.23, -0.34$]	$\beta = -0.13$ [$-0.08, -0.19$]
TD	$\beta = 0.22$ [$0.19, 0.25$]	$\beta = 0.42$ [$0.34, 0.5$] $p = 0.03$	xx	$\beta = 0.23$ [$0.14, 0.35$]	xx	$\beta = 2.05$ [$1.19, 2.14$]	xx	$\beta = 0.10$ [$0.04, 0.14$]
ASD+E	$\beta = 0.18$ [$0.11, 0.26$]	$\beta = 0.20$ [$0.17, 0.23$]	xx	$\beta = -0.14$ [$-0.10, -0.19$]	xx	xx	$\beta = 0.16$ [$0.11, 0.23$]	$\beta = 0.08$ [$0.02, 0.14$]

Table 6 Detail of performance in standard and self-collected database

Feature input	Type of dataset	Sensitivity (%)		Specificity (%)		Accuracy (%)		AUC	
		SVM	KNN	SVM	KNN	SVM	KNN	SVM	KNN
AD+CC+Q	I	97.9	85.5	94.5	81.2	96.2	82.6	0.901	0.858
CC+GE+Q+EC	ASD versus TD	99.3	87.7	96.4	84.9	97.85	86.4	0.946	0.901
GE+SW+CPL+Q+AD+LE		100	89.2	98.2	86.6	99.5	88.7	0.978	0.919
Q+EC	II	96.3	91.5	94.6	87.4	95.3	89.4	0.977	0.914
AD+GE+Q	ASD versus TD	98.4	93.4	96.3	89.7	97.2	90.7	0.989	0.921
CC+SW+Q+EC		97.6	92.3	94.4	90.5	95.4	91.6	0.966	0.937
GE+SW+CC+Q+AD		98.7	95.6	96.3	92.4	97.8	93.5	0.982	0.947
AD+Q	III	99.1	95.3	97.5	92.5	98.7	94.8	0.998	0.968
SWvCPL+EC	E versus TD	99.3	94.7	96.9	96.3	98.3	95.1	0.994	0.973

Table 7 Evaluation of proposed findings & existing diagnostic studies

Database	Reference	Accuracy (%)
Dataset I (ASD Vs TD)	Djemal et al.	99.1
	Present Study	**99.5**
Dataset II (E vs TD)	Supriya et al.	100
	Mohammadpoory et al.	97
	Present Study	**99.3**
Dataset I & II ASD versus E versus TD	Ibrahim et al.	92.94
	Present Study	**98.4**

abnormalities. High connectivity and integration over the left-hemisphere than right-hemisphere is observed in ASD+E and ASD than TD. It favours literature revealing poor right lobe connectivity responsible for poor cognition and automatic processing in ASD+E and ASD [4]. Thus, comparing ASD and ASD+E reveals additional variations in the right hemisphere compared to left hemispherical connections.

The ASD+E group has a higher $AD^w, LE^w, CPL^w, Q^w, CC^w, EC^w$ whereas GE^w and the SW index was inferior to ASD. On associating ASD+E and E groups, reduced connectivity in the leftover right hemisphere is observed. A higher degree and lesser modularity redirect poor connectivity in sub-network; lower EC^w and GE^w reflect reduced global connectivity; lesser LE^w reflect poor data-segregation in the brain network in the frontal area. The higher CC^w, lower GE^w, LE^w and CPL in the temporal lobe compared to ASD and E group reflect poor strength in the temporal (right) lobe. Our finding favours concerning actions in ASD+E with low stimulation in the occipital lobe and more hubs in the right parietal, reflecting visual imagery loss

[8]. Such is the prime reason for ASD and Epilepsy co-existence with the impaired performance of affected individuals favouring [5, 7, 13]. Our results are consistent with the relevant research [12] reporting deviant global connectivity, local connectivity, and partial presence of small-world structure in a specific cohort. The well-designed overlap recommends that common brain areas among the three disorders lead to misdiagnosis if not measured during the valuation process. The commonality can thoroughly elucidate the heterogeneity of disorder and co-existing settings during diagnosis.

The deviation of complex metrics with age has suggestively assisted characterising the groups through functional brain topology marks. In ASD, for age <11 years, a hyper-connectivity is found in several regions, but during growth (11–18 years), the ASD individuals do not change considerably from TDs within-network connectivity. Nevertheless, the hypo-connectivity across the brain network imparts provision to an atypical global connectivity model. The result helps conclude poor brain connectivity over the whole brain network in ASD [9, 10]. For the epileptic group, dissimilarity in the brain persists, and adulthood does not change their brain topology. It appears that maturity affects and mends the brain functioning of individuals. Thus, the functional abnormality associated with ASD and epilepsy is not uniform throughout life. The present chapter can go afar the studies suggesting under- and over-connectivity in ASD or epilepsy [6]. Furthermore, the VG concept has removed the threshold criterion, which boosted detection sensitivity while calculating connectivity variations.

6 Conclusion

An association between ASD and epilepsy exists as per the evidence from the literature, whereas the underlying mechanism of both disorders is unravelled. Although different factors cause ASD and epilepsy, simultaneously, both conditions develop together and are interrelated. The present chapter reworked ASD-epilepsy classification to extract mechanisms related to the ASD+E condition. Considering resting-state EEG, we investigated whether brain functional topology describes ASD and epilepsy and their relationship. The weighted VG approach is employed to build a brain network connectivity matrix. Different graph metrics were calculated to investigate both cohorts' varying and overlapping brain functional mechanisms. The statistical investigations showed that ASD+E affect brain network topology amongst frontal, temporal, and parietal areas. However, it illustrates functional overlap with ASD(49%) and epilepsy (55%). The complex network metrics variations validate the atypicality and uniformities of functional brain connectivity in three conditions. Combining complex metrics (AD^w, LE^w, CPL^w, Q^w) decides topology in ASD+E to distinguish disorders with higher accuracy (98.7%) from other cohorts. The variation in brain topology from (5–11 years) age group to (11–18 years) leads to heterogeneity and unexplained behavioural abnormalities. Contrary to theoretical works, the present work quantitatively ruled-out ASD+E condition via tracing changes in brain regions and network topology. In the future, considering gender and IQ with age leads to a better understanding of disorder-related changes in functional brain connectivity.

References

1. Ahmadlou M, Adeli H, Adeli A (2012) Improved visibility graph fractality with application for the diagnosis of autism spectrum disorder. Physica A 391(20):4720–4726
2. Andrzejak RG, Lehnertz K, Mormann F, Rieke C, David P, Elger CE (2001) Indications of nonlinear deterministic and finite-dimensional structures in time series of brain electrical activity: Dependence on recording region and brain state. Phys Rev E 64(6):061907
3. Bajestani GS, Behrooz M, Khani AG, Nouri-Baygi M, Mollaei A (2019) Diagnosis of autism spectrum disorder based on complex network features. Comput Methods Programs Biomed 177:277–283
4. Caeyenberghs K, Leemans A (2014) Hemispheric lateralization of topological organization in structural brain networks. Hum Brain Mapp 35(9):4944–4957
5. Capal JK, Carosella C, Corbin E, Horn PS, Caine R, Manning-Courtney P (2018) EEG endophenotypes in autism spectrum disorder. Epilepsy Behav 88:341–348
6. Coben R, Mohammad-Rezazadeh I, Bsc PM, Cannon RL (2014) Using quantitative and analytic EEG methods in the understanding of connectivity in autism spectrum disorders: a theory of mixed over-and under-connectivity. Front Hum Neurosci 8:45
7. Fang H, Wu Q, Li Y, Ren Y, Li C, Xiao X, Xiao T, Chu K, Ke X (2020) Structural networks in children with autism spectrum disorder with regression: a graph theory study. Behav Brain Res 378:112262
8. Kakkar D (2019) Influence of emotional imagery on risk perception and decision making in autism spectrum disorder. Neurophysiology 51(4):281–292
9. Keown CL, Datko MC, Chen CP, Maximo JO, Jahedi A, Müller RA (2017) Network organization is globally atypical in autism: a graph theory study of intrinsic functional connectivity. Biological Psychiatry: Cognitive Neurosci Neuroimaging 2(1):66–75
10. Lamb GV, Green RJ, Olorunju S (2019) Tracking epilepsy and autism. Egyptian J Neuro Psychiat Neurosur 55(1):1–8
11. Lacasa L, Luque B, Ballesteros F, Luque J, Nuno JC (2008) From time series to complex networks: the visibility graph. Proc Natl Acad Sci 105(13):4972–4975
12. Ma K, Yu J, Shao W, Xu X, Zhang Z, Zhang D (2020) Functional overlaps exist in neurological and psychiatric disorders: a proof from brain network analysis. Neuroscience 425:39–48
13. Viscidi EW, Johnson AL, Spence SJ, Buka SL, Morrow EM, Triche EW (2014) The association between epilepsy and autism symptoms and maladaptive behaviors in children with autism spectrum disorder. Autism 18(8):996–1006
14. Wadhera T, Kakkar D (2020) Conditional entropy approach to analyse cognitive dynamics in autism spectrum disorder. Neurol Res 42(10):869–878

AI in Mental Health

Computational Intelligence in Depression Detection

Md. Rahat Shahriar Zawad (ID), **Md. Yeaminul Haque** (ID),
M Shamim Kaiser (ID), **Mufti Mahmud** (ID), **and Tianhua Chen** (ID)

Abstract According to the World Health Organisation, depression is the prime contributor to mental disability worldwide. Depression is a severe threat to people's public and private lives because it causes catastrophic alterations in feelings and emotions. The recent rise in mental health issues and major depressive disorder has spurred many depression detection studies. Computational intelligence-based depression detection has piqued the scientific community's interest due to its increased efficiency and low mistake rate. This work presented a systematic review of recent works on computational intelligence-based depression detection based on their detection models, preprocessing, and data types. Discussing the findings, frameworks for social media, smartphone data, image/video and biosignal based depression detection were suggested. Finally, challenges and future research scopes in depression detection using computational intelligence have also been discussed.

Md. Rahat Shahriar Zawad · Md. Yeaminul Haque
Bangladesh University of Professionals, Dhaka, Bangladesh
e-mail: rahatshahriar06@gmail.com

Md. Yeaminul Haque
e-mail: yeaminulhaque1997@gmail.com

M. S. Kaiser (✉)
Institute of Information Technology, Jahangirnagar University, Savar, Dhaka 1342, Bangladesh
e-mail: mskaiser@juniv.edu

Applied Intelligence and Informatics Lab, Wazed Miah Science Research Centre (WMSRC), Jahangirnagar University, Savar, Dhaka 1342, Bangladesh

M. Mahmud (✉)
Department of Computer Science, Nottingham Trent University, Nottingham NG11 8NS, UK
e-mail: muftimahmud@gmail.com; mufti.mahmud@ntu.ac.uk

Computing and Informatics Research Centre, Nottingham Trent University, Nottingham NG11 8NS, UK

Medical Technologies Innovation Facility, Nottingham Trent University, Nottingham NG11 8NS, UK

T. Chen
Department of Computer Science, University of Huddersfield, Huddersfield HD1 3DH, UK
e-mail: T.Chen@hud.ac.uk

T. Chen et al. (eds.), *Artificial Intelligence in Healthcare*, Brain Informatics and Health,
https://doi.org/10.1007/978-981-19-5272-2_7
145

1 Introduction

Mental health disorder refers to a wide array of disorders affecting one's mood, thinking and behaviour towards others. It directly affects the emotional stability and reasoning capabilities of a person. Constant case of mental illness results in social inabilities leading to a series of consequences in society. Nowadays, people's minds are preoccupied with constant thoughts of competitiveness, incompleteness, and negative ideas. With the rise of modern technological society, the social interaction among peoples has decreased drastically, and society has moved to digital space. Casing regular life to be more hectic and prone to mental illness[1].

Depression or major depressive disorder is a widespread phenomenon in recent times. It is a severe case of mental illness where the feeling of a person's life and interaction with daily activity such as sleeping or working is hampered. A depressed person fails to feel any happiness and zeal in life. Usually, the constant missing of ideal feelings for two weeks is regarded as depression. The symptoms of depression can range from very mild to extreme. Being in mild depression may be normal and usually feels persistently low in energy, whereas the extreme case of depression can go up to the feeling of suicidal tendencies.

Depression can lead to many health problems and extreme tendencies. Depression is reported as one of the most significant causes of mental health conditions globally, and almost 300 million people around the globe are affected by it. According to a survey by World Health Organisation from 2015, it is noted that suicide is the most common reason for death for the world population ranging between the age of 15 and 29, and depression is the prime cause behind suicide [2].

Depression has the potential to be fatal. Early discovery of these diseases, on the other hand, can be efficiently treated with medication or psychotherapy [3]. Computational intelligence and machine learning-based techniques can significantly improve the experience of detecting depression. Using advanced statistics and probabilistic methods for machine learning can result in useful advancements in predicting mental health. Many researchers can extract useful information from data, deliver personalised experiences, and develop automated intelligent systems as a result of it [4].

This study aims to review existing research in the depression detection field and provide useful insights. The main contributions of this study can be summarised as follows:

- Provides detailed analysis of earlier research on depression detection using computational intelligence.
- Discusses techniques used by earlier researchers using the different data domains to detect depression using computational intelligence.
- Provides research gaps and challenges for research on the field, including future research scopes.

The sections of this chapter are organised as follows. The literature review section follows the introduction and contains an overview of previous research publications on depression detection. The next section goes over how to recognise depression in traditional healthcare settings and how machine learning can help. The section after discusses approaches for detecting depression using various data sources. The penultimate section discusses research gaps and their future potential. Finally, the conclusion section brings this chapter to a close.

2 Literature Review

Computational intelligence, in particular, machine learning (ML) and Deep Learning (DL) have been adopted popularly in diverse application areas including anomaly detection [5–10], disease detection [11–19] and smart data analytics [20–28]. Focusing on depression, as it has become a major concern for modern society with an increasing number of people are diagnosed with it, there has been significant effort to detect the same at the earliest onset. However, the alarming fact that only half of the population suffering from depression are detected. The primary purpose of depression detection systems is to provide accurate and quick identification of depression levels in people and, if possible, effective treatment. Several of the most recent state-of-the-art studies for depression identification have been discussed.

Lin et al. [29] proposed an approach named "SenseMood" for revealing the psychological state of users in social media using a deep multimodal learning approach. CNN-based classifier and Bert were applied to extract the deep features from the pictures and text posted by users in publicly available datasets. The system classified the users with depression and normal users through a neural network and achieved an accuracy of 0.884 with precision, recall and F1-score to be 0.903, 0.870, and 0.936, respectively.

Narziev et al. [30] created the "Short-Term Depression Detector (STDD)" platform, which consisted of a smartphone and a wearable device that continuously reported depression group classification metrics. The authors used the Diagnostic and Statistical Manual of Mental Disorders (DSM-5) to extract five characteristics that influence depression: physical activity, mood, social activity, sleep, and food consumption. They collected data from 20 people belonging to four different depression groups based on the Patient Health Questionnaire 9 (PHQ-9). They used Support Vector Machines (SVM) and Random Forest (RF) to create a machine learning (ML) model that could automatically classify depression categories in a short amount of time. With a 96.00% accuracy, their system established the viability of group classification.

Hussain et al. [31] created the Socially Mediated Patient Portal (SMPP), a data-driven tool that uses machine learning classification algorithms to detect depression markers in Facebook users. They studied 4350 users who had their depression assessed using the Center for Epidemiological Studies (CES-D) scale. The authors identified a collection of variables that may distinguish between people with and without depression using a Lexicon-based classifier, SVM, Deep Canonical Correlation Analysis (DCCA), Ensemble learning (voting), Naïve Bayes (NB), and Decision Tree

(DT). Using their devised framework, they conducted a correlation analysis between Facebook features and CES-D scale scores. It was discovered through the investigation that certain Facebook features could distinguish persons with and without depression in a cost-effective manner.

Chiong et al. [32] investigated whether ML techniques might be used to detect depression in social media users by analysing posts, particularly when such posts did not contain specific keywords like "depression" or "diagnostic." The authors looked into Tokenisation, stop word removal, POS tagging, and negative word processing, among other text preprocessing and textual-based featuring methods. They used publicly available datasets to train and test machine learning models such as SVM, LR, Multilayer Perceptron, DT, RF, Adaptive Boosting, and Gradient Boosting with 10-fold cross-validation. Their recommended approaches achieved the best accuracy of 99.80%.

To obtain a better interpretation of the depression detection, Alghowinem et al. [33] conduct a complete analysis of feature selection techniques in the context of depression behaviour from different family groups of feature selection techniques. They created a system that used 38 feature selection techniques from several categories to identify the most promising features for modelling depression detection. The primary dataset used in their research is real-world data collected at the Black Dog Institute as part of an ongoing investigation. The authors additionally employed the University of Pittsburgh depression dataset (Pitt) and the Audio/Visual Emotion Challenge Depression Dataset (AVEC) to help with generalisation. Their findings suggested that the main distinguishing features of the depression detection model are speech behaviour features (such as pauses).

Wu et al. [34] introduced a depression detection method called Deep Learning-based Depression Detection with Heterogeneous Data Sources (D3-HDS), which analysed an individual's living environment, behaviour, and social media activity to predict the depression label. The authors used the CES-D questionnaire to collect data from 1453 people who often used Facebook from 58 Taiwanese universities. To compute each individual's social media representation, they recommended using a Recurrent Neural Network (LSTM). Deep Neural Networks are used to blend the representations with additional non-textual features to predict the individual's depression label. With precision (83.3%), recall (71.4%), and F1 score (76.9%), their model outperformed earlier depression detection methods by a significant margin.

To improve depression identification accuracy, Zhu et al. [35] introduced a content-based ensemble technique (CBEM). They used two biomarkers, eye tracking and resting-state EEG, collected in two studies at Lanzhou University Second Hospital, each with 36 and 34 patients. The authors separated the data sets into subsets based on the experiment's context and then used a majority vote technique to assign labels to the subjects. On the datasets, the authors utilised both static and dynamic CBEM methods, achieving an accuracy of 82.5% and 92.65%, respectively.

Shah et al. [36] created a hybrid model that analyses users' textual social media posts to predict depression. The authors used a Reddit dataset that was previously published for a pilot study called Early Detection of Depression in CLEF eRisk 2017. They used Deep Learning algorithms trained using the training data and then evaluated using the test data. The writers' employed different feature sets, including Trainable Embed Features, Glove Embed Features, Word2VecEmbed, Glove Embed features, and Metadata Features. With an F1-score of 0.81 and latency of only 0.59, Bidirectional Long Short-Term Memory (BiLSTM) with Word2VecEmbed and metadata features worked well.

Lin et al. [37] suggested a method for detecting depression based on voice signals and textual data collected from patient interviews. The model they developed comprised of three components, a Bidirectional Long Short-Term Memory (BiLSTM) network with an attention layer, a One-Dimensional Convolutional Neural Network (1D CNN), and a fully connected network incorporating the outputs of the previous two models to assess the depressive state. They tested their model using two publicly available datasets, the DAIC-WoZ and the Audio-Visual Depressive Language Corpus (AViD-Corpus) and found that their method outperforms existing methods. The proposed 1D CNN model scored 0.81 (F1-Score), 0.92 (Recall), 0.73 (precision), 4.25 (MAE), and 5.45 (RMSSE) on the F1-Score, 0.92 (Recall), 0.73 (precision), 4.25 (MAE), and 5.45 (RMSE). Proposed BiLSTM model achieved 0.83 (F1-Score), 0.83 (Recall), 0.83 (precision), 3.88 (MAE), 5.44 (RMSE). and proposed multi-modal fusion network achieved 0.85 (F1-Score), 0.92 (Recall), 0.79 (precision), 3.75 (MAE), 5.44 (RMSE).

Zeberga et al. [38] suggested a unique methodology for identifying depression and anxiety-related posts quickly and effectively. They proposed using a BERT framework (bidirectional encoder representations from transformers) to extract a large amount of highly relevant depression and anxiety data from Twitter and Reddit. They also suggested a strategy for transferring knowledge from a big pre-trained model (BERT) to a smaller model called knowledge distillation. Finally, the authors conducted comprehensive experiments utilising principal component analysis (PCA) and several deep learning/ML models, with the findings compared to those of other similar ones. Their model outperformed the earlier models, with an accuracy of 98% after numerous hyperparameter tweaks.

Mustafa et al. [39], suggested a L based classification approach for detection of depression levels in social media users. They collected data from 179 Twitter users who have been tested for depression. From that data, they used Term Frequency-Inverse Document Frequency (TF-IDF) and Linguistic Inquiry and Word Count (LIWC) to select the most used words and classify the words into emotions. They used SVM, 1DCNN and RF to classify the depression levels in the participants and achieved 91% accuracy with the 1DCNN classifier. Arun et al. [40] illustrated clinical data from MYsore studies of Natal effects on Aging and Health (MYNAH) to develop a novel approach for detecting depression. Participants in the MYNAH had undergone a thorough examination for cognitive function, mental health, and cardiometabolic disorders. They suggested a model that was created with XGBoost. It assisted in the diagnosis of depression in the MYNAH sample by utilising classification techniques on the available data of assessments and resulting in an accuracy of 97.70%.

Arora et al. [41] described strategies to use a variety of sensory signals like EEG, triode electromyogram, photoplethysmography, skin conductance, hall effect respiration, Galvanic Skin Response, heart rate and temperature within a BodyMedia SenseWear Armband to calculate physiological responses and other necessary patterns. By collecting data signals from those sensors, the authors proposed machine learning techniques such as SVM, K-nearest neighbour (KNN), K-mean, FC-Mean and a PNN classifier. The SVM classifier achieved the highest performance.

Dong et al. [42] suggested pre-trained classifiers to extract deep speaker recognition (SR) and speech emotion recognition (SER) features and then fused the two deep audio features to detect depression between the voice and emotional variations of the speaker. For depression detection, the Feature Variation Coordination Measurement (FVCM) technique was presented to capture the coordination aspects of continuous change among extensive voice feature spaces. The authors proposed a new hierarchical depression detection model where multiple fuzzy layers were trained, and that was tested on the AVEC 2013 and AVEC 2014 benchmark databases. This model helped them get an F1 score of 0.824 and avoid overfitting problems. For future work, they decided to consider using interaction databases to verify the model's generalisation ability.

Alsagri et al. [43] used machine learning approaches to identify whether a Twitter user is depressed or not based on their network activities and tweets. They gathered 111 user-profiles and more than 300,000 tweets. They tried different machine techniques like DT, NB and SVM to identify the depression level, from which SVM-linear achieved the best results with the accuracy and F-measure of 82.5 and 0.79, respectively. As it was a binary classification problem, they managed a total number of 500 users with more than 1M Tweets, from which 334 users were classified as depressed.

Hosseini et al. [44] introduced customised multinomial Naïve Bayes algorithms to the domain of depression identification in social media based on cognitive and psychoanalytic observations. The feature extraction resource they used consisted of 21 categories of symptoms and behaviours that are mainly clinically abstracted during psychoanalytic cognitive therapy of depressed patients. They used a subset of the CLEF/eRsik dataset, which consisted of 340 examples, and among them, only 40 positive examples were considered. With those obtained features, they applied a Bayesian classifier based on the multinomial Naïve Bayes algorithm to classify whether the user is depressed or not and got an F1 score of 82.75%.

Hui et al. [45], proposed a novel framework for major depressive disorder detection using CNN. They collected EEG data for public datasets where 30 healthy and 34 MDD patients were recorded. The authors preprocessed the collected data using short-time Fourier transform (STFT) and fed the data to their CNN model. The results showed an accuracy of 99.58%, precision, sensitivity, specificity, and F1-score 99.40%, 99.70%, 99.48%, and 99.55%, respectively. This approach obtained higher performance than earlier frameworks in the field.

To discover the highest accuracy and recall for depression identification, Bai et al. [46] tested machine learning algorithms based on EEG signal characteristics. The researchers used 7 separate subchannels to acquire EEG data from 213 healthy volunteers. The preprocessing work was done with a bandpass filter. SVM, KNN, DT, NB, RF, and Logistic Regression were employed as machine learning methods. Using the RF model with Power Spectral Density features achieved the best accuracy of 66.95% with a recall of 90.13% on the Gamma band. The RF model had the highest accuracy of 76.97% and the highest recall of 89.54% for models that incorporated all features.

Lu et al. [47], proposed a depression detection method using gait data from video image collected using kinetic camera. They collected data from 95 individuals using a Microsoft Kinetic camera and used an ordinary least square and Gaussian filter for preprocessing the data. They used Fast Fourier transform for feature extraction and SVM, KNN and LDA to evaluate their dataset's performance. Their proposed machine learning models achieved the best accuracy of 88.89%.

Xie et al. [48] proposed a novel approach for depression detection suing SDS questionnaire and video recording. They collected Self-Rating Depression Scale (SDS) questionnaire data and video recordings from 200 individuals approved by Guandong Medical University. They used 3D CNN and redundancy-aware self-attention (RAS) for framework construction, achieving an accuracy of 0.925 ± 0.004%, the sensitivity of 0.907 ± 0.006% and specificity of 0.924 ± 0.005%.

Figure 1 shows a word cloud presenting most used words from titles of the articles reviewed in this section. Table 1 presents A summary of Datatype, Models, Preprocessing, and performance of recent computational intelligence based depression detection researches.

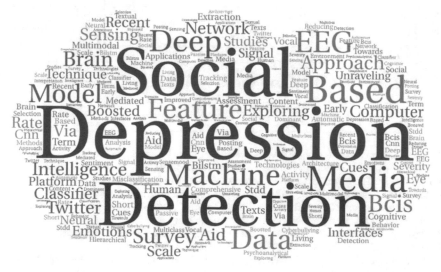

Fig. 1 The word cloud depicting retrieved keywords from the article titles representing recent works on depression detection

Table 1 A summary of datatype, models, pre-processing, and performance of recent computational intelligence based depression detection researches

Refs.	Datatype	Model	Pre-processing	Performance
[29]	Image and text	CNN, Bert	Bert	Acc: 0.884, pre: 0.903, recall: 0.870 and f1-score :0.936
[30]	Smartphone data	SVM, RF	–	Acc: 96%
[31]	Text	LbC, SVM, DCCA, Ensemble learning (voting), NB, and DT	–	Identified features for depression detection
[32]	Text	SVM, LR, MP, DT, RF, AB, and GB	Tokenisation, stop word removal, POS tagging, and negative word processing	Acc: 99.80%
[33]	Audio, Video	Group SAOLA, SAOLA, RF, GB, t-score, Chi square, LASSO, GA, SVM	–	Identified speech behaviour features best suitable for depression detection
[34]	Text, Smartphone data	DNN & LSTM	–	Pre: 83.3%, Recall: 71.4%, and F1 score: 76.9%
[35]	Biomarker	CBEM	–	Static CBEM: 82.05% (Acc) and dynamic CBEM 92.65% (Acc)
[36]	Text	BiLSTM	Trainable embed features, Glove embed features, Word2VecEmbed, Glove embed features	F1-score: 0.81 and latency: 0.59
[37]	Audio, Video	CNN-BiLSTM	–	0.85 (F1-Score), 0.92 (Recall), 0.79 (precision), 3.75 (MAE), 5.44 (RMSE)
[38]	Text	BiLSTM	Bert, Word2Vec	Acc 98%
[39]	Text	SVM, 1DCNN, RF	TF-IDF and LIWC	Acc 91%
[40]	Biosignal	XGBoosting		Acc 97.70%
[41]	Biosignal	SVM, kNN, K-mean, FC-Mean and a PNN	–	SVM: Acc 92%
[42]	Audio	Fuzzy	–	F1 score of 0.824
[43]	Text	DT, NB and SVM	–	SVM- 82.5 (Acc) and 0.79 (F1-score)
[44]	Text	NB	–	82.75 F1
[45]	Biosignal	CNN	STFT	Acc: 99.58%
[46]	Biosignal	SVM, KNN, DT, NB, RF, LR	Band pass filter	Acc: 76.97% (RF)
[47]	Video	SVM, KNN and LDA	FFT	Acc: 88.89%
[48]	Video, Text	3DCNN	–	Acc: 0.925 ± 0.004

Legend

In Model Column: SVM—Support Vector Machine, LR—Linear regression, RF—Random forest; KNN—K-Nearest Neighbor; LbC—Lexicon-based classifier; AB—AdaBoost; NB–Naïve Bayes; DT–Decision tree; 1DCNN—1 Dimensional Convolutional Neural Network; BiLSTm—Bidirectional Long Short-Term; MP—Multilayer Perceptron; Memory; CBEM—content-based ensemble technique; PNN—Probabilistic Neural Network; DCCA—Deep Canonical Correlation Analysis; AB—Adaptive Boosting; GB—Gradient Boosting

In Pre-processing Column: TF-IDF—Term Frequency-Inverse Document Frequency; LIWC—Linguistic Inquiry and Word Count, STFT—Short Time Fourier transform

In Performance Column: Acc—Accuracy; Pre—Precision; RMSE—Root Mean Square Error; MAE—Mean Absolute Error

3 Depression Detection

Depression is regarded as the most common mental health problem encountered by people in today's society. Unfortunately, only half of the people suffering from depression get the opportunity to avail proper medication for their depression. It can be due to the lack of awareness and all. But mostly due to the lack of detection of depression.

World health organisation (WHO) reports different barriers to detecting mental health problems around the globe in their reports to encourage research to work on the issue [49]. Many research and steps have been taken to develop a straightforward process for the detection of depression quickly. Usually, it works with marking symptoms, medical history and going through some questionnaire. There have been a significant number of research that try to investigate the movement of the face to identify depression [50]. Depression usually starts in adulthood, although children and adolescents have been identified with depression nowadays almost regularly. Sometimes anxiety and depression of adults have a more severe effect on the children they are involved with, causing more severe depression in them. There have been some risk factors identified as indulging with the cause of depression:

- Genetics: Family history of depression is one reason children have depression issues.
- Stress: Work or life-related loads can result in overstress, resulting in severe depression.
- Poor nutrition: Lack of nutrition in the body affects a person's daily life, resulting in depression.
- Other physical health issues: Having physical issues or illnesses that are hard to cure can cause depression in a person's mind.
- Having an addiction to drugs: Drug addiction is one of the prime causes of depression.
- Imbalanced brain chemistry: Imbalance in brain chemistry happens when there are missing neurotransmitters in a person's brain. Which results in greater complications and even depression.

Depression is typically diagnosed by healthcare professionals using a variety of questionnaires, and self-reporting [51]. Figure 2 presents a relational diagram showing the prime causes behind people suffering from depression.

4 Computational Intelligence in Depression Detection

According to the National Institute of Mental Health, depression affects one out of every 15 adults (6.7%) each year. One in every six people (16.6%) will suffer from depression at some point in their lives [52]. As a result, detecting depression

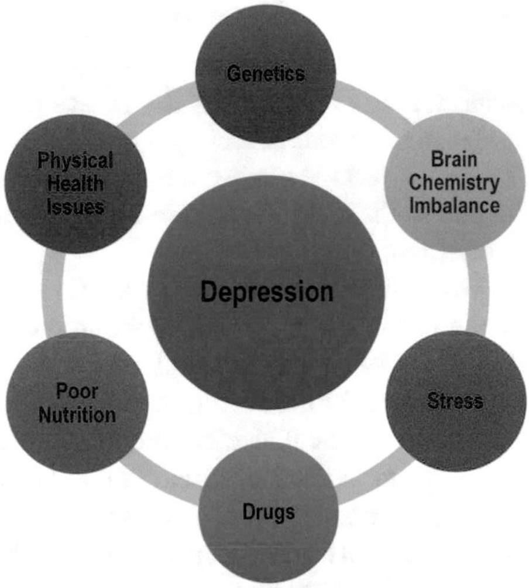

Fig. 2 Relational diagram showing the prime causes behind a people suffering from depression

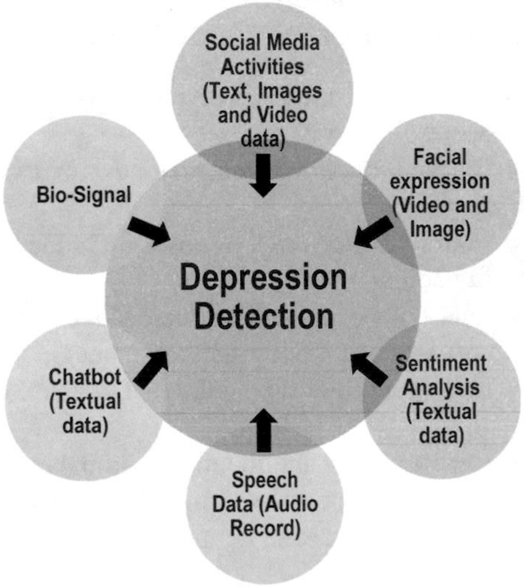

Fig. 3 Datatypes used in researches for depression detection

is increasingly seen as a particularly significant issue for people's safe and satisfied existence. With their fast and efficient detection capabilities, computational intelligence-based depression detection systems could represent a breakthrough in this area. Researchers have employed heterogeneous data from sources such as social media, image, and video data, BioSignal, and smartphone data to diagnose depression. These strategies and their algorithms and feature extraction methods are briefly discussed in this section. Figure 3 presents Datatypes used in researches for depression detection.

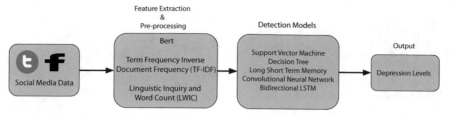

Fig. 4 A general diagram representing social media based depression detection

4.1 Depression Detection from Social Media Data

The posts, photographs, and data regarding relationships and flow between persons, groups, and other identities in social networks are commonly referred to as social media data. Most people use social networking sites to express themselves and post about their daily lives in today's environment. As a result, social media has become the most investigated area for detecting depression and mental health disorders. Term Frequency Inverse Document Frequency (TF-IDF) and Word2Vec have been common feature extraction strategies, according to a study of recent publications on depression diagnosis using textual and social media data [51]. TF-IDF determines the relevance of words based on their existence in a document and the frequency inverse of the present documents. Word2Vec, on the other hand, is a neural network model that learns word connections from a broad corpus of text. These two strategies greatly aid the performance of detection models. SVM and BiLSTM are two higher-performing models for textual data detection methods. Because SVM can categorise any encoded vector and BiLSTM can work on both previous and future data sequence input, they are complementary. Figure 4 presents a general diagram representing social media-based depression detection.

4.2 Depression Detection from Image/Video Data

Images and videos are more expressive datatypes considering they can shadow the movement and expressions of a person. As depression is a mental health issue, several research in recent times has considered using the image and video data for depression detection systems. Usually, for image/video data preprocessing, Principal component analysis (PCA) is considered the most used feature extraction technique [53]. As PCA uses principal components to decrease the data size, it is suitable for image data. In the case of machine learning algorithms, CNN has been the better performing algorithm as it can develop a lighter representation of a two-dimensional image. Figure 5 presents a general diagram representing image/video-based depression detection.

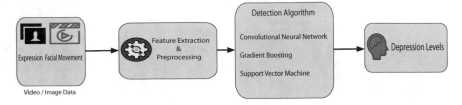

Fig. 5 A general diagram representing image/video based depression detection

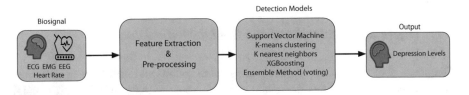

Fig. 6 A general diagram representing biosignal based depression detection

4.3 Depression Detection from Bio Signal

The human body is built on a complex web of interconnected organs and metabolic activities. Even little problems with any of the organs might alter the entire balancing scenario in the human body. Depression, as a mental health disorder, has been linked to abnormalities in human biological functioning. Based on this notion, many studies have used biosignals such as ECG, EMG, EEG, and HR to diagnose depression. EEG measures, in particular, have been extensively used in most recent studies for the diagnosis of depression, as EEG depicts the electrical form of brain activity. Deep learning-based depression identification from EEG output has been a hot topic in recent years, according to Safayari et al. [54]. Because EEG signals are electric, they require artefact and noise removal, which is primarily accomplished using various types of bandpass filters and quick feature extraction using Fast Fourier Transform. Convolutional layers or the Fourier transform have been widely used. The detection models used in most studies in this area are DCNN or LSTM. Figure 6 presents a general diagram representing biosignal based depression detection.

4.4 Depression Detection from Smartphone Data

Smartphones have now become an integral part of people's daily lives. They take their smartphones with them everywhere they go. As a result, smartphones can keep track of important aspects of a person's life, such as sociability, health, and even mental health. Many studies on smartphone-based data collection approaches for depression identification have been conducted. Sleep, physical activity, circadian rhythm, socia-

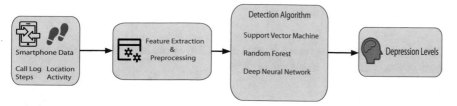

Fig. 7 A general diagram representing smartphone based depression detection

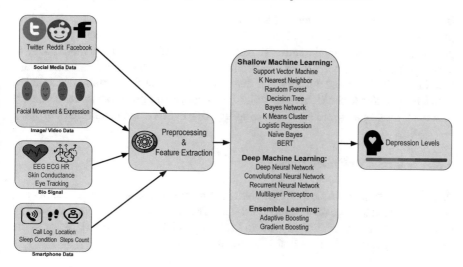

Fig. 8 A general depression detection framework. Data collected from different sources such as social media, bio-trackers, smartphones are pre-processed and provided into detection models consisting of computational intelligence algorithms, which detects the depression levels in patients

bility, location, and phone use are all variables that can be utilised to detect depression and other mental health disorders in people [55]. The strength and quality of these markers gathered via smartphone sensors have been utilised to categorise a person's depression state using SVM and DNN based algorithms. Figure 7 presents a general diagram representing smartphone-based depression detection. Figure 8 presents a general framework for depression detection using computational intelligence.

5 Challenges and Research Direction

Challenges and limitations of earlier research can become crucial for future researchers as they provide decision-making guidelines. This section includes the research gaps and challenges of earlier research, including the future scopes of the field.

5.1   Gaps in the Literature

This section includes the research gaps of earlier works in depression detection and some of the challenges of this research work.

5.1.1   Size and Quality of Data

It's worth noting that the number and quality of the data available for any Computational Intelligence application significantly impact the model's or algorithm's performance. With a small number of samples and data, the model is more likely to overfit and perform poorly in testing scenarios. However, the amount of data available in the field of mental health and depression detection is substantially smaller, which may be due to the higher expenditure on data collection due to the involvement of human participants and the ever-changing criteria of mental health markers [56].

5.1.2   Lack of Validation Data

As the size of samples in the field of mental health-related data is low, the consequence is a lack of data to validate developed models. The availability of external validation data sources is also exceptionally low in the field, which creates the risk factor of the models being not suitable for real-life scenarios and testing.

5.1.3   Generalisation of the Models

The performance and prediction of computational intelligence research depend entirely on the features employed in algorithm development. However, depending on how the features are chosen, the models may become overly reliant on a specific circumstance or group of people. Because this is a mental health-related study, the outcomes of these investigations should also be compared with clinical diagnosis accuracy rather than just the likelihood of correct prediction [57].

5.1.4   Lack of Multiclass Classifiers

Because binary classification models are easier to build, most machine learning models are binary classifiers. However, in the instance of depression detection, this can lead to forecasts that do not accurately reflect the severity of the problem. Only detecting depression or regular can lead to a mildly sad or momentarily depressed individual mistakenly diagnosed as seriously depressed and prescribed incorrectly, resulting in long-term health consequences.

5.1.5   Highly Imbalanced Data

The datasets in the field of depression detection are highly imbalanced in many cases and less marking of rare events. As a result, the models' build-up using them tends to miss the rare event while predicting which can cause unexpected outcomes in medication or treatment. The number of samples being depressed in the datasets is also a reason for the wrong prediction.

5.1.6   Lack of Deep Learning Models

In the case of the healthcare domain, deep learning models have been extraordinarily successful in the prediction or detection of health problems. But, notably, there has been a significant increase in the number of research using deep learning models for depression detection. Exploring deep learning models can become crucial in the correct prediction of depression in people.

5.2   Future Research Scopes

Next, this section highlights the specific approaches that could help develop research on the effectiveness of computational intelligence-based depression detection.

5.2.1   Exploration of Deep Learning Approaches

The success of deep learning approaches in the case of healthcare applications has been highly accepted. The ability of deep learning approaches to predict or classify complex data makes them very suitable for depression detection and prediction. In future research in depression detection, using deep learning techniques can open up more opportunities for correct detection and medication for solving depression issues in human beings.

5.2.2   High-Quality Dataset

A better dataset is a must to make a more suitable and accurate depression detection algorithm. A larger sample size and diversified class of people can create a much more acceptable and highly accurate depression detection model, which can be built through collaboration or participation of a large group of people in dataset making.

5.2.3 Transfer Learning

The technique of employing a model designed for one purpose to detect the desired scenario is known as transfer learning. Such adaptable models can often produce considerably better performance and outcomes in the long run. If depression is detected, the transfer learning strategy should be tested. Because of the variability in the input data, flexible algorithms will become the key difficulty in mental health research.

5.2.4 Models with Continual Learning

Continual learning lets machine learning models learn continuously from the incoming data stream. As the available data in the healthcare sector, particularly in the case of depression detection, is low, continual learning can be a way to better models and results. The ever-changing scenario of data in this particular section can open up new opportunities.

6 Conclusion

Mental health is one of the most significant features of a well-balanced life that requires to be given a great amount of emphasis. Depression is the most common and serious mental health issue that negatively affects a person's behaviour and way of thinking. So, a cheaper and more accurate depression detection system must be made available to the greater society. Thus, more research is required to be done on depression detection to aid society.

Many different algorithms and techniques have been proposed to detect depression and other mental health issues. Every year many new frameworks and ways are also being introduced. However, there has still been a significant number of issues to be sorted and marked in depression detection. Healthcare data being complex and heterogenous has affected the growth of expert systems in depression detection.

In recent years, computational intelligence has experienced substantial growth and development. Computational intelligence's contribution to depression detection has the potential to change the game forever. Expert systems can be used to make automatic detection and possible suggestions for treating this clinically curable disease using computational intelligence. This study aimed to highlight recent successes and research in the field of depression detection and identify research gaps and potential future research areas for researchers. Only human creativity and sound decisions and study can offer great triumphs in this field in the future of computational intelligence-based depression detection systems.

Acknowledgements MM is supported by the AI-TOP (2020-1-UK01-KA201-079167) and DIVERSASIA (618615-EPP-1-2020-1-UKEPPKA2-CBHEJP) projects funded by the European Commission under the Erasmus+ programme.

References

1. Chung J, Teo J (2022) Mental health prediction using machine learning: taxonomy, applications, and challenges. Appl Comput Intell Soft Comput 2022
2. World Health Organization (2019) Global status report on alcohol and health 2018. World Health Organization
3. Cuijpers P, Sijbrandij M, Koole SL, Andersson G, Beekman AT, Reynolds CF III (2013) The efficacy of psychotherapy and pharmacotherapy in treating depressive and anxiety disorders: a meta-analysis of direct comparisons. World Psychiatry 12(2):137–48
4. Jordan MI, Mitchell TM (2015) Machine learning: trends, perspectives, and prospects. Science 349(6245):255–60
5. Fabietti M et al (2020) Artifact detection in chronically recorded local field potentials using long-short term memory neural network. In: Proceedings of the AICT 2020, pp 1–6
6. Al Nahian MJ, Ghosh T et al (2020) Towards artificial intelligence driven emotion aware fall monitoring framework suitable for elderly people with neurological disorder. In: Proceedings of the brain information, pp 275–286
7. Fabietti M, Mahmud M, Lotfi A (2021) Anomaly detection in invasively recorded neuronal signals using deep neural network: effect of sampling frequency. In: Proceedings of the AII, pp 79–91
8. Al Nahian MJ et al (2021) Towards an accelerometer-based elderly fall detection system using cross-disciplinary time series features. IEEE Access 9:39413–31
9. Fabietti M, Mahmud M, Lotfi A (2022) Channel-independent recreation of artefactual signals in chronically recorded local field potentials using machine learning. Brain Inform 9(1):1–17
10. Lalotra GS, Kumar V, Bhatt A, Chen T, Mahmud M (2022) iReTADS: an intelligent real-time anomaly detection system for cloud communications using temporal data summarization and neural network. Secur Commun Netw 2022:9149164
11. Mahmud M et al (2018) Applications of deep learning and reinforcement learning to biological data. IEEE Trans Neural Netw Learn Syst. 29(6):2063–79
12. Biswas M et al (2021) An XAI based autism detection: the context behind the detection. In: Proceedings of the brain information, pp 448–459
13. Mahmud M, Kaiser MS, McGinnity TM, Hussain A (2021) Deep learning in mining biological data. Cogn Comput 13(1):1–33
14. Deepa B et al (2022) Pattern descriptors orientation and map firefly algorithm based brain pathology classification using hybridized machine learning algorithm. IEEE Access. 10:3848–63
15. Mammoottil MJ, Kulangara LJ, Cherian AS, Mohandas P, Hasikin K, Mahmud M (2022) Detection of breast cancer from five-view thermal images using convolutional neural networks. J Healthc Eng 2022:4295221
16. Kumar I et al (2022) Dense tissue pattern characterization using deep neural network. Cogn Comput 1–24. [ePub ahead of print]
17. Paul A et al (2022) Inverted bell-curve-based ensemble of deep learning models for detection of COVID-19 from chest X-rays. Neural Comput Appl 1–15
18. Prakash N et al (2021) Deep transfer learning COVID-19 detection and infection localization with superpixel based segmentation. Sustain Cities Soc 75:103252
19. Ghosh T et al (2021) Artificial intelligence and internet of things in screening and management of autism spectrum disorder. Sustain Cities Soc 74:103189
20. Watkins J, Fabietti M, Mahmud M (2020) Sense: a student performance quantifier using sentiment analysis. In: Proceedings of the IJCNN, pp 1–6
21. Satu M et al (2020) Towards improved detection of cognitive performance using bidirectional multilayer long-short term memory neural network. In: Proceedings of the brain information, pp 297–306
22. Faria TH et al (2021) Smart city technologies for next generation healthcare. In: Data-driven mining, learning and analytics for secured smart cities, pp 253–274

23. Ghosh T et al (2021) An attention-based mood controlling framework for social media users. In: Proceedings of the brain information, pp 245–256
24. Biswas M, Tania MH, Kaiser MS et al (2021) ACCU3RATE: a mobile health application rating scale based on user reviews. PLoS ONE 16(12):e0258050
25. Nawar A, Toma NT, Al Mamun S et al (2021) Cross-content recommendation between movie and book using machine learning. In: Proceedings of the AICT, pp 1–6
26. Ghosh T et al (2021) A hybrid deep learning model to predict the impact of COVID-19 on mental health form social media big data. Preprints 2021(2021060654)
27. Satu MS et al (2021) TClustVID: a novel machine learning classification model to investigate topics and sentiment in COVID-19 tweets. Knowl-Based Syst 226:107126
28. Al Banna MH et al (2021) Attention-based bi-directional long-short term memory network for earthquake prediction. IEEE Access 9:56589–603
29. Lin C, Hu P, Su H, Li S, Mei J, Zhou J et al (2020) Sensemood: depression detection on social media. In: Proceedings of the 2020 international conference on multimedia retrieval, pp 407–411
30. Narziev N, Goh H, Toshnazarov K, Lee SA, Chung KM, Noh Y (2020) STDD: short-term depression detection with passive sensing. Sensors 20(5):1396
31. Hussain J, Satti FA, Afzal M, Khan WA, Bilal HSM, Ansaar MZ et al (2020) Exploring the dominant features of social media for depression detection. J Inf Sci 46(6):739–59
32. Chiong R, Budhi GS, Dhakal S, Chiong F (2021) A textual-based featuring approach for depression detection using machine learning classifiers and social media texts. Comput Biol Med 135:104499
33. Alghowinem SM, Gedeon T, Goecke R, Cohn J, Parker G (2020) Interpretation of depression detection models via feature selection methods. IEEE Trans Affect Comput
34. Wu MY, Shen CY, Wang ET, Chen AL (2020) A deep architecture for depression detection using posting, behavior, and living environment data. J Intell Inf Syst 54(2):225–44
35. Zhu J, Wang Z, Gong T, Zeng S, Li X, Hu B et al (2020) An improved classification model for depression detection using EEG and eye tracking data. IEEE Trans Nanobiosci 19(3):527–37
36. Shah FM, Ahmed F, Joy SKS, Ahmed S, Sadek S, Shil R (2020) Early depression detection from social network using deep learning techniques. In: IEEE region 10 symposium (TENSYMP). IEEE, pp 823–826
37. Lin L, Chen X, Shen Y, Zhang L (2020) Towards automatic depression detection: a bilstm/1d cnn-based model. Appl Sci 10(23):8701
38. Zeberga K, Attique M, Shah B, Ali F, Jembre YZ, Chung TS (2022) A novel text mining approach for mental health prediction using Bi-LSTM and BERT model. Comput Intell Neurosci 2022
39. Mustafa RU, Ashraf N, Ahmed FS, Ferzund J, Shahzad B, Gelbukh A (2020) A multiclass depression detection in social media based on sentiment analysis. In: 17th international conference on information technology–new generations (ITNG 2020). Springer, pp 659–662
40. Arun V, Prajwal V, Krishna M, Arunkumar B, Padma S, Shyam VA (2018) Boosted machine learning approach for detection of depression. In: IEEE symposium series on computational intelligence (SSCI). IEEE, pp 41–47
41. Arora A, Joshi A, Jain K, Dokania S, Srinath P (2018) Unraveling depression using machine intelligence. In: 2018 3rd international conference on communication and electronics systems (ICCES). IEEE, pp 1029–1033
42. Dong Y, Yang X (2021) A hierarchical depression detection model based on vocal and emotional cues. Neurocomputing 441:279–90
43. AlSagri HS, Ykhlef M (2020) Machine learning-based approach for depression detection in twitter using content and activity features. IEICE Trans Inf Syst 103(8):1825–32
44. Hosseini-Saravani SH, Besharati S, Calvo H, Gelbukh A (2022) Depression detection in social media using a psychoanalytical technique for feature extraction and a cognitive based classifier. In: Mexican international conference on artificial intelligence. Springer, pp 282–292
45. Loh HW, Ooi CP, Aydemir E, Tuncer T, Dogan S, Acharya UR (2022) Decision support system for major depression detection using spectrogram and convolution neural network with EEG signals. Expert Syst 39(3):e12773

46. Bai R, Guo Y, Tan X, Feng L, Xie H (2021) An EEG-based depression detection method using machine learning model. Int J Pharma Med Biol Sci 10:17–22
47. Lu H, Shao W, Ngai E, Hu X, Hu B (2021) A new skeletal representation based on gait for depression detection. In: 2020 IEEE international conference on E-health networking, application and services (HEALTHCOM). IEEE, pp 1–6
48. Xie W, Liang L, Lu Y, Wang C, Shen J, Luo H et al (2021) Interpreting depression from question-wise long-term video recording of sds evaluation. IEEE J Biomed Health Infor
49. Funk M et al (2016) Global burden of mental disorders and the need for a comprehensive, coordinated response from health and social sectors at the country level. Accessed on 2016;30
50. Diederich J, Al-Ajmi A, Yellowlees P (2007) Ex-ray: data mining and mental health. Appl Soft Comput 7(3):923–8
51. Babu NV, Kanaga E (2022) Sentiment analysis in social media data for depression detection using artificial intelligence: a review. SN Comput Sci 3(1):1–20
52. Major Depression (2022). https://www.nimh.nih.gov/health/statistics/major-depression
53. Ashraf A, Gunawan TS, Riza BS, Haryanto EV, Janin Z (2020) On the review of image and video-based depression detection using machine learning. Indonesian J Electr Eng Comput Sci (IJEECS) 19(3):1677–84
54. Safayari A, Bolhasani H (2021) Depression diagnosis by deep learning using EEG signals: a systematic review. Med Novel Technol Dev 12:100102
55. De Angel V, Lewis S, White K, Oetzmann C, Leightley D, Oprea E et al (2022) Digital health tools for the passive monitoring of depression: a systematic review of methods. NPJ Digital Med 5(1):1–14
56. Vabalas A, Gowen E, Poliakoff E, Casson AJ (2019) Machine learning algorithm validation with a limited sample size. PLoS ONE 14(11):e0224365
57. Park SH, Han K (2018) Methodologic guide for evaluating clinical performance and effect of artificial intelligence technology for medical diagnosis and prediction. Radiology 286(3):800–9

Investigating Mental Wellbeing in the Technology Workplace Using Machine Learning Techniques

Tahmid Alam, Tianhua Chen, Magda Bucholc, and Grigoris Antoniou

Abstract With the technology industry becoming steadily more and more populated, professionals within the field are finding themselves prone to suffering from different mental health issues. This is accompanied with more willing to share and discuss the issue as well as more resources put available to support sufferers. Bearing the aim to understand better the mental wellbeing of those working in the technological workplace, this paper utilise machine learning techniques to analyse questionnaire survey data acquired from a non-profit corporation of Open Source Mental Illness (OSMI), whereby unsupervised machine learning was used to identify clusters and potential patterns shared between the OSMI respondents; wile artificial neural network was used to analyse whether it's possible to establish, based on the survey responses, if an individual suffers from mental health problems.

Keywords Mental Wellbeing · Mental health · Machine learning · Clustering · Artificial neural network

1 Introduction

The technology field of work is one that is ever-changing and growing. With constant innovation regarding emerging technologies, along with greater public-exposure as time progresses, the number of people opting for a career in the general technological field is consequently steadily increasing. This increase in the workforce comes with its own problems; job saturation is making potential tech careers more tumultuous for young professionals, leading to a sense of unstable job security [1]. This, coupled with the rapidly evolved emerging technologies can lead to technical professionals spending their out of work hours completing further training/studying, subsequently

T. Alam · T. Chen (✉) · G. Antoniou
Department of Computer Science, University of Huddersfield, Huddersfield, UK
e-mail: T.Chen@hud.ac.uk

M. Bucholc
Intelligent Systems Research Centre, School of Computing and Engineering and Intelligent Systems, Ulster University, Londonderry, UK

T. Chen et al. (eds.), *Artificial Intelligence in Healthcare*, Brain Informatics and Health,
https://doi.org/10.1007/978-981-19-5272-2_8

165

leaving them overworked and stressed. This scenario may be further amplified by the COVID-19 pandemic that has led to worsen mental wellbeing [2] as a result of more fierce competition in the job market.

Whilst stress alone may not be a cause for concern considering it can be found in almost any workplace, it can potentially be a precursor to much more severe mental health issues, such as anxiety and depression if the levels of stress are continuously high [3]. Needless to say, suffering from any of the aforementioned mental health issues can be debilitating for the individual at hand, but it can also have ramifications on the company that employs them. Employees suffering from mental health disorders such as depression have been noted to suffer from lower levels of productivity in the work place [4] while workplaces with a higher number of those suffering from mental health disorders generally have a lower employee-retention rate, coupled with lower employee satisfaction. Therefore, identifying earlier indicators on whom may be suffering, as well as devising effective plans and resources to limit the strain on mental health would be beneficial both for the employee and the employer.

Recent advancement of Artificial Intelligence (AI) and machine learning in particular has witnessed a number of successful transformations in the healthcare domain [5–8]. As the machine learning techniques enable to learn automatically from data, they can potentially offer new insights for extracting patterns of human behaviour and identifying mental health symptoms and risk factors [9], which has observed numerous successes for mental disorders such as the attention deficit hyperactivity disorder and autism [10–12]. In the specific area of mental wellbeing in the workplace, it's also common a theme to utilise machine learning techniques to predict whether an individual would require mental health treatment and to identify factors that could significantly contribute to worsen mental health. While it's more common to see machine learning applied in the general workplace [13], the research on these techniques in the tech industry is more limited, though there also existed research which aimed to establish what the strongest predictors of mental health are within the technological workplace [14], where only statistical methods were utilised instead of machine learning techniques to assess the predictors, which is the focus of our research instead.

A research study carried out in 2019 by Open Source Mental Illness (OSMI), a non-profit corporation that aims to raise awareness and support for mental wellness, involved the researchers at hand conducting various forms of supervised machine learning on the survey responses to assess how they can be at predicting whether an individual would require mental health treatment [15]. Regarding the data used, the participants answered the original OSMI survey all worked within the technological workplace. The survey itself consisted of 80 predictors and over 1500 responses. The methods utilised included Logistic Regression, Support Vector Machine (SVM) and Decision Trees, where it was found that the Decision Trees yielded the best results with an accuracy score of 84% and precision of 0.84.

A similar body of research was conducted where the researchers at hand also utilised supervised ML techniques to predict whether or not an individual would require mental health treatment, off the given data [16]. The data used in this study was also provided by OSMI, where the participants in the original survey worked in the tech workplace, but with over 750 responses. A similar research was conducted by [16]. Despite also using prevalent methods such as Logistic Regression, Random Forest and Decision Trees, the decision tree classifier applied in this study only resulted in a considerably lower accuracy of just under 70%, whereas the boosting, which is an ensemble method, resulted in the highest level of accuracy with 75.13%. A possible cause for performance difference possibly result from the different subjects that exhibit different human behaviour and characteristics as well as the feature selection methods employed. The use of clustering that is able to establish the possible relations and underlying knowledge in a unsupervised manner has also been integrated with supervised learning approach resulting in as high as 90% accuracy [17].

Whilst building a model of high accuracy to predict whether someone does in fact require mental health treatment is a prevalent theme, due to the amount of factors that may affect such a result, along with the general 'noise' that may come with the data, identifying features that are significant in contributing towards the worsen mental wellbeing is another important topic for early prevention and effective monitoring. For instance, both [15, 16] explore decision tree models that are underpinned by computing feature significance such as entropy and gini index to grow the tree. It was concluded in [16] that gender and family history were the factors which held the highest influence on stress and mental health; while the history of mental health along with family history contribute most towards disorder prediction in [15]. This is consistent with conclusion drawn by [13] that summarises having family with mental health disorders can be a somewhat effective predictor [13]. With study by [15] also including workers who are not necessarily technical professionals within the tech industry, they found that those that do work in the tech field are slightly more at risk of developing stress and mental health Problems, even if the role itself is not technology based.

In line with the increasingly popular trend of employing machine learning and data science with application to study the mental health of those working in the technological field, this paper aimed to carry out both unsupervised Machine Learning, in efforts to identify any possible trends and significant factors in those who suffer from mental health problems, as well as building predictive models through supervised learning to establish whether or not an individual with certain characteristics may suffer from mental health problems.

2 Materials and Methods

2.1 The Data

The data source used for this study was retrieved from Kaggle but was originally created by Open Sourcing Mental Illness (OSMI), a company which is centered around raising awareness and providing resources to support mental wellness within the Tech and open source communities. OSMI has been a key source of information for previous studies [13, 15, 16] and has an extensive range of information in the form of survey responses.

2.2 Data Preprocessing

The original data came from a questionnaire survey for investigating the mental wellbeing in tech industry. It contained 1433 observations across 63 features. Whilst the questions in the survey ranged from personal questions (such as 'what is your age?', 'Which city do you live in?', 'What is your gender'?), the majority of questions related to their profession or the company for which they worked at. Many of the questions involved a direct approach in questioning the participant on their own outlook on their mental health.

Whilst most of the features were categorical, age was numeric as well as questions such as those asking the individual to expand on the previous question that were open-space as opposed to drop down answers, therefore resulting in a multitude of string based responses. Regarding the feature which asks the respondent of their preferred gender, due to the vast range of answers given, these were mapped to the values of 'male', 'female' and 'other'.

In terms of missing values, there were almost 22000 instances of 'Not Applicable' Values, which may partly be due to that several question are not applicable to the respondents, such as the follow-up questions where the prior question didn't apply to them either. To combat this, any attributes which contained 50% (or more) of its values as Na were empirically dropped. For the remainder, to avoid a considerable amount of data dropped, imputations were ran to replace Na values with the Mode response of the respective predictor, though more advance interpolation technique [18] may be explored in future.

As mentioned earlier, the majority of the data was categorical, therefore it was necessary to encode the values into numeric form for subsequent computation. For this, two methods were chosen: *One Hot Encoding* (OHE) and *Ordinal Encoding* (OE). OHE assigns a group of bits among which the legal combinations of values are only those with '1' and all the others '0'. OE on the other hand involves mapping each unique label to an ranked integer value based on the known relationship between the categories of the underlying variable. After conducting OHE, this produced an updated dataset which now consisted of 555 features (one for each question and its possible response). As OE merely converts the responses to numeric equivalents, the feature number remained the same (55).

2.3 Flowchart

As shown in Fig. 1, the proposed methodology took place over several stages, which is denoted with the varying colours in the flowchart. In red, the 'Data Gathering' stage refers to the acquisition of the initial data, which in this case refers to collecting the survey responses from the 2016 OSMI survey from Kaggle. This was then followed by the preprocessing steps, which are represented by the yellow nodes in the figure. 'General Preprocessing' refers to the main 'clean up' of data, i.e. dealing with NA values, followed by feature transformation through Ordinal Encoding.

Once the data was appropriately preprocessed, the machine learning tasks (represented by the green nodes) then followed, where they were done independently of each other. The unsupervised learning part required an additional step of cluster (number) evaluation to be conducted, after which we then carried out the cluster analysis itself. The cluster number evaluation consisted of 2 methods to establish the appropriate number of clusters: the *Elbow Method* and the *Silhouette Methods*, which will be discussed in Sect. 3A.

For the supervised investigation, an extra stage of preprocessing was introduced: Data Splitting. We chose to split the data via a 66:33 ratio for the training and testing data respectively, after which a neural network (NN) model was created to test the prediction accuracy when using the feature 'Do you currently have a Mental Health disorder?' as the target feature.

Fig. 1 Flowchart of proposed methodology

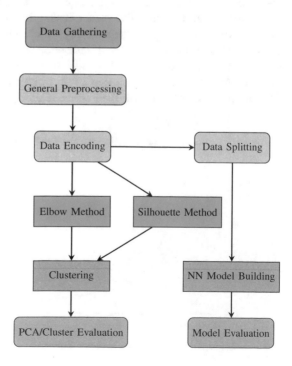

After both machine learning tasks had been completed, evaluation was then conducted individually, represented by the orange nodes. For the unsupervised task, this came in the form of dimension reduction techniques (namely PCA) which in turn allowed us to produce cluster visualisations. We evaluated the supervised task by measuring (and visualising) the accuracy and loss for both the training and test data.

3   Experimentation and Discussion

3.1   Cluster Analysis

Once the preprocessing and encoding of the raw data, the popular k-means clustering was first applied, with the aim to find any potential hidden patterns or data groupings. However, the number of clusters K is a important hyper-parameter to explore; hence two popular methods are used to determine an appropriate of clustering, including the *Elbow Method* [19] and *Silhouette Analysis* [20].

The premise of the Elbow Method is to run the KMeans clustering on the chosen dataset across a range of different K values (in this case 1–15), where upon each value of K, the sum of squared errors (SSE) was calculated. As the number of K increases, the SSE (or 'distortion') decreases, where (hypothetically) the decrease in SSE will dramatically level off after a specific number of K. When conducted on the encoded data, as can be seen in Fig. 2, the optimal K value may be set to 4.

To further validate the value of K chosen, Silhouette Analysis was undertaken. This involves measuring the 'separability' of clusters; both within and between the clusters themselves. It calculates the mean distance within a cluster (known as the intra-cluster distance (a)), and also the mean distance between a sample and its nearest clusters which it's not a part of (known as the nearest-cluster distance (b)). The silhouette coefficient can then be calculated using the Eq. 1, where 'a' is the

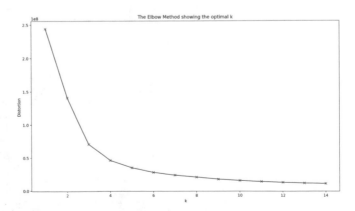

Fig. 2   SSE results on encoded data to detect 'Elbow'

Table 1 Average silhouette scores for each K values from 2–6

Number of clusters	Average silhouette score
2	0.426
3	0.537
4	0.542
5	0.543
6	0.522

mean intra-distance cluster distance, 'b' is the mean nearest-cluster distance and 's' is the silhouette score. Silhouette scores can range between 1 to –1, where a score of 1 is best as it suggests that the data point (o) is 'compact' within its respective cluster, and thus far away from other. A score of 0 implies it's overlapping and scores close to –1 therefore suggest inaccuracy. Analysis was conducted for K values ranging from 2–6, where the average silhouette score for each iteration with its respective number of clusters can be seen in Table 1. The most promising values were in case of K = 4 and K = 5, where the individual visualisation for each can be seen in Figs. 3 and 4.

To further reinforce previous findings, these cluster may allude to the notion that certain demographics/groups of people may be prone to suffering from mental health issues. Whilst previous studies have concluded that factors such as family history with mental health and occupation may affect the mental wellbeing [13, 16], further

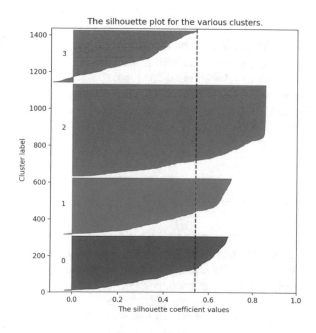

Fig. 3 Silhouette score visualisation for K = 4

Fig. 4 Silhouette score
visualisation for K = 5

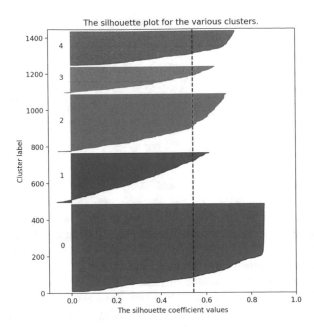

analysis would need to be conducted to establish which traits are shared amongst those within the same cluster, and whether it differs or aligns from previous findings.

$$s = (b - a)/max(a, b) \tag{1}$$

With the above exploration, the K number was finally chosen to be 5 from this point forward as it resulted in the highest average silhouette score, but when comparing the visualisations, the scores dipped into negative comparatively less (overall) compared to when K = 4, where the 4th cluster contains a considerable negative element. It is also worth noting that the hierarchical clustering was also attempted (namely the *Agglomerative* approach), however when validating the number of clusters via the silhouette method, the respective average silhouette scores dropped considerably.

3.2 Visualisation

Considering the ordinal encoded data contained numerous features (55 for the OE data and 555 for the OHE data), it's extremely difficult to visualise the clusters in their current form. Therefore, dimension reduction in the form of Principle Component Analysis (PCA) was conducted. PCA aims to summarise the present data in the form of *Principal Components* (PC) to lower the dimensionality, with the potential trade off of losing some of the original data. As the aim here was to reduce the dimensions down to 2–3 (for visualisation purposes), when conducting PCA on the OHE data,

Fig. 5 2D visualisation of clusters using 2 Principal Components from OE data

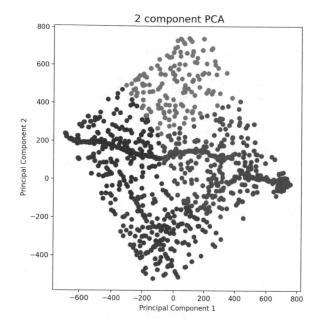

the cummulative variance explained by 2 PC was only 24%, therefore a majority of the data's variance was lost. Even as the number of PC was increased to 10, this still only accounted for 47% of the data's cummulative variance. On the other hand, when PCA was conducted on the OE data for 2 PC, 99% of the cumulative variance was retained. Once the data was reduced successfully, it was then possible to visualise the clusters in a 2D manner.

In Fig. 5 we can see for example distinct clusters with minimal overlap, suggesting that there may indeed be shared features which are represented across the 2 principal components. Considering these 2 components are an amalgamation of the features present within the survey however, the clusters themselves therefore may represents multiple features each which in turn may attribute to one's mental health situation.

Whilst we also carried out supervised machine learning afterwards, we considered these steps to be independent of each other. As mentioned earlier, this was done as we aimed to first simply test whether there are indeed underlying patterns to be found within the data, i.e. any shared features between those who do suffer from mental health problems. This was then separately followed by testing to see if it's possible to predict whether an individual actually suffers from mental health problems.

After the clusters had been determined and visualised, the next task was to assess which conditions applied to the clusters at hand. Ordinarily there would be several different approaches where this could be done, such as plotting Parallel Coordinate Plots (PCP) or utilising supervised learning such as Decision Trees or Random Forest to understand the rules that are applied to the data points in the clusters. Due to the highly dimensional nature of the data at hand, along with the fact that the data itself is almost made up of entirely of categorical data, PCP would be uninformative as the graph produced would become tied, resulting in a spaghetti plot.

Other than cluster analysis, Feature Importance was also conducted with the pseudo-target being the question '*Do you currently have mental health disorder?*'. After applying and fitting a Random Forest Classifier to the model and choosing the top 10 features of highest perceived 'importance' being centered around the individual's current and previous mental state; more specifically—if they *did* have mental health disorders and it *did* affect their work when it wasn't treated properly, along with whether or not they had mental health disorders in the past.

3.3   Building a Predictive Model Using Artificial Neural Networks

The aforementioned field of '*Do you currently have a mental health disorder?*' was used as the target variable when creating a Neural Network model to establish whether it's possible to accurately predict the response, from the previous responses given. The model itself was tuned over time and the final parameters/details can be see in the Table 2.

As we reduced the dataset further to contain 50 features, in efforts to reduce the dimensionality. The feature '*Do you currently have a mental health disorder?*' was used as the target, allowing us to test and train the model on the remaining 49 features. We empirically partitioned the data into 67:33 splits for the training and testing data respectively. The target has three possible values of classification ('yes', 'no' or 'maybe'), and considering the task at hand was that of classification, the output layer thus had a shape of 3. The final results for the accuracy and loss (based on the validation data) averaged 76.8% and 0.78% respectively. The results in comparison to the training data can been seen in Figs. 6 and 7. Increasing the Epoch number further led to increased divergence between the training and test accuracy and loss, suggesting that the model was over-fitting, which in turn may be somewhat resultant of the dataset's small size.

Whilst the validation data resulted in a similar accuracy to that of the testing data, overall the accuracy struggled to increase above 77%. Similarly the loss value can be seen to reach roughly 0.8 at epoch 5 and decreases only slightly for the remaining epochs; a loss value which is arguably still too high to be ideal.

Table 2 Model parameter/hyperparameter tuning

Parameter/hyperparameter	Number
Number of layers	4
Number of epochs	40
Batch size	1
Number of neurons (per layer)	40

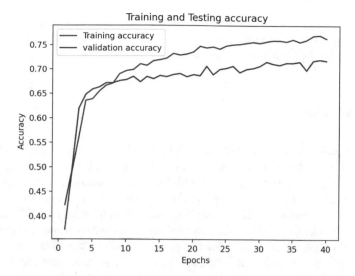

Fig. 6 Training and testing accuracy

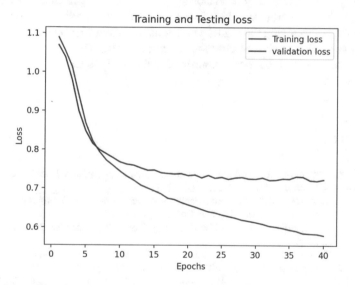

Fig. 7 Training and testing loss

Whilst the results of the supervised learning weren't as high as we'd hoped, they still show promise. In comparison to some of the studies mentioned earlier, the accuracy of this particular model falls roughly within the same bandwidth, with [16] achieving an accuracy of 75% when using boosting algorithm for prediction on a similar premise and data. Predicting whether or not an individual may be suffering from a mental health problem would be invaluable in terms of providing treatment and creating a safe workplace, but in order to create an adequate model, a larger dataset may be required to train the model.

4 Conclusion

This study has aimed to study the mental health characteristics exhibited by those working in the technological workplace through machine learning techniques. With the use of Kmeans clustering, along with feature extraction technique of PCA, it was possible to visualise the clusters in the data, while the number of clusters were established to 5 through the Elbow Method and Silhouette Analysis. With the use of supervised learning through artificial neural networks, we were able to further reinforce the notion that there may indeed be grounds to identify/predict if an individual is suffering from mental health issues, strictly from the answers they provide. Whilst our results fall within the range of previous studies [15, 16], further improvement in accuracy could potentially be achieved by advanced feature engineering through calculating their importance, which in turn may aid the selection of more informative features in improving the model's performance. To further build upon this work, analysis can be also conducted to establish transparent rules to the clusters in question to unlock the implicit influence of contributing factors for a deeper understanding of mental wellbeing.

References

1. Nayak RD (2014) Anxiety and mental health of software professionals and mechanical professionals. Int J Human Soc Sci Invent 3(2):52–56
2. Chen T, Lucock M (2022) The mental health of university students during the covid-19 pandemic: an online survey in the UK. Plos One 17(1):e0262562
3. Cohen JI (2000) Stress and mental health: a biobehavioral perspective. Issu Mental Health Nurs 21(2):185–202
4. Burton WN, Schultz AB, Chen C-Y, Edington DW (2008) The association of worker productivity and mental health: a review of the literature. Int J Workplace Health Manag
5. Chen T, Shang C, Su P, Keravnou-Papailiou E, Zhao Y, Antoniou G, Shen Q (2020) A decision tree-initialised neuro-fuzzy approach for clinical decision support. Artif Intell Med 111:101986
6. Su P, Chen T, Xie J, Zheng Y, Qi H, Borroni D, Zhao Y, Liu J (2020) Corneal nerve tortuosity grading via ordered weighted averaging-based feature extraction. Med Phys
7. Chen T, Keravnou-Papailiou E, Antoniou G (2021) Medical analytics for healthcare intelligence - recent advances and future directions. Artif Intell Med 112:102009
8. Oyeleye M, Chen T, Titarenko S, Antoniou G (2022) A predictive analysis of heart rates using machine learning techniques. Int J Environ Res Public Health 19(4):2417
9. Thieme A, Belgrave D, Doherty G (2020) Machine learning in mental health: A systematic review of the hci literature to support the development of effective and implementable ml systems. ACM Trans Comput-Human Interact (TOCHI) 27(5):1–53

10. Tachmazidis I, Chen T, Adamou M, Antoniou G (2021) A hybrid ai approach for supporting clinical diagnosis of attention deficit hyperactivity disorder (adhd) in adults. Health Inform Sci Syst 9(1):1–8
11. Chen T, Antoniou G, Adamou M, Tachmazidis I, Su P (2021) Automatic diagnosis of attention deficit hyperactivity disorder using machine learning. Appl Artif Intell 1–13
12. Stirling J, Chen T, Adamou M (2021) Autism spectrum disorder classification using a self-organising fuzzy classifier. In: Fuzzy logic. Springer, pp. 83–94
13. Laijawala V, Aachaliya A, Jatta H, Pinjarkar V (2020) Classification algorithms based mental health prediction using data mining. In: 2020 5th international conference on communication and electronics systems (ICCES). IEEE, pp 1174–1178
14. Aggreh M, Akinsiku T, Ewuzie A, Hessings F, Jones W, McLaverty D, Mugoma WE, Obed V, Oduala E, Mental health in the tech workplace: what are the strongest
15. Katarya R, Maan S (2020) Predicting mental health disorders using machine learning for employees in technical and non-technical companies. In: 2020 IEEE international conference on advances and developments in electrical and electronics engineering (ICADEE). IEEE, pp 1–5
16. Reddy US, Thota AV, Dharun A (2018) Machine learning techniques for stress prediction in working employees. In: 2018 IEEE international conference on computational intelligence and computing research (ICCIC). IEEE, pp 1–4
17. Srividya M, Mohanavalli S, Bhalaji N (2018) Behavioral modeling for mental health using machine learning algorithms. J Med Syst 42(5):1–12
18. Chen T, Shang C, Yang J, Li F, Shen Q (2020) A new approach for transformation-based fuzzy rule interpolation. IEEE Trans Fuzzy Syst. https://doi.org/10.1109/TFUZZ.2019.2949767
19. Yuan C, Yang H (2019) Research on k-value selection method of k-means clustering algorithm 2(2):226–235
20. Kaufman L, Rousseeuw PJ (2009) Finding groups in data: an introduction to cluster analysis. Wiley

Computational Intelligence in Detection and Support of Autism Spectrum Disorder

Sabbir Ahmed ⓘ, Silvia Binte Nur ⓘ, Md. Farhad Hossain ⓘ,
M Shamim Kaiser ⓘ, Mufti Mahmud ⓘ, and Tianhua Chen ⓘ

Abstract Autism Spectrum Disorder (ASD) refers to a spectrum of conditions characterised mainly by impairments in social interaction, speech and nonverbal communication, and restricted—repetitive behaviour. The lack of physical testing, done primarily via behaviour analysis, makes ASD diagnosis more difficult. The emergence of Computational Intelligence techniques has resulted in the development of a variety of fast and early ASD diagnosis methods based on multiple input modalities. The premise of computational intelligence (CI) and its efficiency in detecting and monitoring ASD has been examined in this chapter, which has recently advanced. Two

S. Ahmed · S. B. Nur · Md. Farhad Hossain · M. S. Kaiser
Institute of Information Technology, Jahangirnagar University, Savar, Dhaka 1342, Bangladesh
e-mail: sabbir.iit.ju@gmail.com

S. B. Nur
e-mail: binteashfinur@gmail.com

Md. Farhad Hossain
e-mail: farhadiitju@gmail.com

M. S. Kaiser (✉)
Applied Intelligence and Informatics Lab, Wazed Miah Science Research Centre (WMSRC),
Jahangirnagar University, Savar, Dhaka 1342, Bangladesh
e-mail: mskaiser@juniv.edu

M. Mahmud (✉)
Department of Computer Science, Nottingham Trent University, Nottingham NG11 8NS, UK
e-mail: muftimahmud@gmail.com; mufti.mahmud@ntu.ac.uk

Computing and Informatics Research Centre, Nottingham Trent University, Nottingham NG11 8NS, UK

Medical Technologies Innovation Facility, Nottingham Trent University, Nottingham NG11 8NS, UK

T. Chen
Department of Computer Science, University of Huddersfield, Huddersfield HD1 3DH, UK
e-mail: T.Chen@hud.ac.uk

© The Author(s), under exclusive license to Springer Nature Singapore Pte Ltd. 2022   179
T. Chen et al. (eds.), *Artificial Intelligence in Healthcare*, Brain Informatics and Health,
https://doi.org/10.1007/978-981-19-5272-2_9

types of studies have been discussed in this article. Several aspects of ASD screening, including questionnaires, eye scan paths, movement tracking, behavioural analysis from video, brain scans, and more, have been discussed using machine learning and deep learning. Secondly, ASD detection and monitoring applications have been studied extensively in the past year, with significant advances. Finally, a discussion has been made on the challenges faced in ASD detection and management with future research scopes.

1 Introduction

Autism spectrum disorder (ASD) is a complicated, irreversible developmental condition that usually manifests in early infancy and negatively influences a person's social skills, communication, relationships, and self-control. According to the fifth edition of the diagnostic and statistical manual of mental disorders [1], ASD is a neurodevelopmental disease characterised by deficits in social communication as well as the occurrence of repetitive and restricted patterns of activities, behaviour, or interests. Deficits in social-emotional reciprocity, nonverbal communicative behaviours during social interactions, and difficulty in developing, maintaining, and understanding relationships are the primary indicators of impairments in social communication. Some of the signs that manifest restricted and repetitive patterns of behaviour and activities in people with ASD include stereotyped or repetitive motor movements, insistence on sameness, inflexible adherence to routines, ritualised verbal or nonverbal behavioural patterns, hyper- or hypo-reactivity to sensory inputs, and unusual interest in sensory aspects of the environment. These signs have been used in identifying the varieties of ASD. Faras et al. [2] have termed ASD as a Pervasive Developmental Disorder (PDD) and categorised to: Autistic Disorders (AD), Asperger's Syndrome (AS), Childhood Disintegrative Disorder (CDD), Pervasive Developmental Disorder-Not Otherwise Specified (PDD-NOS) and Rett Syndrome (RS).

A clinical study suggests that toddlers who got early intensive therapy not only had functional gains but also required fewer services than those who received "treatment as usual" during a two to three-year follow-up period, which resulted in overall cost savings [3]. As a result, early intervention-and, by implication, early diagnosis-have the potential to enhance function while lowering societal costs [4]. Early identification of children with impairments and their treatment has been found to improve child outcomes for the developmental disorder (DD), and autism [5]. Developmental monitoring (also known as developmental surveillance by the American Academy of Pediatrics) is promoted by the World Health Organization [6] as a procedure for the early diagnosis of developmental difficulties, particularly in low, and middle-income countries (LMIC). In comparison to relying solely on clinical diagnosis, evidence from high-income countries (HIC) suggests that providing screening instruments in routine healthcare visits can result in earlier and more accurate identification of children in need [7]. Regular screening for ASD or DD during healthcare visits is an effective way to detect the condition early and allows any referral for additional diagnosis and intervention. Despite its significance, however, early diagnosis remains a hurdle in both HIC and LMIC [8]. In early life, when developmental changes are fast, early symptoms are typically subtle, and this makes the identification difficult [9]. In general, ASD diagnosis is a complex procedure due to the disorder's developmental and widespread nature. Many of the signs of ASD, such as delayed expressive language development, poor social responsiveness, behavioural issues, and repetitive behaviour, can also be found in other disorders and syndromes. The presence of intellectual disabilities further complicates the differential diagnosis process, especially in very young children whose impairments in interpersonal interactions must be separated from the ones produced by other cognitive impairments. Professionals use a variety of official and informal ASD screening techniques. These might be anything from casual observations to official evaluations.

The Modified Checklist for Autism in Children, Revised (M-CHAT) is a common 20-question assessment designed for children aged 16–30 months [10]. The Ages and Stages Questionnaire (ASQ) [11] is a broad developmental screening method that focuses on developmental issues at distinctive ages. The ASQ consists of 40 questions on reciprocal social interaction (such as social smiling, willingness to participate with other children, and trying to offer comfort to others), language and communication (including the use of traditional gestures, interpersonal conversation, and generalising utterances), and repetitive and stereotyped behavioural patterns. The ASQ also contains a question concerning self-injurious conduct and another about the individual's present language functioning [11]. Autism Diagnostic Observation Schedule (ADOS) contains semi-structured observational questions. The examiner assesses the child's answers to various familiar and unusual circumstances, looking for ASD-related behaviours. ADOS consists of several subtasks whose goal is to determine social capabilities, such as eye contact and social smiling [12]. Autism Diagnostic Interview, Revised (ADI-R) is a semi-structured questionnaire for family caregivers to diagnose ASD by interpreting parents' observations about their children's everyday activities [13]. Because the ADI-R evaluation depends on caregiver reports, it does not allow for direct observation of children's social behaviours. Instead of relying solely on psychoanalysis or other theoretical assumptions, Childhood Autism Rating Scale (CARS) is based on direct behavioural observation. The CARS is beneficial for research and administrative classification and for generating a comprehensive explanation of a child's unusual behaviour [14]. The following are some popular techniques for controlling and monitoring ASD systems: at the outset, ASD symptoms must be discovered, which may be done in various ways, such as utilising questionnaires to identify the most prevalent ASD signals. Once this step is complete, we may use the Internet of Things (IoT)-based devices that use different sensors to track an individual's everyday actions. We can monitor individuals' behaviour and how they respond to diverse circumstances by deploying these technologies. After identifying it, we can develop a system to monitor or ease their behavioural cycle. We can utilise a variety of apps or web-based platforms to do it. Thus, we can train them and improve their lives by providing diverse approaches, equipment, and other resources.

2 Computational Intelligence

Computational intelligence (CI) as a domain aims in creating intelligent systems to solve complicated problems. In real-life optimisation, classification, or regression problems, all the possible states or outcomes are too large to compute using the most sophisticated computer systems. The scarcity of deterministic methods has led to the development of nature-inspired methods to find valuable solutions and heuristics from uncertain, incomplete databases. These methods, also driven by utilising learning methods from experiments and data, can provide approximate solutions for many NP-hard problems using fewer computations and resources. Thus CI refers to utilising learning methods from experiments and data [15]. The main key point for CI algorithms is the trade-off between accuracy and computational time. Again using learning parameters that are set as constants for these algorithms allows leading to the desired solution more quickly.

The scope of CI is quite vast and includes fuzzy computing, neural networks, and evolutionary computing. Over time, these learning methods evolved, and machine learning and neural networks have received extensive attention lately. A vast amount of methodology has been derived from these branches. According to Kruse et al., CI consists of neural networks, fuzzy logic, evolutionary algorithms, and Bayes networks [16]. Swarm intelligence is also mentioned as a core part of CI by Engelbrecht et al. [15]. In terms of applications, techniques pertaining to these diverse areas have been applied in a wide range of problem domains including anomaly detection [17–22], disease detection [23–31] and smart data analytics [32–40].

2.1 Neural Networks

Neural networks are inspired by the learning methods of our brain, and by simulating the brain's functioning, computers can learn and process various heuristics. This is mainly done by creating artificial neurons and connecting them so that they can mimic the brain's functioning. At the artificial level, each neuron responds conditionally to convey some information or not. When many such artificial neurons are connected, they create a network for learning subtle patterns that solve complex problems. Until recently, putting together a large neuronal network and making them learn required significant computational. However, currently, it is possible to experiment with deeper structures of such Artificial Neural Networks (ANN) due to the recent advancements in hardware technologies and programming libraries [41]. Common examples of such large scale artificial neural networks include Convolutional Neural Networks (CNN) for image classification and processing, recurrent neural networks and Long Short Term Memory (LSTM) for analysing time-series data, and Generative Adversarial Networks (GAN) for synthetic data generation. Modern trends towards self-supervised learning, federated learning, and deep reinforcement learning are also increasing.

2.2 Fuzzy Logic

Fuzzy logic has been attributed to human decision-making, which takes advantage of our ability to reason with relatively incomplete or approximate data [42]. Instead of placing true or false conditioning, the approach utilises a continuous rating for making decisions. Thus it works well with partial reasoning and tries to duplicate human cognition. This approach of intermediate truth allows a fuzzy set to contain a wide range of values between 0 and 1. These properties made fuzzy logic ideal for scenarios with incomplete and imprecise data, such as natural language processing or control engineering. Exploiting this approach of low power computation, many modern systems like temperature controlling, washing machines, and gear selection in automobiles utilised fuzzy logic. Fuzzy logic is based on the if-then rule, variables and membership functions. The fuzzy membership functions are employed to transform the initial raw input supplied to a fuzzy system. Fuzzy logic does not work on its own; instead, it describes the relationship of the If-then rules using the membership function. A rudimentary fuzzy system could categorise input data before applying if-then rules to different continuous variables with predefined ranges. The initial if-then description is applied as if some variable has a specific range of values, then the variable changes. However, this type of initial logic is given by humans and may contain errors, imprecision and false data. Hence, fuzzy logic allows comprehension in an unconventional environment to better understand the relevance of the insights.

2.3 Evolutionary Computation

Evolutionary computation is a discipline of soft computing and AI that consists of optimisation algorithms based on biologically inspired methods. Overall, in the techniques, stochastic optimisation is achieved through the nature-inspired population using trial and error methods [43]. By replicating the behaviour of natural elements, evolution or mathematical changes occur on a step by step basis. A preliminary collection of possible solutions is developed and continually revised for an optimal solution in evolutionary computing. In each iteration, lesser desirable information is stochastically discarded through randomised modifications. An explicit fitness function is used to compute the necessary statistical correctness of each solution. Nature-inspired selection criteria are then applied to a set of possible solutions toward finding the optimised solution. Again these solutions work as the base for the subsequent iterations. Hence a sub-optimal solution is reached with relatively less computational power.

3   Computational Intelligence in Autism Detection

Various sensing technology embedded within wearable devices, such as micro-
phones, heart rate, motion, accelerometer, and pulse oximeter, provide a better insight
into the ailments and symptoms of a patient. Similarly, video, simulation, eye tracking, and virtual reality-based scenarios contribute to the accurate assessment of ASD
diagnosis rather than the questionnaire-based ones [44]. These devices can collect
critical patient information, which then can be analysed using machine learning (ML)
and deep learning (DL) algorithms to extract relevant information [24, 45–49]. Initial
diagnosis of ASD based on data from IoT devices might perhaps assist professionals.
Moreover, IoT and ML systems allow for mass primary diagnosis with little or no
health professional involvement. Therefore, the datasets play an essential role in the
diagnosis of ASD.

3.1   Datasets and Methods

Many researchers have conducted studies with different modalities of data to identify
biomarkers and traits among ASD and neurotypical people. Multiple studies in the
literature have reported various data acquisition techniques to find differences in
biomarkers among ASD, neurodegenerative and neurotypical patients. Labelling
these key biomarker-based features in each dataset provides future research scope
for researchers of different backgrounds. Since creating a dataset is a tedious task
requiring multidisciplinary contribution, several datasets have been made publicly
available, covering a range of modalities from structured data to image, audio, and
video data.

The ASD screening in children dataset consists of a total of 20 features(10
behavioural features and 10 individual characteristics) that are utilised to classify
ASD cases [50]. A further innovative way of ASD detection using the Scanpath
Trend Analysis is the use of eye movement from the web [51]. An eye-tracking
dataset featuring visualisations of eye-tracking Scanpaths focusing on ASD allows
identifying the condition from eye-movements [52]. Carette et al. [53] proposed
an eye movement tracking based ASD detection system using LSTM. A total
of 17 ASD and 15 neurotypical patients were studied with an accuracy of 83%.
Elbattah et al. [54] suggested an eye-tracking Scanpath method for ASD classification using the K-mean clustering algorithm and reported maximum accuracy with the
k value set at four. Similarly, Carette et al. [55] presented a technique that converts an
eye-tracking Scanpath into an image and then classifies the image for ASD screening. They experimented with Random Forest (RF), Support Vector Machine (SVM),
Linear Regression (LR), Naïve Bayes (NB), and ANN algorithms and obtained a
maximum AUC of 90%. Tao et al. [56] classified ASD utilising eye Scanpath using
saliency mapping from Convolutional Neural Network (CNN) generator and dis-
criminator part with encoder, decoder. An image has been given to the patient to

capture their eye Scanpath, then utilising a CNN-LSTM algorithm for classification. In an interesting review work, Chita-Tegmark et al. [57] reviewed 38 eye-tracking and eye Scanpath based ASD detection methods. They considered eight factors to measure the effectiveness of each method.

Data were collected using a mobile app called ASDTests to form another structured dataset to test autism in toddlers [58]. In addition, datasets consisting of 300 images from 28 individuals with and without ASD [59] and video clips of children with ASD performing reach-to-grasp activities [60] have also been reported.

Goal et al. [61] proposed a modified Grasshopper Optimisation Algorithm (GOA) for feature selection in the AQ10 questionnaire-based data set, which improved the classification accuracy of RF, LR, NB and KNN and achieved 100% accuracy for child and adolescence datasets. In another work, Pratama et al. [62] applied SVM, RF, and ANN on the AQ10 dataset with 10-fold cross-validation without any feature selection. Thabtah and Peebles [63] proposed a new rule-based architecture for detecting ASD on several ASD datasets. During this, the bagging, rule induction, boosting, and decision trees methods were empirically assessed, with RML outperforming the others. Kupper et al. [64] prepared an ADOS questionnaire and conducted a survey in Germany. They minimised the feature of ADOS into only five attributes. Then classification was applied using SVM with an AUC of 82%. Levy et al. [65] proposed techniques to extract features from the ADOS questionnaire and applied 17 different supervised learning models. Their extracted feature set also contained information related to sex and age and could differentiate ASD from non-ASD reliably. The ML techniques include LR, Lasso, SVM, ADTree, RF, Ridge, Elastic net, LDA, AdaBoost, etc.

Oh et al. [66] proposed an EEG based ASD detection system where they used Marginal Fisher Analysis and Student's t-test for selecting features that were classified using an SVM classifier. Data from 37 children were classified with an accuracy of 98%. Similar EEG-based classification using transfer learning and pre-trained models were used by Bygin et al. [67]. For feature extraction, they used local binary pattern and short-term Fourier transform. The features were transformed into image format for classification. Khodatars et al. [68] reviewed deep learning-based methods suitable for neuroimaging-based diagnosis and rehabilitation of ASD. Challenges related to ASD detection and management were also addressed in this article. Classifiers such as SVM and K-means have also been utilised for ASD detection. Parvathi et al. [69] categorised children below three years old with ASD and achieved 96% accuracy using SVM. In another work, Jagota et al. [70] applied an ANN-based approach to detect ASD patients. Structural Magnetic Resonance Imaging (sMRI) has also been utilised to analyse the brain functionality of ASD patients. To classify ASD Mishra et al. [71] extracted surface and volumetric morphometric features of sMRI to classify with SVM, RF, K-Nearest Neighbours (KNN), and Extra Trees (ET) ML models. They also provided a comparative analysis for each of the ML classifiers. Raj et al. [72] used three publicly accessible datasets to compare the performances of LR, SVM, NN, NB, and CNN.

Rule-based ML methods have also been applied to ASD screening to provide more insight into the models' decision-making process to the clinical experts. Thabtah et al. [73] devised and evaluated such approaches on datasets from adults, adolescents, and toddlers. Omar et al. [74] merged classification and regression tree-random forest (RF-CART) with RF-ID3 and implemented it in a mobile app. Hossain et al. [75] examined 25 machine learning classifiers on a collected ASD dataset and found that SVM based on Sequential minimum optimisation (SMO) performs best in their experiment setting. Though individual screening systems like questionnaires, eye tracking, neuroimaging, genetic data, and electronic health records provide adequate results, the combination of these methods yields greater accuracy. A multimodal screening system consists of each screening method, as mentioned earlier, and then summarises each prediction into a final prediction. Multiple ML classifiers run parallelly with a final classifier that takes each of the first stage classifiers as input. In this manner, several ASD symptoms can be analysed for diagnosis [76] (Table 1).

4 Computational Intelligence in Autism Management

Since ASD is correlated to physiological changes associated with negative emotions in people, monitoring these emotional changes can provide caregivers with a real-time picture of what these people are going through. An effective monitoring system may raise caregivers' awareness of a person's emotional condition, allowing them to take the appropriate steps to reduce stress symptoms and encourage the individual to use better stress coping skills.

This section will look at how IoT-based and wearable gadgets might aid individuals with ASD by detecting their actions using various sensors. Then we'll look at the applications and websites that can be used to monitor their behaviour.

Anxiety problems are common in children and adolescents with ASD, with an estimated incidence rate of 40% [77]. Various physiological indicators and markers are considered for physiological and emotional evaluations. Heart Rate Variability (HRV) is a helpful metric that computes the time intervals between two successive R peaks in an ECG signal obtained by an ECG sensor. Jansen et al. found some evidence of heart rate arousal variability in response to public speaking stresses [78]. The total number of breaths, or respiratory cycles, that occur each minute is known as the respiratory rate (RR). The respiration rate might alter owing to disease, stress, and other factors. The respiratory centre, which is located inside the Medulla Oblongata of the brain, regulates breathing rate. The rate of respiration has been proved to be an effective stress indicator [79]. The conductivity of the skin is measured by the Galvanic Skin Response (GSR). The GSR may be measured by inserting two electrodes on the skin's surface, one of which injects a small amplitude AC into the skin, and the other uses Ohm's Law to calculate the skin's impedance given a certain voltage. GSR has been suggested as a potential stress indicator [80].

Wearable gadgets for physiological and, to a lesser extent, emotional monitoring are widely available on the market. Cabibihan et al. [81] conducted a review of the academic literature on several sensing technologies that might be used for ASD screening and treatments. Eye trackers, movement trackers, physiological activity monitors,

Table 1 Review of recent literature

Author	Methodology	ML model	Data type	Dataset size	Evaluation matric	Limitation	Year
Carette [53]	An automated technique using on LSTM neural nets that focuses on the saccade portion of eye during reading	LSTM	Eye trackng	ASD 17, Non 15	Accuracy 83%	Exclusion of comparison with other NN	2017
Carette [55]	Using color gradients, cohesively represent eye motions into an image-based manner while preserving the dynamic features of eye movement	RF, SVM, LR, NB, ANN	Eye trackng	ASD 29, Non 30	AUC 90%	NA	2019
Elbattah [54]	A eye tracking scanpath method for ASD classification using K-mean clustering algorithm, and find maximum accuracy with the k value set at four,	Grayscale, PCA, t-SNE, Autoen-coder Features, K-Means Clustering	Eye trackng	ASD 29, Non 30	Accuracy 94%	NA	2019
Tao [56]	Eye scan path by saliency mapping from CNN generator and discriminator part with encoder, decoder utilising a CNN-LSTM algorithm for classification	SalGAN, CNN-LSTM	Eye tracking	ASD 14,Non 14	Accuracy 74.22%	NA	2019
Goel [61]	Optimization algorithm GOA for accelerating ML algorithm	GOA, LR, NB, KNN, RF-CART-ID3, BACO	AQ-10, Question-naire	1100	Accuracy of near 100%	Low con-vergence speed for GOA	2020
Thabtah [63] and Peebles	On several ASD datasets, bagging, rule induction, boosting, and decision trees methods were empirically assessed, with RML outperforming the others	RIDOR, None, RIPPER, RML, Bagging, CART, PRISM, C4.5	AQ-10, Q-CHAT, Question-naire	ASD 189, Non ASD 515	F1 Score more than 90%	Not applied to any toddler dataset	2020

(continued)

Table 1 (continued)

Author	Methodology	ML model	Data type	Dataset size	Evaluation matric	Limitation	Year
Kupper [64]	ADOS questionnaire based data, minimizing features into only five attributes, classification using SVM	Recursive feature selection, kohen cappa, SVM	ADOS, Question-naire	ASD 385, Non ASD 288	AUC of 82%	Affect of different ML algorithm in selected feature is known	2020
Levy [65]	Collected separate data for child and adult, applied 17 supervised ML algorithms, 10 features from ADOS and SVM, LDA gained most AUC	LR, Lasso, SVM, ADTree, RF, Ridge, Elastic net, Nearest shrunken centroids, LDA, AdaBoost, Relaxed Lasso	ADOS, Question-naire		AUC of 95%	Impure source and survey of data	2017
Pratama [62]	SVM, RF, ANN applied into AQ-10 dataset with 10 fold cross validation	SVM, RF, ANN	AQ-10, Question-naire	4189 ASD	Sensitivity of 87.89%	Absence of feature selection	2019

tactile sensors, voice prosody and speech detectors, and sleep quality assessment devices were among the sensing technologies studied. The devices' advantages and usefulness in assisting the treatment of various symptoms of people with ASD, as well as their limits, were evaluated. Tang et al. [82] focused on the integration of a realistic multi-sensory environment (including a facial expression detection module through Kinect V2's HD Face API) to assist in 'reading' the emotions of ASD youngsters. They integrated four sorts of 'meters' in their design to collectively sense users' behavioural patterns, and individual and group emotions as detailed below:

1. Individual physiological (bio-sensory) data: pulse rate, sweat (through a set of Microsoft Band 2 to be worn by the target player).
2. Individual behavioural meters: head, hands, and upper-body movements, gestures and motions (through touch and pressure sensors), and face expression (not included in the present system architecture).
3. Sociometers with integrated sensors, low-cost depth sensors, and RGB-B sensors (two sets of Kinect V2).

Notenboom et al. [83] used physiological signals to evaluate autistic people's emotions, and they created recommendations based on the target group's user requirements. Because the target population is sensitive to stimuli and has difficulty adjusting, certain design criteria are important. As possible designs, a smartwatch, a patch, and an infrared camera were considered. The recommendations were developed as a result of the examination of these designs. The smartwatch came out on top, followed by the patch. An infrared camera isn't the best option. The principles can be utilised to create a wearable that measures autistic children's physiological signals. Northrup et al. [84] created a combination of tailored features in a wearable sensor and mobile app that analyses stress reactivity in children with autism in real-time and sends on spot notifications to a caregiver through a mobile portable device. Below are some example apps which have been made available aiming at this vulnerable group.

4.1 Apps and Platforms for Supporting People with Autism

LetMeTalk

The free AAC talker [85] software, which is accessible for both Android and iOS, assists in the creation of intelligible phrases by aligning graphics. This row of photographs may be interpreted as a phrase if the images are linked together in a meaningful way. This program, they believe, is appropriate for autism symptoms, Asperger syndrome, and Autism Spectrum Disorder. AAC stands for aligning images (Augmentative and Alternative Communication). LetMeTalk's picture library includes over 9,000 easy-to-understand photos from ARASAAC (http://arasaac.org). Additionally, the built-in camera may be used to add existing photographs from the device or to capture new ones. Considering ASD patients have a hard time interacting with neurotypicals or other peers in society, this type of software can be huge assistance in expressing their emotions.

Coughdrop

Symbol based AAC [86] is another AAC app. The history of building Coughdrop is quite interesting. Brian Whitmer, a software engineer and entrepreneur, was looking for an effective communication method for his daughter who had been diagnosed with Rett Syndrome when he came up with Coughdrop. He was disappointed by bad design decisions and outdated technology because of his experience in usability, so he teamed with around 30 Speech-Language Pathologists, Occupational Therapists, and IT specialists to create something better. CoughDrop was the outcome. Brian soon met Scot Wahlquist, whose son had autism and was nonverbal, and the two collaborated to improve CoughDrop for people with any communication requirement. They believed that too many suppliers were attempting to "lock in" clients through proprietary solutions and expensive costs, and they sought to change that. As a result, CoughDrop was made open-source and included open-licensed materials such as free symbols and community-generated boards, as well as all of our word sets, which are all provided under a Creative Commons license. This software is accessible on the App Store, Google Play, and Amazon, and it may also be accessed through web browsers and Windows. This software allows you to communicate with friends and family in a personalised way across numerous devices. With a simple interface and enough support and teaching, one may gradually increase one's vocabulary. It operates offline with a cloud backup, making switching devices a breeze if something goes wrong. It's also possible to share boards with others and open-license them for usage by anybody, across classes, and make access management easier. Individuals may plan a successful approach using built-in goal-tracking tools and gain recommendations for how to strengthen communication tactics from community experts. License consumption may be readily tracked and data can be viewed across rooms, buildings, or teams. People may easily travel between classrooms, and access constraints can be simplified.

Applied Behaviour Analysis (ABA)

ABA is a behaviour treatment based on learning and behavioural science. ABA treatment applies what we know about behaviour to real-life settings. The objective is to encourage positive behaviours while reducing detrimental or learning-inhibiting behaviours. Behaviour analysis approaches have been used and researched for decades. They've aided a wide range of learners in gaining new abilities, from living a healthier lifestyle to learning a new language. Therapists have used ABA to assist children with autism and other developmental issues. Many strategies for analysing and modifying behaviour are used in Applied Behaviour Analysis. ABA flashcards and games—emotion [87] is a useful program for applied behaviour analysis (ABA) therapists and other professionals who work with students with autism and similar problems. This software is only accessible in the app store and is completely free. Telehealth mode for distance learning is one of the app's features. Designed specifically for intense instruction sessions, create your own flashcards or use the built-in activities. Use photographs from your gallery or look for pictures and gif animations on the internet. Data collecting and automatic grading Multiple student profiles are supported.

Autism Read and Write

Autism Read and Wright is available through a Google Play store app that is primarily developed to enable ASD children in learning the fundamentals of reading and writing. To get started with the reading lessons, click on 'Start—Reading' lessons and 'Start—Writing' lessons to get started with writing. The reading and writing classes are of varying degrees of difficulty. Change the levels by going to Settings—Reading level or Settings—Writing level.

Social Story Creator Educators

Social story creator educators [88] is an iOS device software that can assist children with Autism to better learn how to deal with various social events, as well as allow them to create tales about various occurrences. Autism is linked to reciprocal behaviours, making it difficult for persons with autism to react appropriately to a circumstance. As a result, this sort of tool can assist people who are unaware of how to handle these circumstances.

Rethink Ed

Rethink Ed [89] is a web-based platform that offers autistic children social-emotional learning, mental health awareness, and special education. It guarantees that autistic children have access to the most effective educators who can provide them with a high-quality education. Rethink Ed offers scalable professional development for students with autism, including video models, high-quality lesson plans, and a curriculum. Communication and social skills are emphasised to help individuals with ASD fully engage in their education.

AsDetect
AsDetect [90] is a screening application for people with ASD. This software is a useful tool for detecting ASD early on. It is straightforward to use; simply sign up for the app, then enter the patient's information and complete an evaluation. After completing these procedures, one may check the results and determine whether or not a person has ASD. They created a demographic questionnaire by administering assessments such as The Bayley Scales of Infant Development (BSID)- Third Edition, The Autism Diagnostic Observation Schedule (ADOS), 2nd Edition, The Autism Diagnostic Interview-Revised (ADI-R), and the Modified Checklist for Autism in Infants and Toddlers (M-CHAT).

Mental Imagery Therapy for Autism
The goal of Mental Imagery Therapy for Autism (MITA) [91] aims to provide language therapy for children with autism. It aims to create unique, digital apps based on proven, evidence-based early-intervention therapies designed specifically for very young children with ASD. These apps have the potential to significantly narrow the gap between the quantity of therapy prescribed and the amount of therapy actually received by children with ASD while also improving care quality. MITA's activities use a systematic way of teaching the skill of responding to many cues. The most distinctive characteristic of these exercises is their ability to deliver instruction outside of the verbal realm, which is critical for children with ASD who are either nonverbal or just marginally spoken. While these youngsters may not be able to follow a spoken command (such as "pick up the red crayon beneath the table"), preliminary findings from the pilot research show that they can obey a command provided visually rather than vocally. MITA helps children develop their creativity and linguistic skills. The visual activities are organised methodically to help your youngster learn to notice many characteristics of an item. MITA begins with easy tasks that educate kids to focus on only one aspect of a situation, such as size or colour. The tasks become increasingly challenging with time, requiring your youngster to focus on two things at once, such as colour and size. After the kid has practised paying attention to two features, the program progresses to puzzles that need the child to pay attention to three features, such as colour, size, and form, and finally to problems that require the child to pay attention to an ever-increasing number of qualities.

The Jade
The Jade [92] Autism app aids in the development of cognitive skills by increasing information and improving development. It can act as a mediator in acquiring skills and abilities such as attention and logical reasoning and assisting in problem-solving, strategic thinking, and decision-making. Activities are categorised into degrees of difficulty within each category. Each phase is only unlocked based on the child's performance, following the natural flow of learning and respecting each child's pace and personality.

5 Challenges and Future Research

The increase of overall ASD cases worldwide has prompted the search for cost-effective ASD evaluation tools. The deployment of rapid and accurate assessment measures based on computationally intelligent techniques, including machine-learning algorithms, have addressed that need. Despite considerable attempts to develop ML-based ASD evaluation tools utilising fMRI, eye tracking, and genetic data, the promising results based on behavioural data necessitate additional investigation. Sustaining correctness, assuring balance data, employing a benchmark dataset, and lowering diagnosis duration are all critical concerns in ASD classification. Despite this, the lack of sufficient dataset size remains a key challenge in CI-inspired detection and support of ASD. Because the symptoms of ASD patients vary and the number of patients who agree to participate in data gathering methods is still low, the amount of data representing each variation of ASD is also very low. Most of the studies are based on data collected from 50 to 300 ASD patients at most, the size of publicly available datasets [50–52, 58–60] are significantly smaller than other healthcare-related datasets. Data augmentation is also common in various approaches to increase data instances. Again most of the datasets are based on questionnaires which may not be adequate to capture the subconscious behaviour and social deficits of ASD patients. Due to the limited amount of data, deep learning techniques have limited implementations and a low success rate in detecting ASD accurately. Again to further reduce time and computational complexity, feature reduction and selection algorithms are also employed. ASD detection has been used with several modalities such as questionnaire, EEG, ECG, MRI, eye tracking, eye scan path, simulation and task completion, facial imaging, Neuroimaging, behaviour analysis, body movement, video and audio analysis, genetics, and more. Though numerous attempts have been made for classification from the modalities mentioned above, most of the study consists of classification from only one or two modalities. Again due to the scarcity of data, only shallow ML and DL models have been utilised in most studies. Even though numerous wearable devices can detect and monitor various physiological changes, some apps can detect ASD and track various features. These aren't complete; instead, they serve as a supplement to one another. There is a dire need for a comprehensive platform that can be used to detect, manage, and monitor people with ASD. Mobile and online applications are frequently device-specific, requiring a specific device to function. Robust integration and sharing management systems are also necessary to work with various wearable devices. Although there are some downsides, research in this scope is vast and proper implementation as the product can eliminate most of them.

6 Conclusion

Autism spectrum disorder (ASD) is a complex developmental condition that involves persistent challenges in social interaction, speech and nonverbal communication, and restricted/repetitive behaviours. The effects of ASD and the severity of symptoms are different in each person. And in some cases, some people are not diagnosed until they are adolescents or adults. Complex characteristics and symptoms of developmental and cognitive disorders add complications to classifying in clinical decision-making and deterministic computational methods. Computational intelligence algorithms have been utilised broadly to solve developmental disorders, specifically ASD. In this study, the basis of computational intelligence and its effectiveness in detecting and monitoring ASD has been discussed with recent advancements. Screening result is critical in the research of ASD and, therefore, can be improved to properly and early diagnose the specific criteria of ASD. Early and fast detection with more data-centric approaches can be facilitated by generating large benchmark datasets from multiple modalities. The CI methods can still be improved for performance and reliability to be implemented in real-life scenarios. Management and monitoring applications mostly require proprietary wearable devices, which are yet to be openly available for mass use. Again, most of these applications are at the research stage, limiting their usability for actual consumers. Consumer-grade monitoring devices with open standards to aid ASD patients are also needed. Several such mechanisms were discussed in this study with their accomplishments and limitations. Still, much research is needed to diagnose ASD with better accuracy and develop support systems suitable for the mass population without heavy human interactions.

Acknowledgements MM is supported by the AI-TOP (2020-1-UK01-KA201-079167) and DIVERSASIA (618615-EPP-1-2020-1-UKEPPKA2-CBHEJP) projects funded by the European Commission under the Erasmus+ programme.

References

1. Association AP, et al (2013) Diagnostic and statistical manual of mental disorders (DSM-5®). American Psychiatric Publisher
2. Faras H, Al Ateeqi N, Tidmarsh L (2010) Autism spectrum disorders. Ann Saudi Med 30(4):295–300
3. Dawson G, Rogers S, Munson J, Smith M, Winter J, Greenson J et al (2010) Randomized, controlled trial of an intervention for toddlers with autism: the Early Start Denver model. Pediatrics 125(1):e17-23
4. Cidav Z, Munson J, Estes A, Dawson G, Rogers S, Mandell D (2017) Cost offset associated with Early Start Denver Model for children with autism. J Am Acad Child Adolesc Psychiatry 56(9):777–83
5. Berlin LJ, Brooks-Gunn J, McCarton C, McCormick MC (1998) The effectiveness of early intervention: examining risk factors and pathways to enhanced development. Prev Med 27(2):238–45

6. Organization WH et al (2012) World health statistics: a snapshot of global health. In: World health statistics: a snapshot of global health
7. Hamilton S (2006) Screening for developmental delay: reliable, easy-to-use tools: win-win solutions for children at risk and busy practitioners. J Fam Pract 55(5):415–23
8. Barton ML, Dumont-Mathieu T, Fein D (2012) Screening young children for autism spectrum disorders in primary practice. J Autism Dev Disord 42(6):1165–74
9. Mukherjee SB, Aneja S, Krishnamurthy V, Srinivasan R (2014) Incorporating developmental screening and surveillance of young children in office practice. Indian Pediatr 51(8):627–35
10. Robins DL, Casagrande K, Barton M, Chen CMA, Dumont-Mathieu T, Fein D (2014) Validation of the modified checklist for autism in toddlers, revised with follow-up (M-CHAT-R/F). Pediatrics 133(1):37–45
11. Berument SK, Rutter M, Lord C, Pickles A, Bailey A (1999) Autism screening questionnaire: diagnostic validity. Br J Psychiatry 175(5):444–51
12. Lord C, Risi S, Lambrecht L, Cook EH, Leventhal BL, DiLavore PC et al (2000) The autism diagnostic observation schedule-generic: a standard measure of social and communication deficits associated with the spectrum of autism. J Autism Dev Disord 30(3):205–23
13. Lord C, Rutter M, Le Couteur A (1994) Autism diagnostic interview-revised: a revised version of a diagnostic interview for caregivers of individuals with possible pervasive developmental disorders. J Autism Dev Disord 24(5):659–85
14. Schopler E, Reichler RJ, DeVellis RF, Daly K (1980) Toward objective classification of childhood autism: Childhood Autism Rating Scale (CARS). J Autism Develop Disord
15. Engelbrecht AP (2007) Computational intelligence: an introduction. Wiley
16. Kruse R, Borgelt C, Braune C, Mostaghim S, Steinbrecher M, Klawonn F et al (2011) Computational intelligence. Springer
17. Fabietti M et al (2020) Artifact detection in chronically recorded local field potentials using long-short term memory neural network. In: Proceedings of the AICT 2020 (2020), p 1–6
18. Al Nahian MJ, Ghosh T, et al (2020) Towards artificial intelligence driven emotion aware fall monitoring framework suitable for elderly people with neurological disorder. In: Proceedings of brain information (2020), pp 275–286
19. Fabietti M, Mahmud M, Lotfi A (2021) Anomaly detection in invasively recorded neuronal signals using deep neural network: effect of sampling frequency. In: Proceedings of the AII (2021), pp 79–91
20. Al Nahian MJ et al (2021) Towards an accelerometer-based elderly fall detection system using cross-disciplinary time series features. IEEE Access 9:39413–31
21. Fabietti M, Mahmud M, Lotfi A (2022) Channel-independent recreation of artefactual signals in chronically recorded local field potentials using machine learning. Brain Inform 9(1):1–17
22. Lalotra GS, Kumar V, Bhatt A, Chen T, Mahmud M (2022) iReTADS: an intelligent real-time anomaly detection system for cloud communications using temporal data summarization and neural network. Secur Commun Netw 2022:9149164
23. Mahmud M et al (2018) Applications of deep learning and reinforcement learning to biological data. IEEE Trans Neural Netw Learn Syst 29(6):2063–79
24. Biswas M, Kaiser MS, Mahmud M, Al Mamun S, Hossain MS, Rahman MA (2021) An XAI based autism detection: the context behind the detection. In: Mahmud M, Kaiser MS, Vassanelli S, Dai Q, Zhong N (eds) Proceedings of the brain informatics, LNAI, vol 12960. Springer, pp 448–459
25. Mahmud M, Kaiser MS, McGinnity TM, Hussain A (2021) Deep learning in mining biological data. Cogn Comput 13(1):1–33
26. Deepa B et al (2022) Pattern descriptors orientation and MAP firefly algorithm based brain pathology classification using hybridized machine learning algorithm. IEEE Access 10:3848–63
27. Mammoottil MJ, Kulangara LJ, Cherian AS, Mohandas P, Hasikin K, Mahmud M (2022) Detection of breast cancer from five-view thermal images using convolutional neural networks. J Healthc Eng 2022:4295221

28. Kumar I et al (2022) Dense tissue pattern characterization using deep neural network. Cogn Comput 1–24. [ePub ahead of print]
29. Paul A, et al (2022) Inverted bell-curve-based ensemble of deep learning models for detection of COVID-19 from chest X-rays. Neural Comput Appl 1–15
30. Prakash N et al (2021) Deep transfer learning COVID-19 detection and infection localization with superpixel based segmentation. Sustain Cities Soc 75:103252
31. Ghosh T et al (2021) Artificial intelligence and internet of things in screening and management of autism spectrum disorder. Sustain Cities Soc 74:103189
32. Watkins J, Fabietti M, Mahmud M (2020) Sense: a student performance quantifier using sentiment analysis. In: Proceedings of the IJCNN, pp 1–6
33. Satu M, et al (2020) Towards improved detection of cognitive performance using bidirectional multilayer long-short term memory neural network. In: Proceedings of the brain information, pp 297–306
34. Faria TH et al (2021) Smart city technologies for next generation healthcare. In: Data-driven mining, learning and analytics for secured smart cities, pp 253–274
35. Ghosh T et al (2021) An attention-based mood controlling framework for social media users. In: Proceedings of the brain information, pp 245–256
36. Biswas M, Tania MH, Kaiser MS et al (2021) ACCU3RATE: a mobile health application rating scale based on user reviews. PLoS ONE 16(12):e0258050
37. Nawar A, Toma NT, Al Mamun S et al (2021) Cross-content recommendation between movie and book using machine learning. In: Proceedings of the AICT, pp 1–6
38. Ghosh T et al (2021) A hybrid deep learning model to predict the impact of COVID-19 on mental health form social media big data. Preprints 2021;2021(2021060654)
39. Satu MS et al (2021) TClustVID: a novel machine learning classification model to investigate topics and sentiment in COVID-19 tweets. Knowl-Based Syst 226:107126
40. Al Banna MH et al (2021) Attention-based bi-directional long-short term memory network for earthquake prediction. IEEE Access 9:56589–603
41. Mahmud M, Kaiser MS, McGinnity TM, Hussain A (2021) Deep learning in mining biological data. Cogn Comput 13(1):1–33
42. Hájek P (2013) Metamathematics of fuzzy logic, vol 4. Springer Science & Business Media
43. Bäck T, Fogel DB, Michalewicz Z (1997) Handbook of evolutionary computation. Release 97(1):B1
44. Hosseinzadeh M, Koohpayehzadeh J, Bali AO, Rad FA, Souri A, Mazaherinezhad A et al (2021) A review on diagnostic autism spectrum disorder approaches based on the internet of things and machine learning. J Supercomput 77(3):2590–608
45. Sumi AI, Zohora M, Mahjabeen M, Faria TJ, Mahmud M, Kaiser MS, et al (2018) Fassert: a fuzzy assistive system for children with autism using internet of things. In: Wang S, Yamamoto V, Su J, Yang Y, Jones E, Iasemidis L et al (eds) Brain informatics. LNAI, vol 11309. Springer, pp. 403–412
46. Al Banna MH, Ghosh T, Taher KA, Kaiser MS, Mahmud M (2020) A monitoring system for patients of autism spectrum disorder using artificial intelligence. In: Mahmud M, Vassanelli S, Kaiser MS, Zhong N (eds) Proceedings of the brain informatics. LNAI, vol 12241. Springer, pp 251–262
47. Akter T, Ali MH, Satu MS, Khan MI, Mahmud M (2021) Towards autism subtype detection through identification of discriminatory factors using machine learning. In: Mahmud M, Kaiser MS, Vassanelli S, Dai Q, Zhong N (eds) Brain informatics. LNAI, vol 12960. Springer, pp 401–410
48. Ghosh T, Banna MHA, Rahman MS, Kaiser MS, Mahmud M, Hosen ASMS et al (2021) Artificial intelligence and internet of things in screening and management of autism spectrum disorder. Sustain Urban Areas 74:103189
49. Ahmed S, Hossain M, Nur SB, Shamim Kaiser M, Mahmud M et al (2022) Toward machine learning-based psychological assessment of autism spectrum disorders in school and community. In: Proceedings of trends in electronics and health informatics. Springer, pp 139–149

50. Thabtah FF (2017) Autistic spectrum disorder screening data for children data set. UCI Mach Learn Repos
51. Eraslan S, Yesilada Y, Yaneva V, Harper S (2020) Autism detection based on eye movement sequences on the web: a scanpath trend analysis approach. Zenodo. https://doi.org/10.5281/zenodo.3668740
52. Carette R, Elbattah M, Dequen G, Guérin JL, Cilia F (2018) Visualization of eye-tracking patterns in autism spectrum disorder: method and dataset. In: 2018 thirteenth international conference on digital information management (ICDIM). IEEE, pp 248–253
53. Carette R, Cilia F, Dequen G, Bosche J, Guerin JL, Vandromme L (2017) Automatic autism spectrum disorder detection thanks to eye-tracking and neural network-based approach. In: International conference on IoT technologies for healthcare. Springer, pp 75–81
54. Elbattah M, Carette R, Dequen G, Guérin JL, Cilia F, Learning clusters in autism spectrum disorder: image-based clustering of eye-tracking scanpaths with deep autoencoder. In: (2019) 41st annual international conference of the IEEE engineering in medicine and biology society (EMBC). IEEE, pp 1417–1420
55. Carette R, Elbattah M, Cilia F, Dequen G, Guérin JL, Bosche J (2019) Learning to predict autism spectrum disorder based on the visual patterns of eye-tracking scanpaths. In: HEALTHINF, pp 103–112
56. Tao Y, Shyu ML (2019) SP-ASDNet: CNN-LSTM based ASD classification model using observer scanpaths. In: (2019) IEEE international conference on multimedia and expo workshops (ICMEW). IEEE, pp 641–646
57. Chita-Tegmark M (2016) Social attention in ASD: a review and meta-analysis of eye-tracking studies. Res Dev Disabil 48:79–93
58. Thabtah F (2017) Autism spectrum disorder screening: machine learning adaptation and DSM-5 fulfillment. In: Proceedings of the 1st international conference on medical and health informatics 2017, pp 1–6
59. Duan H, Zhai G, Min X, Che Z, Fang Y, Yang X et al (2019) A dataset of eye movements for the children with autism spectrum disorder. Zenodo. https://doi.org/10.5281/zenodo.2647418
60. Zunino A, Morerio P, Cavallo A, Ansuini C, Podda J, Battaglia F et al (2018) Video gesture analysis for autism spectrum disorder detection. In: International conference on pattern recognition (ICPR)
61. Goel N, Grover B, Gupta D, Khanna A, Sharma M et al (2020) Modified grasshopper optimization algorithm for detection of autism spectrum disorder. Phys Commun 41:101115
62. Pratama TG, Hartanto R, Setiawan NA (2019) Machine learning algorithm for improving performance on 3 AQ-screening classification. Commun Sci Technol 4(2):44–9
63. Thabtah F, Peebles D (2020) A new machine learning model based on induction of rules for autism detection. Health Inform J 26(1):264–86
64. Küpper C, Stroth S, Wolff N, Hauck F, Kliewer N, Schad-Hansjosten T et al (2020) Identifying predictive features of autism spectrum disorders in a clinical sample of adolescents and adults using machine learning. Sci Rep 10(1):1–11
65. Levy S, Duda M, Haber N, Wall DP (2017) Sparsifying machine learning models identify stable subsets of predictive features for behavioral detection of autism. Molecul Autism 8(1):1–17
66. Oh SL, Jahmunah V, Arunkumar N, Abdulhay EW, Gururajan R, Adib N et al (2021) A novel automated autism spectrum disorder detection system. Complex Intell Syst 7(5):2399–413
67. Baygin M, Dogan S, Tuncer T, Barua PD, Faust O, Arunkumar N et al (2021) Automated ASD detection using hybrid deep lightweight features extracted from EEG signals. Comput Biol Med 134:104548
68. Khodatars M, Shoeibi A, Sadeghi D, Ghaasemi N, Jafari M, Moridian P et al (2021) Deep learning for neuroimaging-based diagnosis and rehabilitation of autism spectrum disorder: a review. Comput Biol Med 139:104949
69. Parvathi M et al (2021) Early detection support mechanism in ASD using ML classifier. Turkish J Comput Math Educ (TURCOMAT) 12(10):4543–9

70. Jagota V, Bhatia V, Vives L, Prasad AB (2021) ML-PASD: predict autism spectrum disorder by machine learning approach. In: Artificial intelligence for accurate analysis and detection of autism spectrum disorder. IGI Global, pp 82–93

71. Mishra M, Pati UC (2021) Autism detection using surface and volumetric morphometric feature of sMRI with Machine learning approach. In: International conference on advanced network technologies and intelligent computing. Springer, pp 625–33

72. Raj S, Masood S (2020) Analysis and detection of autism spectrum disorder using machine learning techniques. Proc Comput Sci 167:994–1004

73. Thabtah F, Peebles D (2020) A new machine learning model based on induction of rules for autism detection. Health Inform J 26(1):264–86

74. Omar KS, Mondal P, Khan NS, Rizvi MRK, Islam MN (2019) A machine learning approach to predict autism spectrum disorder. In: 2019 international conference on electrical, computer and communication engineering (ECCE). IEEE, pp 1–6

75. Hossain MD, Kabir MA, Anwar A, Islam MZ (2021) Detecting autism spectrum disorder using machine learning techniques. Health Inform Sci Syst 9(1):1–13

76. Zheng ZK, Staubitz JE, Weitlauf AS, Staubitz J, Pollack M, Shibley L et al (2021) A predictive multimodal framework to alert caregivers of problem behaviors for children with ASD (PreMAC). Sensors 21(2):370

77. Van Steensel FJ, Bögels SM, Perrin S (2011) Anxiety disorders in children and adolescents with autistic spectrum disorders: a meta-analysis. Clin Child Fam Psychol Rev 14(3):302–17

78. Jansen L, Gispen-de Wied CC, Wiegant VM, Westenberg HG, Lahuis BE, Van Engeland H (2006) Autonomic and neuroendocrine responses to a psychosocial stressor in adults with autistic spectrum disorder. J Autism Dev Disord 36(7):891–9

79. Vinkers CH, Penning R, Hellhammer J, Verster JC, Klaessens JH, Olivier B et al (2013) The effect of stress on core and peripheral body temperature in humans. Stress 16(5):520–30

80. Viqueira Villarejo M, García Zapirain B. Méndez Zorrilla A (2012) A stress sensor based on galvanic skin response (GSR) controlled by ZigBee. Sensors (Basel) 12(5):6075–6101

81. Cabibihan JJ, Javed H, Aldosari M, Frazier TW, Elbashir H (2016) Sensing technologies for autism spectrum disorder screening and intervention. Sensors 17(1):46

82. Tang TY (2016) Helping neuro-typical individuals to "Read" the emotion of children with autism spectrum disorder: an internet-of-things approach. In: Proceedings of the the 15th international conference on interaction design and children, pp 666–671

83. Notenboom T (2017) Using technology to recognise emotions in autistic people [B.S. thesis]. University of Twente

84. Northrup CM, Lantz J, Hamlin T (2016) Wearable stress sensors for children with autism spectrum disorder with in situ alerts to caregivers via a mobile phone. Iproceedings 2(1):e6119

85. (haftungsbeschraenkt) AU. LetMeTalk (2014). https://apps.apple.com/us/app/letmetalk/id919990138

86. Coughdrop. https://www.coughdrop.com/

87. Nival. ABA cards (2020). https://apps.apple.com/us/app/aba-cards/id1507765578

88. Autism T (2015) Social story creator educators. https://apps.apple.com/us/app/social-story-creator-educators/id998334331

89. Rethink ed. https://www.rethinked.com/edu/

90. Mozolic-Staunton B, Donelly M, Yoxall J, Barbaro J (2020) Early detection for better outcomes: universal developmental surveillance for autism across health and early childhood education settings. Res Autism Spectrum Disord 71:101496

91. Language therapy for children with autism (mita) - apps on Google Play. Google. https://play.google.com/store/apps/details?id=com.imagiration.mita

92. Jade - apps on Google Play. Google. https://play.google.com/store/apps/details?id=com.jadeautism.jadeautism&hl=en&gl=US

AI for COVID-19

A Case Study of Using Machine Learning Techniques for COVID-19 Diagnosis

Marco Dinacci, Tianhua Chen, Mufti Mahmud, and Simon Parkinson

Abstract The Coronavirus disease (COVID-19) is a worldwide pandemic that has lead to millions of death and is affecting every corner of the society. The industrial and scientific communities are continuously working to curb the spread of the pandemic, with efforts in numerous areas including disease detection and diagnosis, virology, vaccine and drug development. As a powerful technique, Artificial Intelligence (AI) and machine learning techniques have been widely incorporated in COVID-19 related research and development. With the aim to establish a use case of machine learning techniques for COVID-19 diagnosis, this paper applies the XGBoost machine learning technique, while examining a number of hyperparameters and data preprocessing techniques, to identify an accurate predictive model, followed by the use of Shapley value to study predictors that are most informative of the diagnosis. Evaluated on a collection of anonymised patients data collected out of the standard Reverse Transcriptase Polymerase Chain Reaction (RT-PCR) and additional laboratory test results, the best model obtained demonstrates high diagnostic performance.

1 Introduction

Coronavirus disease (COVID-19) is an infectious disease caused by the SARS-CoV-2 virus. As of 27 January 2022, the World Health Organisation has reported over 356 million confirmed cases and 5.6 million deaths across the globe [24]. The associated restrictions as a result of the rising incidence also result in from school closures, devastated industries and millions of jobs lost, to worsen public mental welling and undermined progress on global poverty and clean energy [3, 10, 15]. Even with the

M. Dinacci · T. Chen (✉) · S. Parkinson
Department of Computer Science, School of Computing and Engineering, University of Huddersfield, Huddersfield, UK
e-mail: T.Chen@hud.ac.uk

M. Mahmud
Department of Computer Science, Nottingham Trent University, Nottingham, UK

© The Author(s), under exclusive license to Springer Nature Singapore Pte Ltd. 2022
T. Chen et al. (eds.), *Artificial Intelligence in Healthcare*, Brain Informatics and Health,
https://doi.org/10.1007/978-981-19-5272-2_10

advent of vaccines and the gradual ending of lockdowns, the social, economic and cultural effects of the pandemic will cast a long shadow into the future.

The development of Artificial Intelligence (AI) techniques have been accelerated as a result of recent advances in machine learning and data analytics [9], which has led to numerous successful applications in various domains including the healthcare [7, 12, 19, 20]. In the context of the COVID-19, AI has been widely used in disease detection and diagnosis, virology and pathogenesis, drug and vaccine development, and epidemic and transmission prediction [6].

In particular, the diagnosis of virus infection is a significant part of COVID-19 research and practice. The current detection methods used for COVID-19 disease mainly include nucleic acid testing, serological diagnosis, chest X-ray and CT image inspection [6]. Bearing high sensitivity and specificity, the real-time Reverse Transcriptase Polymerase Chain Reaction (RT-PCR) is the current standard detection technology in diagnosing the COVID-19 virus. Isothermal nucleic acid amplification and blood testing methods are also commonly used for rapid screening of SARS-CoV-2. Medical imaging inspection is another widely used clinical approach for COVID-19 detection and diagnosis, which generally includes chest X-ray and lung CT imaging.

The existing testing and detection methods in medical practice also underpin recent research of utilising AI and machine learning techniques to develop more robust and accurate computer-assisted techniques as a complementary solution to medical analysis [18, 21]. While results such as blood test, CT and X-ray scans, respiratory sound and RT-PCR have been extensively applied, researchers have also experimented diagnosing with only a questionnaire survey and without any physiological analysis [25]. Despite numerous efforts in the wide AI scientific community, a recent study [18] suggested overly optimistic performance based on observations of methodological pitfalls and biases out of the analysis of a large number of papers.

In working towards demonstrating a use case of machine learning techniques for the diagnosis of COVID-19, this paper aims to establish an effective model for its automatic diagnosis. Utilising the XGBoost, a powerful machine learning technique, this paper examines a number of model hyperparameters and data preprocessing techniques, followed by the use of Shapley value to identify predictors that are most informative of the diagnosis. With application to a collection of anonymised patients data of the SARS-CoV-2 RT-PCR and additional laboratory test, the best model obtained demonstrates high diagnostic performance and point out factors that might worth further clinical attention.

The remainder of this chapter is structured as follows. Section II reviews the related work of machine learning for COVID-19 diagnosis in recent literature. Section III presents the experimental settings, results and discussions. Section IV concludes the chapter and points out potential future works.

2 Literature Review

Depending on the use of source materials used for diagnosis, this section therefore reviews popular machine learning methods applied to COVID-19 predictions, which can generally include the use of medical imaging, blood tests, and respiratory sound.

For research based on medical imaging, two most common imaging techniques are chest X-Rays and chest Computed Tomography (CT). In [16] a deep learning network based on the popular ResNet50 architecture was used to predict COVID-19. The model produces features from a series of CT slices and combines them into a max-pooling operation, which is then fed to a fully connected layer and a softmax activation function to obtain a probability score for each diagnostic category, i.e., COVID-19, Community Acquired Pneumonia (CAP), non-pneumonia. Evaluated on an independent testing set made of 10% of the original image files, the model is able to achieve the area under the curve of the receiver operating characteristics (AUROC) of 0.96 from a dataset consisting of 4356 chest CT examinations of 3322 patients. It is however worth noting that limitations of research include that patients affected by COVID-19 might show similar imaging characteristics as pneumonia caused by different viruses, where CAP was the only type of pneumonia used as comparison. The second limitation is the difficulty in interpreting the results produced by the neural network, which is a common issue to most deep learning methods, though it may be significant in this area where predictions may have an direct impact on human life.

On the other hand, due to being cheap and widespread, there is a lot of interest in the clinical community in using Chest X-rays (CXR) to discriminate COVID-19. In [22], an empirical evaluation is conducted for the evaluation of pre-training and transfer learning of standard CNN models including ResNET, COVID-Net, DenseNet) through six datasets among which COVID Radiographic imaged Data-set for AI (CORDA), created out of 386 patients that were screened for COVID-19. Whist promising, the study concluded that the CXR data needed to determine whether CNNs can be effectively used as an aid in the fight against COVID-19 pandemic, need to be scaled up by a factor of two, or more. This is also consistent with findings from a recent survey that concludes being short of large-scale data sets is the main challenge that hinders the implementation of AI-based imaging inspection [6].

Apart from medical imaging, the diagnosis of COVID-19 may be significantly facilitated with routine blood tests, which are able to provide numerous important indicators that may correlate with patients of COVID-19 [1]. For instance, [2] has opted for an interpretable model based on decision trees in order to obtain more insights and concluded that parameters such as white blood cells (WBC), C-reactive protein (CRP), neutrophils (NEU), lymphocytes (LYM), monocytes (MONO), eosinophils (EOS), basophils (BAY), aspartate and alanine aminotransferase (AST and ALT, respectively), lactate dehydrogenase (LDH) and others have shown high correlations in patients diagnosed with COVID-19. A similar study by [4] identified prognostic serum biomarkers in patients at greatest risk of mortality from COVID-19, where a model was developed to predict whether a patient would expire within 48 hours. Despite achieving 91% sensitivity and 91 % specificity on a held-out testing dataset with support vector machine (SVM), Shapley additive explanations (SHAP) was further implemented in order to be able to capture the contribution of each feature to the model's output, though the results may be limited by a unbalanced sample with a relative minority of positive mortalities from a single institution of source.

There are alternative uses of machine learning for COVID-19 diagnosis. For instance respiratory sounds have been collected aiming to diagnose COVID-19 using audio such as breath and cough of a potential patient. In a recent study [13], where the data is crowd-sourced by allowing individuals to download a phone app that enables to record a small audio of a user breathing and coughing, a CNN model was then trained over 355 patients to detect symptomatic and asymptomatic COVID-19 cases through these recordings, with a AUROC performance of 0.846. Such innovation is able to address a significant issue of small data sample, though the senior participants may be under-represented due to their less familiarity with the app.

Despite massive efforts have been spent to develop ML models to help fight against COVID-19, [18] concludes that all papers analyzed have methodological pitfalls and biases, leading to overly optimistic performance. The main issues identified are reproducibility, following of best practices, and the lack of external validation. Models performance is generally biased due to small sample sizes, due to the sensitivity nature of clinical data for which there isn't yet a sufficiently large repository of international COVID-19 data that can be used to train more complicated deep models. In addition to the lack of data, another limitation of numerous existing studies rarely provided details on how the AI model predictions were interpreted and tracked, which would have provided more insights to facilitate the understanding and further the treatment and prevention of the disease.

3 Experimentation and Discussion

The following investigative experimentation aims to examine the performance of machine learning for the COVID-19 diagnosis, with application to a open source data set that contains anonymised patients data from the Hospital Israelita Albert Einstein, at São Paulo, Brazil. The samples were collected to perform the SARS-CoV-2 RT-PCR and additional laboratory tests during a visit to the emergency room.

A high-level view of the steps taken during the experiment is illustrated in Fig. 1. The loops in the diagram are meant to explain that hill-climbing was done by a combination of different data sampling approaches and hyper-parameters configurations.

Fig. 1 Experiment flowchart

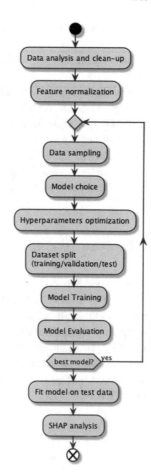

3.1 Data Preprocessing

The dataset is made of 111 features and 5644 entries. The vast majority of features are derived from standard blood tests, such as number of red blood cells, platelets, leukocytes, lymphocites, hematocrytes, but also the presence of other viruses such as Influenza A and B, Rhinovirus, including coronaviruses such as Coronavirus229E and CoronavirusOC43. About 15% of the features, such as number of urobilinogen, ketone bodies, esterase, and others, are obtained from urine samples.

In terms of missing values, approximately 25% of the attributes have less than 1% of values. Some attributes have a large percentage of invalid values (up to 100%), so we removed any column where most values were encoded as "Not a Number" (NaN).

Some columns that weren't relevant to the task were therefore removed. These are `'Patient admitted to regular ward'`, `'Patient admitted to semi-intensive unit'` and `'Patient admitted to intensive care unit'`.

Before using the dataset for training, all the values in Portuguese were converted English, such as "Ausentes" which was translated to "absent". The translation was done using Google Translate. Some of the Boolean features were represented with a mix of strings such as "true" or "false" and some with 0s and 1s. We converted these features to use a native Boolean representation. String and object based features have been encoded as integers, which helps normalize labels so that they contain only values between 0 and n_classes-1.

3.2 Data Sampling

As shown in Fig. 2, the dataset is highly imbalanced since most of the patients resulted negative to COVID-19 after the tests. It contains 5086 negative use cases and 558 positive ones. To achieve reliable results, the dataset was re-balance through sampling, including the random oversampling from the minority class and random undersampling from the majority one. We then simply removing the rows from the negative use cases which contained multiple null values. In over-sampling, we randomly duplicated examples from the minority class and added them to the training dataset. With under-sampling we did the opposite by randomly removing samples from the majority class.

After balancing the dataset it was split into train (70%), test (15%) and validation (15%) datasets. The validation set was used to evaluate the model hyperparameters, the test set was used to evaluate the predictive power of the model against data it hadn't seen before (Table 1).

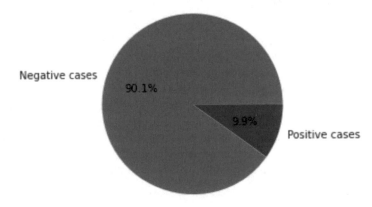

Fig. 2 Negative versus positive cases

Table 1 Sampling experiments

Sampling technique	Area under curve	F1 score
Random oversampling	0.6695	0.73
Random undersampling	0.5431	0.55
Nulls removal (threshold = 10)	0.8865	0.85
Nulls removal (threshold = 20)	0.9541	0.95
Nulls removal (threshold = 23)	0.9533	0.96
Nulls removal (threshold = 30)	0.9522	0.95

3.3 Model Selection

The prediction model was developed using XGBoost that belongs to the family of gradient boosting algorithms [8], for its being a very efficient and flexible distributed method that has found numerous successful application [23]. The XGBoost can be used for both regression and classification and produce a model composed of an ensemble of decision trees.

XGBoost is particularly effective at dealing with imbalanced datasets since it does not make any assumptions on the data distribution nor about the relationships among features, and can be configured using the `scale_pos_weight` hyperparameter to scale the gradient's weights for the positive (minority) class during training. Changing the scale of the weights between positive (minority) and negative (majority) classes has the effect to over-correct the errors made by the model on the positive class, ultimately resulting in a better model.

The prediction scores of each individual tree are summed up to get the final score, in the form:

$$\hat{y}_i = \sum_{k=1}^{K} f_k(x_i), \ f_k \in \mathcal{F} \tag{1}$$

where K is the number of trees, f is a function in the functional space of F, which is the set of all possible CARTs (classification and regression trees). In XGBoost, the objective function is:

$$\text{obj} = \sum_{i=1}^{n} l(y_i, \hat{y}_i^{(t)}) + \sum_{i=1}^{t} \Omega(f_i) \tag{2}$$

where the first operand is the training loss function and the second the regularization one which helps the model to avoid overfitting.

Tree boosting is fundamentally similar to Random Forests as both techniques use tree ensembles as their models. A Random Forests classifier could have also been a possible choice, but according to Chen [5], there is a high probability that a bootstrap sample (the data points from the training data from which a decision tree is fitted) contains few or even none of the minority class, resulting in a tree with poor performance for predicting the minority class. This isn't a good choice since the minority class is represented by the positive COVID-19 cases which is the main class to predict.

3.4 Hyperparameters Optimization

The XGBoost can be configured with a large number of hyperparameters. In order to find a good combination, we used a grid search with cross validation, which enables to evaluates all possible combinations of the given parameter values.

The grid search was customised with five parameters. We used a range of values for the number of estimators (the decision trees), the maximum tree depth (6, 7 and 9) and sub-samples ratio, which is used to train the classifier at each interaction on a sub-sample of the training data. This technique combines gradient boosting with bootstrap averaging (bagging) and is described in [14]. The summary of grid search hyperparameters is presented in Table 2. This is integrated with a k-fold (k = 10 in our case) cross-validation to split the data into multiple groups to reduce bias and variance.

3.5 Evaluation

To evaluate the model we considered both precision and recall, but considering a false negative mistake that incorrectly miss diagnose a positive case, the metric of recall is potentially more significant than precision, as it can be more affordable to take more tests to find out whether one is actually positive than missing any positive case which could potentially put more people under risk.

On the other hand, patients who were incorrectly classified as having COVID-19 might have a different illness (in [16] the authors have highlighted the ambiguity between predictions of COVID-19 and various types of different pneumonias), so we can't simply discard precision.

Table 2 Summary of grid search hyperparameters

Hyperparameter	Range of values	Best value
Estimators count	[100, 300, 500, 700]	100
Sub-sample ratios	[0.5, 0.7, 1.0]	0.5
Max tree depth	[6, 7, 9]	9
Cross-validation	10-fold	N/A
Metric	ROC AUC score	N/A

Table 3 Results from best model

Model	Precision	Recall	F1 score	ROCAUC
XGBoost	96.15%	94.94%	96.00%	95.33%

A good trade-off between recall and precision is the F1 score, which is the harmonic mean of recall and precision, i.e.

$$F_1 = \frac{\text{Precision} \times \text{Recall}}{\text{Precision} + \text{Recall}}$$

In order to understand how well the model can separate the two classes, we also computed the *Area Under the Receiver Operating Characteristic Curve* (ROC AUC) from the prediction scores in order to determine whether the model can rank a random positive case of COVID-19 higher than a random negative case.

We experimented with different thresholds and removing columns which contained at least 23 null values produced the model with the best ROCAUC and F1 score, as reported in Table 1.

The best results are presented in Table 3, which is able to high F1 score, with close capacity in both precision and recall. To better visualize how the model can separate the two classes, the ROC probabilistic curve is depicted in Fig. 3, which far outperform the random guess of the diagonal line.

Fig. 3 ROC curve

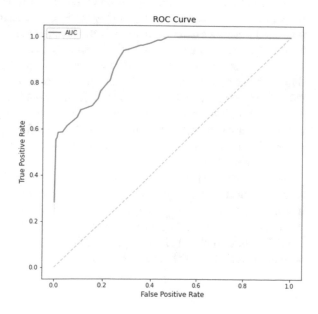

Fig. 4 Confusion matrix

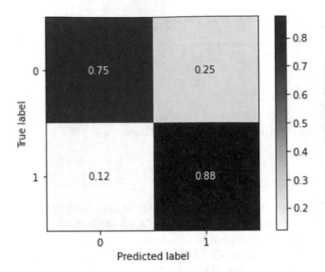

In general, the results are very encouraging as we have obtained an F1 score of 0.96 score and 95.33% on AUC measured on a held out test set composed of 15% of the original data. The imbalance in the dataset was addressed by removing the rows from the negative use cases which contained multiple null values. This simple approach was more effective than oversampling from the minority class and undersampling from the majority class.

To visually assess the quality of the classifier we plotted a confusion matrix and inspected the results. As we can see in Fig. 4 the model performed well, but incorrectly predicted a negative outcome instead of the positive outcome 22 times, and predicted 53 times a positive outcome instead of a negative one.

Furthermore, in order to identify the subset of predictors that are more informative and contributes more towards the decision, the **SH**apley **A**dditive ex**P**lanations (SHAP) value [17] is utilised which is a concept used in game theory to represent the average of all the marginal contributions to all possible coalitions (features in this case). It enables to explain the prediction of a classifier by computing the `Shapley` value of each feature in order to determine how much a feature contribute to the classifier prediction.

The top 20 most important features are plotted in Fig. 5. The most important features identified are the patient age quantile and a high count of white cells (leukocytes, eosinophils, monocytes, lymphocytes), which is clearly a sign that a patient's body is reacting to a pathogen. This is in line with some of the results we discovered in the literature such as [2] where positive COVID-19 cases were strongly correlated with an increased white blood cells count.

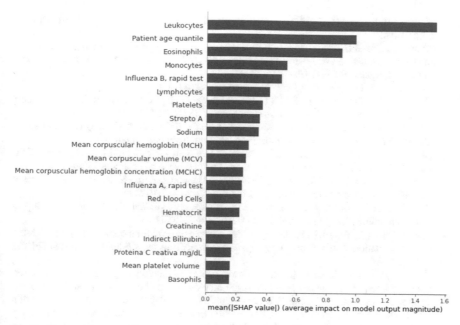

Fig. 5 20 most important features

4 Conclusion

COVID19 is an unprecedented global pandemic against which various strands of research and practice have been invested to fight. In line with recent trends of employing machine learning techniques to facilitate its diagnosis, this paper has engineered a predictive model through data sampling and the hyperparameters that achieves promising diagnostic accuracy on anonymised results of over 5600 entries. Whilst promising, additional improvements could be provided by experimenting with alternative sampling techniques, and to explore advanced interpolation techniques [11] in response to the existence of numerous missing values.

References

1. Alves MA, Castro GZ, Oliveira BAS, Ferreira LA, Ramírez JA, Silva R, Guimarães FG (2021) Explaining machine learning based diagnosis of covid-19 from routine blood tests with decision trees and criteria graphs. Comput Biol Med 132:104335
2. Alves MA, Castro GZ, Oliveira BAS, Ferreira LA, Ramírez JA, Silva R, Guimarães FG (2021) Explaining machine learning based diagnosis of covid-19 from routine blood tests with decision trees and criteria graphs. Comput Biol Med 132:104335. Accessed from https://www.sciencedirect.com/science/article/pii/S0010482521001293. https://doi.org/10.1016/j.compbiomed.2021.104335

3. Barbier EB, Burgess JC (2020) Sustainability and development after covid-19. World Develop 135:105082
4. Booth AL, Abels E, McCaffrey P (2021). Development of a prognostic model for mortality in covid-19 infection using machine learning. Modern Pathol 34(3):522–531. Accessed from https://doi.org/10.1038/s41379-020-00700-x
5. Chen C (2004) Using random forest to learn imbalanced data
6. Chen J, Li K, Zhang Z, Li K, Yu PS (2021) A survey on applications of artificial intelligence in fighting against covid-19. ACM Comput Surv (CSUR) 54(8):1–32
7. Chen T, Antoniou G, Adamou M, Tachmazidis I, Su P (2021) Automatic diagnosis of attention deficit hyperactivity disorder using machine learning. Appl Artif Intell 1–13
8. Chen T, Guestrin C (2016) Xgboost: a scalable tree boosting system. In: Proceedings of the 22nd ACM SIGKDD international conference on knowledge discovery and data mining
9. Chen T, Keravnou-Papailiou E, Antoniou G (2021) Medical analytics for healthcare intelligence - recent advances and future directions. Artif Intell Med 112:102009
10. Chen T, Lucock M (2022) The mental health of university students during the covid-19 pandemic: an online survey in the UK. Plos One 17(1):e0262562
11. Chen T, Shang C, Yang J, Li F, Shen Q (2020) A new approach for transformation-based fuzzy rule interpolation. IEEE Trans Fuzzy Syst. Accessed from https://doi.org/10.1109/TFUZZ.2019.2949767
12. Chen T, Su P, Shen Y, Chen L, Mahmud M, Zhao Y, Antoniou G (2022) A dominant set-informed interpretable fuzzy system for automated diagnosis of dementia. Front Neurosci
13. Coppock H, Gaskell A, Tzirakis P, Baird A, Jones L, Schuller B (2021) End-to-end convolutional neural network enables covid-19 detection from breath and cough audio: a pilot study. BMJ Innov 7(2):356–362. Accessed from https://innovations.bmj.com/content/7/2/356. http://orcid.org/10.1136/bmjinnov-2021-000668
14. Friedman J (2002) Stochastic gradient boosting. Comput Stat Data Anal 38:367–378
15. Kaiser MS, Mahmud M, Noor MBT, Zenia NZ, Al Mamun S, Mahmud KA et al (2021) iworksafe: towards healthy workplaces during covid-19 with an intelligent phealth app for industrial settings. IEEE Access 9:13814–13828
16. Li L, Qin L, Xu Z, Yin Y, Wang X, Kong B, Xia J (2020) Using artificial intelligence to detect covid-19 and community-acquired pneumonia based on pulmonary ct: evaluation of the diagnostic accuracy. Radiology 296(2):E65–E71. Accessed from https://europepmc.org/articles/PMC7233473. https://doi.org/10.1148/radiol.2020200905
17. Lundberg SM, Lee S-I (2017) A unified approach to interpreting model predictions. In: Guyon I et al (eds) Advances in neural information processing systems, vol 30, pp 4765–4774. Curran Associates, Inc. Accessed from http://papers.nips.cc/paper/7062-a-unified-approach-to-interpreting-model-predictions.pdf
18. Roberts M, Driggs D, Thorpe M, Gilbey J, Yeung M, Ursprung S, AIX-COVNET (2021) Common pitfalls and recommendations for using machine learning to detect and prognosticate for covid-19 using chest radiographs and ct scans. Nat Mach Intell 3(3):199–217. Accessed from https://doi.org/10.1038/s42256-021-00307-0
19. Stirling J, Chen T, Bucholc M (2020) Diagnosing alzheimer's disease using a self-organising fuzzy classifier. In: Fuzzy logic recent applications and developments. Springer
20. Su P, Chen T, Xie J, Zheng Y, Qi H, Borroni D, Liu J (2020). Corneal nerve tortuosity grading via ordered weighted averaging-based feature extraction. Med Phys
21. Syeda HB, Syed M, Sexton KW, Syed S, Begum S, Syed F, Yu Jr F (2021) Role of machine learning techniques to tackle the covid19 crisis: systematic review. JMIR Med Inform 9(1):e23811. Accessed from http://medinform.jmir.org/2021/1/e23811/
22. Tartaglione E, Barbano C. A, Berzovini C, Calandri M, Grangetto M (2020) Unveiling covid-19 from chest x-ray with deep learning: a hurdles race with small data. Int J Environ Res Public Health 17(18). Accessed from https://www.mdpi.com/1660-4601/17/18/6933
23. Wang J, Yue-Xin L, Chun-Ying W (2019) Survey of recommendation based on collaborative filtering. J Phys: Conf Ser 1314

24. World Health Organisation (2022) Coronavirus disease (COVID-19) pandemic. https://www.who.int/emergencies/diseases/novel-coronavirus-2019
25. Zoabi Y, Deri-Rozov S, Shomron N (2021) Machine learning-based prediction of covid-19 diagnosis based on symptoms. npj Digit Med 4(1):3. Accessed from https://doi.org/10.1038/s41746-020-00372-6

A Fuzzy Logic Approach to a Hybrid Lexicon-Based Sentiment Analysis Detection Tool Using Healthcare Covid-19 News Articles

Jarrad Neil Morden, Arjab Singh Khuman⊕, Adebamigbe Fasanmade, and Musa Muhammad

Abstract The delivery of unbiased news articles in the healthcare sector is one of the prominent problems in the fight against unvaccinated individuals as Covid-19 causes great skepticism among many groups of people. Companies such as Facebook have already integrated AI models for context to content that is rated by third-party fact-checkers to detect misinformation ("Fonctionnement du programme de vérification tierce de Facebook," Fonctionnement du programme de vérification tierce de Facebook. https://www.facebook.com/journalismproject/programs/third-party-fact-checking/how-it-works?locale = fr_FR (accessed Sep. 06, 2021)). In this paper we use Natural Language Processing (NLP) and Sentiment Analysis to derive the content of news articles, an API is integrated to gather news articles from various sources using the newsapi ("News API – Search News and Blog Articles on the Web," News API. https://newsapi.org (accessed Oct. 28, 2021)). Applying VADER, Text Blob, and Flair rule-based lexicons, we create a hybrid approach from the lexicons and combine each method, we then present a novel Fuzzy-Logic Lexicon Mamdani Rule-Base Multi Inference System (FLLMRBMIF) that can generate a final sentiment from each output of polarity, we then classify into a positive, neutral and negative result. The results demonstrate that it is possible to integrate a tool to classify the sources in real-time allowing more insightful information on biased news stories.

Keywords Sentiment analysis · VADER · Text blob · Flair · Fuzzy-logic · Lexicon · Mamdani · Healthcare · Artificial intelligence · False news · Covid-19

J. N. Morden
School of Computer Science and Informatics, De Montfort University, Leicester, UK
e-mail: P2433071@alumni365.dmu.ac.uk

A. S. Khuman (✉)
School of Computer Science and Informatics, Institute of Artificial Intelligence (IAI), Leicester, UK
e-mail: arjab.khuman@dmu.ac.uk

A. Fasanmade · M. Muhammad
School of Computer Science and Informatics, Cyber Technology Institute (CTI), Leicester, UK
e-mail: adebamigbe.fasanmade@dmu.ac.uk

M. Muhammad
e-mail: musa.muhammad@coventry.ac.uk

© The Author(s), under exclusive license to Springer Nature Singapore Pte Ltd. 2022
T. Chen et al. (eds.), *Artificial Intelligence in Healthcare*, Brain Informatics and Health,
https://doi.org/10.1007/978-981-19-5272-2_11

1 Introduction

Over the last two decades, a sizable anti-vaccination movement has developed, resulting in a decrease in herd immunity among the general population. The fact that websites represent a range of concerns regarding vaccine safety and varying degrees of distrust in medicine has been noted before in this context. These kinds of websites rely heavily on emotional appeal to convey their message, and they have previously been recognized as a source of concern for getting reliable information [3]. Previous research has identified several reasons why people in other countries are hesitant to be immunized against COVID-19, including concerns about efficacy and safety, prior exposure to COVID-19, concerns about the vaccine's novelty, religious beliefs, a lack of trust, a dislike for needles, a belief that COVID-19 is not a risk, a preference for natural immunity, and being infected. [4–7]. On the other hand, as a result of the proliferation of viral social media news stories, celebrities have emerged as a major source of information. When the pandemic of COVID-19 started, it precipitated one of the most divisive vaccination projects in modern history. The World Health Organization labeled the COVID-19 issue an "infodemic" as early as February 2020, stressing the need of improving accurate communications and building local confidence in public health institutions in order to fight the pandemic. The critical role of tailored messaging and delivery strategies in increasing vaccination coverage has been shown [8, 9]. Whether local governments make it easy and enjoyable for residents to get vaccinated at local bars, or partner with trusted and community-based organizations on roll-out and messaging campaigns, this report outlines a variety of ways sentiment data can assist local policymakers in assessing and improving their roll-out and messaging strategies to increase resident vaccination rates.

2 What is Sentiment Analysis?

The word sentiment has at least two different meanings in common English. It is often used to refer to (a) an emotion or anything emotionally charged, as well as (b) a particular subjective perspective. Sentiment Analysis commonly referred to as opinion-mining is a collection of methods for identifying opinion, sentiment, and subjectivity in text [3–5]. Sentiment analysis is usually regarded a branch of computational linguistics and, to a lesser degree, computer science, although it is most closely related to computational linguistics. Social science, on the other hand, views sentiment analysis as a discipline, not a method. Information extraction is an aspect of computational and information science that deals with compressing, summarizing, and making inferences from collections of texts [6–8].

Sentiment analysis in a computer sense gained popularity in the early 2000s within computational linguistics [9]. Research on subjectivity in the wider artificial intelligence paradigm goes back to Lotfi Zadeh's 1965 explanation of Fuzzy Logic, which dates to the 1960s [10] He believed that conventional computer logic could not deal with imprecise or ambiguous data. Sentiment analysis's subjectivity was presented for the first time in 1980's [11], It addressed the subject of research differently than current sentiment analysis and performed a little contribution. In the 1950s, computational linguistics concentrated on addressing a range of problems in human language understanding, with machine translation being the main concern. At first, human language was believed to be just a logical problem, and that if one could create a system that could accurately translate a natural language sentence's syntax and understand the natural language proposition's meaning, that system would be able to effectively interpret and paraphrase sentences. Translation attempts before the proliferation of computer power and sufficient data were very difficult. The technique through which major gains were made was by moving away from deductive reasoning and focusing on machine learning, which is the act of leveraging statistical patterns discovered in natural language data.

In this article, lexicon-based sentiment analysis is used. A sentiment lexicon is a collection of lexical characteristics (e.g., words, phrases, etc.) that have been classified as positive or negative according to their semantic orientation (i.e. subjectivity, polarity) [12]. The sentiment analysis method uses one of the lexicons as a comparison to help detect key terms in the text. The unsupervised machine learning does not rely on adequate annotated training material that humans have assigned; thus, it is able to provide acceptable results. To further address this challenge, we have examined approaches that do not need extensive training data or just require a little amount of it. The lexical approach is used most frequently in sentiment analysis. Their collection of words comes preloaded with connections to certain emotions. Lexicon-based methods are very simple and efficient. A simple method is used to assign a polarity to every document using a sentiment lexicon.

3 Consensus Sentiment Analysis of News Articles Using a Fuzzy Inference System

The objective of this study is to develop a model that can analyse the content of news articles from numerous sources around the globe, moreover, to be able to analyse how biased a news article is compared to another. This model would then form the basis of a computer application which an individual or organisation could use in confidence, furthermore, to develop a timely, and strong representation of perceptions on healthcare news articles, rather than focusing on scaremongering media. The objective of this paper is to analyse the sentiment of the given discourse using Fuzzy logic. The identification and characterization of sentiment as positive, negative and neutral are tackled in this paper. The proposed framework can be seen below in Fig. 1.

Each sentiment analysis model uses its own custom rule-base or framework to determine what sentiment tag is given, these tags are; positive, negative or neutral. An output of the final sentiment from each sentiment analysis model is fed into fuzzy

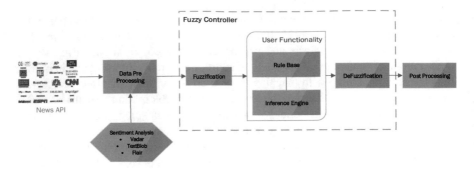

Fig. 1 Proposed framework

opinion model named FLLMRBMIF. Opinion mining system automatically extracts opinionated phrases from POS tagged user reviews and classifies them based on their sentiment. We performed the sentiment analysis on a real-time API that can extract the news articles straight from the source. By combining three 3 sentiment analysis methods and a fuzzy output, the aim to create a new and better model.

The proposed system uses 4 models:

- Vadar Sentiment Analysis
- TextBlob Sentiment Analysis
- Flair Sentiment Analysis
- Fuzzy-Logic Lexicon Mamdani Rule-Base Multi Inference System (FLLM-RBMIS).

4 Data Pre-processing and Sentiment Analysis

Let us assume the inputs are crisp measurements from measuring equipment, rather than linguistic. A pre-processor, conditions the measurements before they enter the controller. Examples of pre-processing are quantization in connection with sampling or rounding to integers; A quantizer converts an inbound measurement to fit it to a discrete universe.

- normalization or scaling onto a particular, standard range;
- filtering in order to remove noise;
- averaging to obtain long-term or short-term tendencies;
- a combination of several measurements to obtain key indicators; and
- differentiation and integration, or their approximations in discrete time.

5 Data Transformation Process

Data gathered from API's require preprocessing to remove noise before the opinion mining process can be performed. These news articles usually contain mistakes in spelling, grammar, use of non-dictionary words such as abbreviations or acronyms of common terms, mistakes in punctuation, incorrect capitalization etc., furthermore, URL cleaning due to special characters need to be removed. These mistakes in the dataset make preprocessing step are essential. In this stage tasks such as spell error correction using a standard word processor, sentence boundary selection and repetitive punctuation conflation is done. Preprocessing steps generate sentences which can be parsed automatically by the linguistic parser. Moreover, each source from the API will use the coronavirus keyword, thus, the only articles featured will be surrounding that topic.

6 Sentiment Analysis Algorithms

This is a pragmatic method to text analysis that does not need training or the use of machine learning models. This technique produces a set of guidelines by which the text is classified as positive/negative/neutral. Additionally, these rules are referred to as lexicons. As a result, the rule-based method is referred to as the Lexicon-based approach. We utilized the Vadar, Text Blob, and Flair lexicons since they are often used for sentiment analysis.

(a) *Vadar*

The Vadar compound score is calculated by adding the valence ratings of each word in the lexicon, adjusting them according to the criteria, and then normalising them to fall between -1 (the most extreme negative) and $+1$ (the most extreme positive) (most extreme positive). This is the most relevant metric if a single unidimensional assessment of a sentence's emotion is required. As outlined below in Fig. 2.

(b) *TextBlob*

TextBlob returns a sentence's polarity and subjectivity. Polarity falls between $[-1, 1]$, where -1 represents a negative sentiment and 1 represents a positive one. Negative expressions invert the polarity. TextBlob has semantic markers that facilitate detailed analysis. For instance, emoticons, the exclamation mark, and emojis. Subjectivity falls between 0 and 1. Subjectivity measures the proportion of personal opinion and factual information in a writing. Greater subjectivity indicates that the content includes more personal opinion than objective facts. Using the same statement aforementioned previously we can see the TextBlob score represented below in Fig. 3.

```
from vaderSentiment.vaderSentiment import SentimentIntensityAnalyzer

def sentiment_scores(sentence):

    sid_obj = SentimentIntensityAnalyzer()
    sentiment_dict = sid_obj.polarity_scores(sentence)

    print("Overall sentiment dictionary is : ", sentiment_dict)
    print("sentence was rated as ", sentiment_dict['neg']*100, "% Negative")
    print("sentence was rated as ", sentiment_dict['neu']*100, "% Neutral")
    print("sentence was rated as ", sentiment_dict['pos']*100, "% Positive")

    print("Sentence Overall Rated As", end = " ")

    # decide sentiment as positive, negative and neutral
    if sentiment_dict['compound'] >= 0.05 :
        print("Positive")

    elif sentiment_dict['compound'] <= - 0.05 :
        print("Negative")

    else :
        print("Neutral")

if __name__ == "__main__" :

    sentence = "This article is considered a positive influence on the vaccination programme"

    # function calling
    sentiment_scores(sentence)
```

```
Overall sentiment dictionary is :  {'neg': 0.0, 'neu': 0.735, 'pos': 0.265, 'compound': 0.5574}
sentence was rated as   0.0 % Negative
sentence was rated as   73.5 % Neutral
sentence was rated as   26.5 % Positive
Sentence Overall Rated As Positive
```

Fig. 2 Vadar sentiment analysis

```
from textblob import TextBlob

def checkscore(compoundscore):
    if compoundscore < 0:
        return "Negative"
    elif compoundscore == 0:
        return "Neutral"
    else:
        return "Positive"

res = TextBlob("This article is considered a positive influence on the vaccination programme")
res1 = float(res.sentiment.polarity)
res2 = float(res.sentiment.subjectivity)
compoundscore = res1 + res2
print(res1, "Polarity")
print(res2, "Subjectivity")
print(compoundscore, "Compound Score")



print("Sentiment is:", checkscore(compoundscore))
```

```
0.22727272727272727 Polarity
0.5454545454545454 Subjectivity
0.7727272727272727 Compound Score
Sentiment is: Positive
```

Fig. 3 TextBlob sentiment analysis

(c) *Flair*

Finally, Flair enables the application of cutting-edge natural language processing (NLP) models to text segments. It operates considerably differently from the preceding models. Flair use a pre-trained algorithm to identify positive or negative remarks and to publish a prediction confidence number in brackets after the

```
from flair.models import TextClassifier
from flair.data import Sentence

classifier = TextClassifier.load('en-sentiment')
sentence = Sentence('This article is considered a positive influence on the vaccination programme')
classifier.predict(sentence)

# print sentence with predicted labels
print('Sentence above is: ', sentence.labels)

2022-06-06 15:45:30,742 loading file C:\Users\          \.flair\models\sentiment-en-mix-distillbert_4.pt
Sentence above is:  ['Sentence: "This article is considered a positive influence on the vaccination programme"'/'POSITIVE' (0.9
954)]
```

Fig. 4 Flair sentiment analysis

label. Flair outputs both the emotion label (positive/negative) and the prediction's polarity (how strongly polarised the statement is, between 0 and 1). See Fig. 4.

7 Fuzzification

The first block inside the FLLMRBMIF controller is *fuzzification interface*, which is a lookup in the membership functions to derive the membership values. The fuzzification block of FLLMRBMIF therefore evaluates the input measurements according to the conjectures of the rules. Each congecture produces a membership grade expressing the degree of fulfilment of the premise.

8 Designing the Fuzzification Interface?

We consider the following important factors and use them to determine the fuzzification interface for the controller.

(1) the specific membership functions—in our case three membership functions are considered
(2) the input universe of discourse for number of fuzzy sets defined—the input universe of discourse is $[-1,1]$.

The Sentiment analysis score is computed with the consensus value that will need to be calculated. The compound score is the sum of positive, negative & neutral scores which is then normalized between -1(most extreme negative) and $+1$ (most extreme positive). The more Compound score closer to $+1$, the higher the positivity of the text. This is the most useful metric if you want a single unidimensional measure of sentiment for a given sentence. An example of the compound score (cs) is computed using the following equation.

$$x = \frac{x}{\sqrt{x^2 + \alpha}} \tag{1}$$

The compound rules (cs) are then set into a multi-classification:

if cs_Vadar is $< 1 = -1$.

if cs_Vadar is $> 1 = 1$.

if cs_Vadar is $= = 1 = 0$.

if cs_TextBlob is $< 1 = -1...$

if cs_Flair is $< 1 = -1...$

Once each compound score is set between -1, 0, and 1, they are weighted by each news source and are given a weight set as a string. We begin to compute this as sum of cs_Vadar + sum of cs_TextBlob + Sum of cs_Flair. Following this formula, it becomes obvious that this range is $[-3, 3]$ which we map to I = { 'EN', VN', 'N', 'Ne, 'P', 'VP', 'EP' }.

The following equations are used to compute the weighted value and normalize $Norm_{I,N}$ the consensus compound score of the news sources to conform to the input universe of discourse.

$[-1, 1]$.

$$W_{N,I} = \sum_N \sum_I Data_{I;N} \tag{2}$$

$$Norm_{I,N} = \frac{W_{N,I}}{Sources_N}, \tag{3}$$

where $Sources_N$ = the number of sources for news source N. Essentially, we can define the fuzzification mapping can be denoted as F:I $\rightarrow$ A.

9 Functionality Block

This section describes the rules base, membership functions and inference engine.

10 Rule-Base

A rule allows for several variables both in the premise and the conclusion. A controller can therefore be multi-input–multi-output (MIMO) or single-input–single-output (SISO). The typical SISO controller regulates a control signal according to an error signal. A controller may apply the *error*, the *change in error*, and the *integral error*, but we will still call it SISO control, because the inputs are based on a single feedback loop. This section assumes that the control objective is to regulate a plant output around a prescribed *setpoint* (*reference*) using a SISO controller.

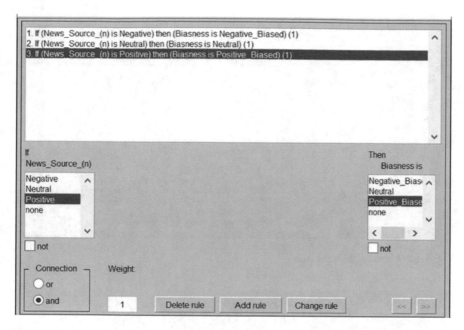

Fig. 5 Rule viewer

A linguistic controller contains rules in the *if–then* format, but they can appear in other formats. Matlab's Fuzzy Logic Toolbox presents the rules to the end-user in a format like the one in Fig. 5.

11 Membership Functions

The final step in creating a fuzzy logic model is to transform the linguistic variables into membership functions that describe the variable in a fuzzy way. Each membership function represents a linguistic variable and defines a fuzzy set that is associated with a particular parameter. Once the fuzzy set is defined, the next step is to define the if–then rules that describe how the fuzzy sets interact. Fuzzy operators are introduced to create connections between the fuzzy sets, namely max (which represents and) and min (which represents or). On completion of the connections, all the propositions are aggregated into the final fuzzy set. This fuzzy set releases a fuzzy number, and this is transformed into a crisp value, through different techniques. See Figs. 6 and 7.

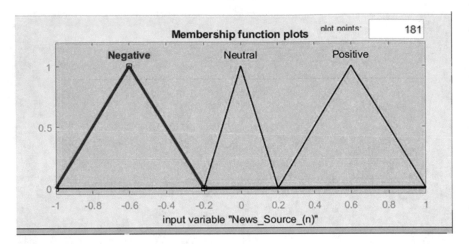

Fig. 6 Input membership functions

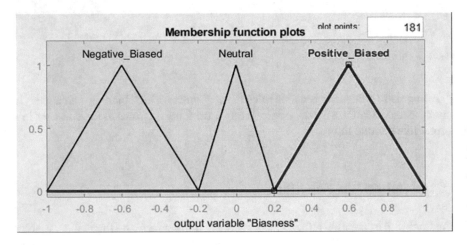

Fig. 7 Output membership functions

12 Multi-inference System

Figure 8 is a graphical construction of the inference, where each of the nine rows represents one rule. Consider, for instance, the first row: if the error is negative (row 1, column 1) and the change in error is negative (row 1, column 2) then the control action should be negative big (row 1, column 3). The chart corresponds to the rule base (3.2). Since the controller combines the error and the change in error, the controller is a fuzzy version of a proportional-derivative (PD) controller.

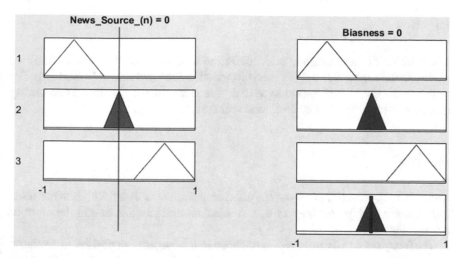

Fig. 8 PD controller

The instances of the error and the change in error are indicated by the vertical lines through the first and second columns of the chart. For each rule, the inference engine looks up the membership value where the vertical line intersects a membership function.

13 Defuzzification

The resulting fuzzy set μA must be converted to a single number in order to form a control signal to the plant. This is *defuzzification*. In Fig. 8 the defuzzified control signal is the x-coordinate marked by the red thick vertical line overlayed on the combined output set. Several defuzzification methods exist.

14 Cogs

The crisp control value uCOG is the abscissa of the centre of gravity of the fuzzy set. For discrete sets, its name is centre of gravity for singletons, COGS. The expression is the membership weighted average of the elements of the set. For continuous sets, replace summations by integrals and call it COG. The method is much used, although its computational complexity is relatively high.

15   Boa

The bisector of area method, BOA, finds the abscissa x of the vertical line that partitions the area under the membership function into two areas of equal size. For discrete sets, uBOA is the abscissa xj that minimizes. Its computational complexity is relatively high. There may be several solutions xj.

16   Mom

An intuitive approach is to choose the point of the universe with the highest membership. Several such points may exist, and it is common practice to take the mean of maxima (MOM).

The fuzzy system, for example, must choose either negative or positive to decide on the appropriateness of a news item; thus, the defuzzifier must choose one (Negative) or the other (Positive), not something in between. These defuzzification methods are indifferent to the shape of the fuzzy set, but the computational complexity is relatively small.

Each source will now contain an output between extremely negative and extremely positive, the problem is that there may not be the same amounted of sources therefore if we compute each extremely negative source from the BBC-News it may differ from the independent news source, therefore each sentiment is then computed and normalised by dividing each sentiment from each source by the total number of sources in the dataset.

Let $hgt(A) = \sup_{x \in A} \mu_A(x)$ be the highest membership degree of A and let $x \in A$: $\mu_A(x) = hgt(x)$ be the set of domain elements with degree of membership equal to $hgt(A)$. Then the first of Maxima is given by $\inf_{x \in A} \{x \in A : \mu_A(x) = hgt(x)\}$ and the last of maxima is given by $\sup_{x \in A} \{x \in A : \mu_A(x) = hgt(x)\}$. Middle of maxima MoM is very similar to first of maxima or last of maxima instead of determining y to be the first or last from all values when S has the maximal membership degree. This method takes the average of these two values formally it is given as:

$$y = \frac{\inf_{x \in A}\{x \in A : \mu_A(x) = hgt(x)\} + \sup_{x \in A}\{x \in A : \mu_A(x) = hgt(x)\}}{2} \qquad (4)$$

17   Post Processing

The final output will be a value of each news source that has combined all three methodologies in a fair and balanced way, therefore, a value of news source will then be further analysed in the Fuzzy Logic Framework to compute a sentiment that handles the subjectivity of the value that is between -1 and 1.

$$F_{Biasssness} = \begin{cases} \text{Positive}, & y \geq 0.45 \\ \text{Negative}, & y \leq -0.45 \\ \text{Neutral}, & \text{otherwise} \end{cases} \quad (5)$$

18 Conclusion

In this chapter, we created a framework for the a Hybrid Lexicon-Based Sentiment Analysis system that can handle data directly from a real-time API. The algorithm may be used to categorize the sentiment of healthcare current events. This can be done across all types of healthcare publications in order to acquire insight on the source of information's biases. The model was able to classify the sentiments using a subjective expert knowledge-rules-base into three outputs, namely Negatively Biased, Neutral, and Positively Biased. Based on this experiment, we can conclude that (n) number of sentiment analysis methods can be used, thereby increasing the accuracy of lexicon-based methods as an alternative to machine learning methods. In the future, we can compare the results of true positives and true negatives with machine learning models. One of the drawbacks of lexicon-based methods is that they require a large amount of "bag of words," or a pre-prepared sentiment lexicon, to score a document by aggregating the sentiment scores of all the words in the document. By combining multiple lexicons, we can avoid gathering an enormous amount of data by combining the sentiment analysis lexicons that already exist.

References

1. Pang B, Lee L Opinion mining and sentiment analysis. p 94
2. Liu B Sentiment analysis and subjectivity. p 38
3. Kasmuri E, Basiron H Subjectivity analysis in opinion mining–a systematic literature review. p 28
4. Jiang J (2012) Information extraction from text. In: Aggarwal CC, Zhai C (eds) Mining text data. Springer US, Boston, MA, pp 11–41. https://doi.org/10.1007/978-1-4614-3223-4_2
5. Piskorski J, Yangarber R (2013) Information extraction: past, present and future. In: Poibeau T, Saggion H, Piskorski J, Yangarber R (eds) Multi-source, multilingual information extraction and summarization. Springer, Berlin, Heidelberg, pp 23–49. https://doi.org/10.1007/978-3-642-28569-1_2
6. Cowie J Information extraction. p 22
7. Dave K, Lawrence S, Pennock DM (2003) Mining the peanut gallery: opinion extraction and semantic classification of product reviews. In: Proceedings of the 12th international conference on World Wide Web. New York, NY, USA, pp 519–528. https://doi.org/10.1145/775152.775226.
8. Zadeh LA (2009) Fuzzy LogicFuzzy logic. In: Meyers RA (ed) Encyclopedia of complexity and systems science. Springer, New York, NY, pp 3985–4009. https://doi.org/10.1007/978-0-387-30440-3_234

9. Carbonell JG (1981) Subjective understanding, computer models of belief systems. UMI Research Press, Ann Arbor, Mich
10. Almatarneh S, Gamallo P (2018) A lexicon based method to search for extreme opinions. PLoS One 13(5):e0197816. https://doi.org/10.1371/journal.pone.0197816
11. Fonctionnement du programme de vérification tierce de Facebook. Fonctionnement du programme de vérification tierce de Facebook. Retrieved September 06, 2021, from https://www.facebook.com/journalismproject/programs/third-party-fact-checking/how-it-works?locale=fr_FR
12. News API—search news and blog articles on the web. News API. Retrieved October 28, 2021, from https://newsapi.org

AI for Cardivascular Diseases

Using Fuzzy Logic to Diagnose Blood Pressure

Natalie Mitchell, Tia Mulholland, and Arjab Singh Khuman(iD)

Abstract This publication documents the research, creation, testing, and critical evaluation of a Fuzzy Inference System (FIS) used to return whether patients have a healthy blood pressure which may aid in prevention of Cardiovascular Disease (CVD). The system aforementioned will utilise public health statistics in order to attempt production of crisp values, those of which point to the likelihood of a patient's blood pressure level. The FIS will take into account those who are aware of their blood pressure value but uncertain of what this means, providing the crisp output and being used to therefore aid them in future steps; and will also contain a more fuzzy logic-oriented calculation regarding the person's lifestyle.

1 Introduction

Logic may be bisected into two main categories; binary, which revolves around absolutes as its basis and allows no degree of membership to other factors outside of true and false, and vagueness, where it is understood that uncertainty must look beyond absolution to accommodate its flexibility and to define all considered possibilities. The latter has adopted the title fuzzy logic; the method of utilising fuzzy sets, models of quantitative or qualitative data, to create conditional degrees of membership towards approximated results. These are then related back into a more human outcome, reflecting our world.

Fuzzy logic is a concept that was emerging as early as the mid-1960s. Lotfi Zadeh's fuzzy set theory describes fuzzy sets as a class of objects holding grades of membership, emphasising that ambiguity and imprecise definition are paramount to human thinking. These sets may be characterised by membership functions which

N. Mitchell · T. Mulholland
School of Computer Science and Informatics, De Montfort University, Leicester, UK

A. S. Khuman (✉)
School of Computer Science and Informatics, Institute of Artificial Intelligence (IAI), Leicester, UK
e-mail: arjab.khuman@dmu.ac.uk

Fig. 1 Union of fuzzy sets within a membership function as modelled by LA Zadeh

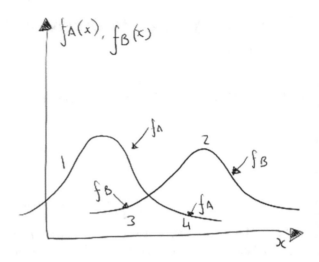

associate a point in the set to a value between zero and one, defining the membership of that point in a nonstatistical manner [1] (Fig. 1).

The subject itself, however, has been in study prior to the writings of Zadeh by Lukasiewicz and Tarski as infinite-valued logic; defined in the early twentieth century as belonging to classes of T-Norm and substructural logics. There are two main categories of FIS; Mamdani and Takagi–Sugeno-Kang (TSK) also known by the simplified title Sugeno [2]. Both are similar, although Sugueno is typically suited towards linearity and systems providing singleton output values and thus focused upon computational efficiency. However, the former is described as highly compatible within medical diagnostics systems where ambiguities are indefinitely present [3]. For this reason, we shall be using a Mamdani FIS as our basis.

One field that can greatly utilise Fuzzy Logic is that of healthcare; namely, to aid within diagnoses and being able to detect potential patterns within those who develop diseases. An area where we struggle to identify illness until it is already present is the cardiovascular system.

Atherosclerosis, the build-up of fatty plaques within the arteries, centralises many of the ailments within Cardiovascular Disease (CVD) alongside many other 'risk factors', with high blood pressure (hypertension) being the most common and thus requiring the earliest possible diagnosis. While there is no cure at this moment in time, there are actions such as lifestyle alterations and medicines like angiotensin converting enzyme (ACE) inhibitors and angiotensin receptor blockers (ARB) that can aid in prevention of worsening condition [7]. Therefore it is worth analysing the chances of someone developing CVD as early as possible so that they may prevent or lower the chances of requiring treatments to ensure a happy and healthy life.

This chapter aspires to articulate the potential design of a system centralised around cardiovascular health wherein, based upon existing attempts at theorising a system in this area, diagnosis of blood pressure levels may be provided as an outcome. Through use of the MATLAB software, three fuzzy inference systems shall be created in a single. m script which shall read data from two Microsoft Excel spreadsheet tables to provide results written to the console and charted on graphs.

2 Literature Review

As previously stated, the practise of fuzzy logic regarding medical diagnostics has great congruency with the Mamdani FIS type.

A Mamdani FIS operates in three stages: fuzzification, aggregation and defuzzification. Fuzzification converts crisp values into fuzzy ones using the knowledgebase and one of three fuzzification methods—gaussian, triangular, or trapezoid—visible in Fig. 2. Aggregation is the application of fuzzy operations in the rule evaluation to determine the fuzzy value result. Defuzzification returns the fuzzy value to a crisp one using one of five methods—bisector, centroid, smallest of maximum (SoM), middle of maximum (MoM), or largest of maximum (LoM).

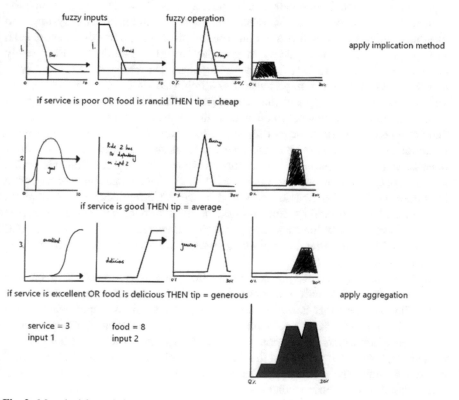

Fig. 2 Mamdani fuzzy inference process

Table 1 Definition of blood pressure levels

Blood pressure category	Systolic mm Hg	And/or	Diastolic mm Hg
Normal	Less than 120	And	Less than 80
Elevated	120–129	And	Less than 80
High blood pressure (Hypertension) stage 1	130–139	Or	80–89
High blood pressure (Hypertension) stage 2	140 or higher	Or	90 or higher
Hypertensive crisis	Higher than 180	And/or	Higher than 120

Blood pressure is measured using systolic and diastolic values: the pressure exerted against artery walls during a beat and while resting. Table 1 below showcases borders for normal, elevated, and high blood pressure using these values [8].

While there is a lot of attention surrounding hypertension because of its incredible risk to our wellbeing, low blood pressure, known as hypotension, should be considered equally when creating a diagnostics system. A chart including what is considered low may be seen below (Fig. 3).

When diagnosing hypertension, only the systolic or diastolic number needs to be higher than expected. This is known as isolated systolic/diastolic hypertension if the number is consistently higher. However, hypotension requires both the systolic and diastolic readings to be below a certain point. It is worth noting that factors such as temperature, stress, and anxiety may impact singular readings [9]. Both rarely cause noticeable symptoms, but some include dizziness, blurry vision, chest pain, and shortness of breath in hypertension and lightheaded/dizziness, nausea, blurry vision, and fainting in hypotension [10, 11]. It is clear to see that, from the given symptoms, not many people would realise they have an irregular blood pressure and would carry on the same as they were. However, this can lead to underlying conditions such as diabetes or in more severe cases strokes, cardiac arrest, kidney disease, and aortic aneurisms. The current treatment for hypertension lies within lifestyle changes to prevent worsening condition. Typical changes include reduction of sodium intake and increased potassium intake, lowering alcohol consumption, weight loss, lowering caffeine consumption, quitting smoking, and good exercise. If your readings reside within stage 2 hypertension, there are medicines such as ACE inhibitors, CCBs, and other forms of blockers and diuretics that can aid in controlling blood pressure levels [12].

Research relating to blood pressure within fuzzy systems goes back to at least the 90 s with Meier et al.'s study into controlling blood pressure during anaesthesia. The publication suggests that during multiple different operations, supervising anaesthetists did not override or intervene with the system, showing that implementation of such controllers have a potential place in operating rooms. At the point of publishing, however, it was stated that further clinical research should be performed before welcoming the system fully. Depth of anaesthesia is measured via blood pressure, heart rate, and other medical signs with blood pressure being the prominent correlation, thus the mean arterial pressure (MAP) was used within the controller. The system was tested rigorously through consultative means initially and performed

Fig. 3 Blood pressure chart

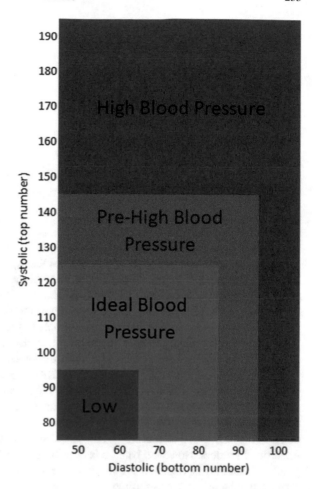

with great robustness shown through the successful live operations. However, it only supported a single form of anaesthetic, and implementations for varying types may have caused inconsistency within the system overall.

As shown above in Fig. 4, gaussian fuzzification was used within the controller, returning the best results thanks to handling marginal error and stabilising the inflow [4]. Our system will not be used to administer medication, but it is worth noting for an existing blood pressure FIS to use gaussian fuzzification to ensure the same outcome. The likelihood of hyper/hypotension may be as gradually measured as possible with moderate overlap in the pre-high range.

Wang et al. produced documented research on the same topic as this chapter: aspiring to present a new non-intrusive continuous blood pressure measuring system using a model-based fuzzy controller. To reduce noise within the system performance, the apparatus' pressure was to remain equal to the MAP where the system provides the counter pressure as compensation. A Synthetic Fuzzy Logic Controller

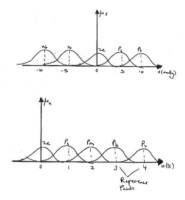

Fig. 4 Membership functions for inflow concentration

(SFLC) controls the micro syringe and is composed of 3 subsystems that process the ascending, descending, and stabilising states of the MAP. A predictor estimates changing tendency in order to trigger one of these respectively [5]. A gaussian-function-type model was used for the tonometer, the device used to detect arterial blood pressure and vessel volume pulse, which is formed of plexiglass which is placed over a superficial artery. The aim of the SFLC was to maintain maximised amplitude of the vessel volume through a close-loop control system.

Thanks to their data found in Fig. 5, the controller shown in Fig. 6 could be broken down into triangular fuzzification methods for the ascending and descending states.

When considering our system's membership functions, it may be that in some cases triangular membership is more effective than gaussian, for example when considering more static data like the blood pressure chart as shown in Fig. 3 with predefined borders. However, when considering one's lifestyle, the border between good and bad may be depicted as gaussian, with more transitional gradients into one another thanks to varying definition.

Nine live experiments were performed on subjects with normotension, and results combined with those of simulated tests gave conclusion towards optimal coupling condition within non-invasive blood pressure measurement, where the MAP was

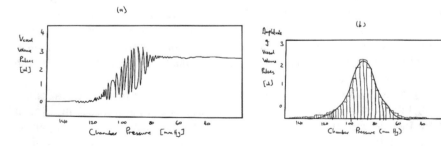

Fig. 5 Static arterial pressure–volume relationship

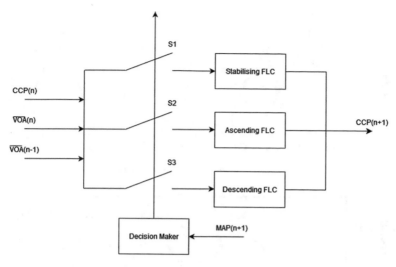

Fig. 6 Using SFLC to stabilise vessel volume amplitude

followed precisely. It was also noted that the regular FLC with PID had lower performance than this SFLC with its linear predictor [5]. We believe that although truthful, a much larger sample would be required to verify these outcomes and will thus aim for a table containing a minimum of 10 patient datasets, which will increase during the testing stage to ensure stability of the system.

Within the field of Artificial Intelligence sits a hybridisation of fuzzy logic and neural networks; a learning fuzzy system gathering its parameters based upon approximation via the latter component. This is known as neuro-fuzzy system, which Melin et al. used to design a hypertension risk diagnosis system, taking inputs of age, risk factors such as parental hypertension and whether subjects smoked, and behavioural blood pressure over a 24-h period via ABPM. The ABPM passes data to three neural network modules consisting of systolic, diastolic, and heart rate to learn behavioural patterns from. Three additional FIS were created based upon heart rate, night profile, and blood pressure of patients to test which architecture would perform best with which membership functions [6]. Looking into similar studies within the field of neural networking for cardiovascular diseases, and the understanding that these modules may be fine-tuned to further increase accuracy, Melin et al. proposed a database of blood pressure readings from different devices. He also decided upon a Mamdani FIS, like ourselves, providing reasoning for the separation of variables into the defined modules, as well as age being independent.

As seen in Fig. 8, triangular membership is once again used, like Wang et al.'s system in Fig. 7, for the blood pressure FIS and contains 24 rules in its rulebase to produce the overall output. Age was defined using trapezoidal membership as this provided them with the best results and may be noted when considering age as an input in our system. Multiple architectures were used to test the network and different memberships were used within the nocturnal profile testing. Then 35 patients were

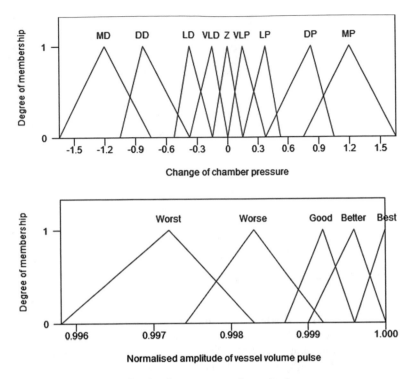

Fig. 7 Membership functions for chamber pressure and vessel volume

used to train the system further and one as a test observation [6]. This yielded a system with around 97% accuracy overall and is a valuable reference source for this project.

3 System Overview

3.1 Approach to the Problem

A person's blood pressure is easy to discern if they have their systolic and diastolic numbers attained from a blood pressure machine. However, not everybody has access to one of these, but blood pressure can still be estimated based on lifestyle and body type. For this reason, the project is comprised of two main systems: one for if a person knows their systolic and diastolic numbers, and one for if they don't. Both systems will be built using the Mamdani style due to its suitability to create rules based on human expert knowledge.

The second system is further split into two to reduce the number of inputs overall. The first calculates a person's BMI and this is then used with lifestyle variables to

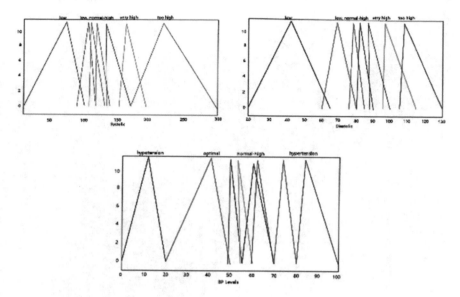

Fig. 8 Blood pressure FIS inputs and output

estimate blood pressure in the second. Typically, for adults, BMI is calculated using only weight and height. However, this variation includes sex and age to make it more precise for the percentage of body fat varies based on these. In general, women have higher body fat than men, and older people more than younger. By including these variables in the calculation, it allows for a better estimation of a person's health rather than just their mass per square meter (Fig. 9).

3.2 System Description

The project has 3 total systems within it. Therefore, each system will be described and justified separately.

This system outputs someone's blood pressure based on their systolic and diastolic numbers. Figure 10 shows a diagram of the system, with Table 2 describing the variables used. Due to the project holding two different systems depending on if these values are known, a variable is used to decide which system to run—Know Sys/Dia—hence it is used as an input here.

Know Sys/Dia is used as an input purely to decide if this system should be run. Due to being a static input (you either know your systolic and diastolic numbers or you don't) the range chosen was 0–4, allowing each variable (yes or no) to be represented by a number. Yes is represented by 1, and no by 3. All rules for this system require this input to be 1, or yes, so if the input is no, or 3, no rules will fire, and the system will not generate an output.

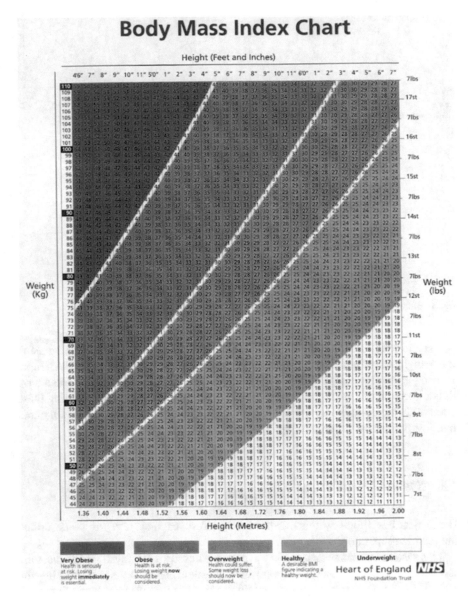

Fig. 9 BMI chart provided by Heart of England NHS

The range for the systolic input is taken from the range that is used in blood pressure charts to calculate the result. Charts do not go above 190 nor do they go below 70. The intervals for this variable were based on final blood pressure readings.

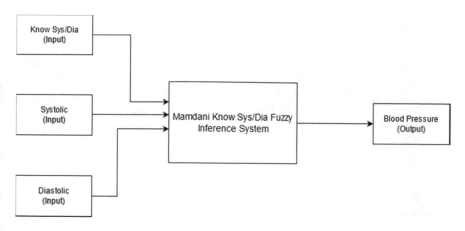

Fig. 10   Diagram of Known Sys/Dia Mamdani FIS

Table 2   Variables used in Known Sys/Dia Mamdani FIS

Variable	Type of variable	Range	Intervals
Know Sys/Dia	Input	0–4	Yes, no
Systolic	Input	70–190	Low, ideal, pre-high, high
Diastolic	Input	40–100	Low, ideal, pre-high, high
Blood pressure	Output	0–100	Low, ideal, pre-high, high

The diastolic variable was created in much the same way as the systolic one; charts for working out blood pressure do not go below 40 or above 100 for diastolic readings. The intervals are also based on final blood pressure readings.

The output of blood pressure is done in the range of 0–100 due to most likelihoods and measurements are done in this range unless a different one is more suitable. It also corresponds with the linguistic intervals; a low number equals low blood pressure. The intervals themselves are taken from the actual readings of blood pressure.

This system calculates a person's BMI; however, it is done slightly different to the traditional way. Normally, BMI for adults does not include gender and age for it is working out a person's mass per square meter. This has no reference to the amount of body fat a person has and is only a guideline to distinguish how healthy they are. Including age and gender morphs the outcome to better reflect a person's health for females tend to have more body fat than males, and the elderly more than the young. Figure 11 shows a diagram of this FIS, with Table 3 describes the variables used.

Height is part of the normal calculation for BMI hence it was chosen as an input. The range is based on the average height of adults (since the system only takes them into account) including average minimum and maximum to get the upper and lower bounds. The intervals are based on people's perception of height; someone is either short, average, or tall when you describe their height.

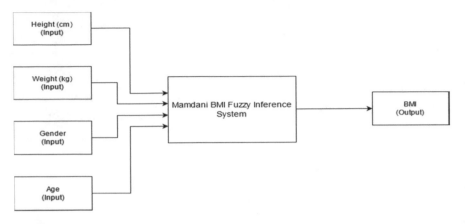

Fig. 11 Diagram of BMI Mamdani FIS

Table 3 Variables used in BMI Mamdani FIS

Variable	Type of variable	Range	Intervals
Height (cm)	Input	147–201	Short, average, tall
Weight (kg)	Input	40–180	Light, average, heavy
Gender	Input	0–4	Male, female
Age	Input	18–120	Young adult, adult, elderly
BMI	Output	9–52	Severely underweight, underweight, ideal, overweight, obese, severely obese

Weight is also part of the normal calculation for BMI. Like height, its range was based on the average for adults; being below 40 kg is highly unlikely, as is being above 180 kg. The intervals are also based on perception of weight.

Gender is not used to calculate an adults BMI but was added into this system to cater it more towards how healthy a person is. Females tend to have more body fat than males who have the same general BMI rating. The range is 0–4 to create two options, male is represented by 1 and female by 3.

Age was added to this FIS for the same reason as gender; to cater it more towards health than mass per square meter. Older people tend to have more body fat than younger with the same BMI rating. The lower boundary is 18 due to BMI being calculated differently for children and teens, so limiting it to only adults reduces the complexity. The upper bound is 120 due to the oldest person to live at present is aged 117, with the oldest person ever recorded was 122.

These variables are used to calculate an adjusted version of a person's BMI which caters more towards their general health. It includes height and weight which are normally the only 2 BMI calculation variables, along with gender and age to adjust it. The output range and intervals come from the NHS BMI scale, which reflects the national standard.

This is the final FIS in the project and calculates someone's blood pressure if they don't have their systolic and diastolic numbers. The system is displayed in Fig. 12 and the variables described in Table 4. This system takes the output of the BMI FIS as an input variable along with general lifestyle data to estimate a person's blood pressure. This is just an estimation; their actual blood pressure reading could be different.

Know Sys/Dia is the same variable that is used in the first FIS to distinguish which system someone's data should be used in. The rules in this system all require the

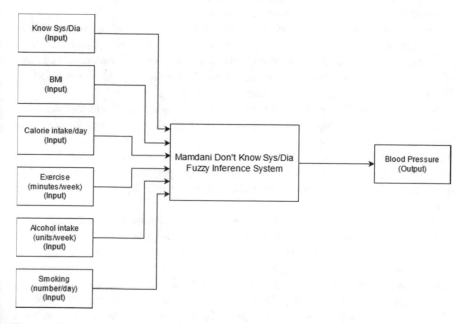

Fig. 12 Diagram of unknown Sys/Dia Mamdani FIS

Table 4 Variables used in Lifestyle/Unknown Sys/Dia Mamdani FIS

Variable	Type of variable	Range	Intervals
Know Sys/Dia	Input	0–4	Yes, no
BMI	Input	9–52	Severely underweight, underweight, ideal, overweight, obese, severely obese
Calorie intake/day	Input	500–6000	Extremely low, low, average, high, extremely high
Exercise (minutes/week)	Input	0–300	Little, average, lots
Alcohol intake (units/week)	Input	0–30	None/low, moderate, high
Smoking (number/day)	Input	0–40	None/light, mild, heavy
Blood Pressure	Output	0–100	Low, ideal, pre-high, high

variable to be 3, or no, whereas in the other system it required them to be 1, or yes. This means that the rules will only fire, and an output generated, if the person doesn't know their systolic and diastolic numbers.

BMI is the output from the second FIS. Its range and intervals come from the NHS BMI scale, reflecting the full range of possible BMI values.

Calorie intake per day is used as an input for your diet influences blood pressure. The range is based on the average for men and woman (2500 and 2000 respectfully) as well as the recommended minimum per day (1200). The upper bound is just over double the recommended amount for men and the lower just under half the recommended minimum to accommodate for extremes.

Exercise helps to keep your blood vessels and heart strong and healthy, as well as to maintain a healthy weight. Both can keep your blood pressure at a normal level and reduce the chance of having high blood pressure. The NHS recommends that adults have roughly 150 min of exercise a week, hence the range is 0 to double this. This is also why it is measured in minutes per week.

Alcohol intake also has an effect, too much can raise your blood pressure. The NHS recommends having no more than 14 units of alcohol a week to not negatively impact your health. The range is 0–30 to accommodate those who do not drink, as well as those who drink in excess with the upper bound being just over double the recommended. The measurement of units per week is used to reflect this recommendation as well as accommodating the fact people don't tend to drink every day.

Smoking damages the heart and blood vessels as well as nicotine in general raises a person's blood pressure. The upper bound of the range was chosen due to there being 20 cigarettes per pack on average, so it is double this to accommodate those who smoke more than a pack a day. The lower bound is set to 0 for not everyone smokes. The intervals where also chosen to reflect this, with the first being None/Light.

The output of Blood Pressure in this system is just an estimation and is not as accurate as the output by the first system (which calculates it based on a person's systolic and diastolic numbers). All the inputs used in this system have an impact on blood pressure. The range reflects the level of blood pressure, with a low number referring to low blood pressure. The intervals are taken from those used to describe the state of a person's blood pressure.

4   System Testing

4.1   Data Collection for Testing

Due to personal data regulations, it will be difficult to gather a large dataset of realistic values, and therefore dummy/placeholder data shall be used until access to raw data is obtained.

4.1.1 Localised Data

To make the systems as accurate as possible, real-life data was collected from friends and family using home blood pressure machines to be used with their consent. Machines used were Omron models M10-IT and MIT5s Connect and SilverCrest SBM 69. The data for not knowing systolic and diastolic readings were also gathered from family and friends with their consent. However, this limited the amount of data entries due to a small sample size. For this reason, along with the real-life data, some entries were fabricated but attempts were made to make them as realistic as possible.

Assumptions were made within the rule base regarding lifestyle, for example a person given an output of Obese would likely not have a low KCal intake or do a high amount of exercise. This created some gaps within the system that may mean specific scenarios would not fire rules, and this would require revising and additional rules in the future. Some data would also become borderline with the intentional design, and it may be that someone is barely over a threshold, thus a default output should have been created ignoring exercise when uncertain.

5 Critical Analysis

The first half of the system, calculating blood pressure based on systolic and diastolic readings, worked incredibly well and was correct almost all the time. Using middle of maximum (MoM) as the defuzzification method resulted in 100% accuracy, with the other methods only getting one or two wrong.

However, the second half of the system, calculating blood pressure based on a person's BMI and lifestyle, wasn't as successful. The calculation of BMI was around 70% accurate, with the highest being centroid defuzzification with 16/19 correct. The ranges of the variables within this FIS were vivid to begin with, and although revised are still not as accurate as they could be due to varying meanings of height and weight. Heaviness had to be split into an additional variable 'very heavy' as it was difficult to define obesity against overweight. On top of this, the system doesn't consider lean BMI limiting its accuracy.

BMI being rather inaccurate fed into the inaccuracy of the lifestyle (don't know sys/dia) fuzzy inference system. The amount the system accurately diagnosed was very similar to the amount the BMI system did. However, it is not completely dependable; BMI could be wrong and blood pressure correct, as well as vice versa. Centroid, bisector and lower of maximum (LoM) were the most precise with 15/19. This inaccuracy is due to the rule base. Harsh assumptions were used to determine the combination of rules, and therefore not allowing for outliers. It was assumed that someone with a high BMI didn't do a lot of exercise and ate more than the average amount of calories per day, therefore rules were only created for these combinations. This resulted in a few data entries firing no rules, for the BMI was calculated as overweight or obese, yet the person did high exercise or ate an average amount. The divisions for smoking and alcohol consumption were also too wide to be properly used to determine the effect on blood pressure. For this to be more accurately measured, more than 3 divisions should have been used for these categories.

6 Conclusion

The premise and design of the system was promising, however the implementation caused it to fall short of expectations. The intricacies and variety of possible outcomes was not taken completely into account when creating its rule base, resulting in several inaccurate calculations. The ranges of several divisions of variables were also inaccurate where there was a lack of research into how to represent them more precisely thanks to varying definitions.

Outside of the system performance, it was highly unlikely that the accuracy of the system alone would reflect a perfect diagnosis; there is more than just lifestyle choices that can affect a person's blood pressure, such as medical conditions like diabetes, which are not considered. Moods such as anxiety also have an effect; if a known sys/dia was taken when the patient was stressed or anxious, this elevates the blood pressure temporarily. Despite the systems underperformance, it does not rule it out from being used in the calculation of blood pressure. With further refinement of variables and a rule base to account for all possibilities, the systems accuracy would be greatly improved.

Acknowledgements Natalie would like to acknowledge Dr Sara Wilford for giving inspiration and guiding early studies into Personal Health Monitoring (PHM) systems and the world of medical computing; her family for undivided support throughout the development of this chapter; and a special acknowledgement to her father Warren Charles Mitchell, for being a loving and dedicated father providing guidance all his life and becoming the driving point for her passion in medical systems regarding CVD.

Tia would like to acknowledge her family and friends, especially those who volunteered their data for use in this project.

Lastly, both authors would like to give acknowledgements and great thanks to Dr Archie Khuman for providing this opportunity after supporting them during their degree and beyond, and for also giving outstanding guidance throughout the lifecycle of the system.

References

1. Department of Electrical Engineering and Electronics Laboratory, University of California (1965) Fuzzy Sets. [online] Berkeley, California, pp 338–342. Retrieved August 15, 2021, from https://www.sciencedirect.com/science/article/pii/S001999586590241X
2. En.wikipedia.org. (n.d.) Fuzzy Logic. [online]. Retrieved August 15, 2021, from https://en.wikipedia.org/wiki/Fuzzy_logic#:~:text=The%20term%20fuzzy%20logic%20was,notably%20by%20%C5%81ukasiewicz%20and%20Tarski

3. Uk.mathworks.com. (n.d.) Mamdani and Sugeno fuzzy inference systems-MATLAB & Simulink-Mathworks United Kingdom. Retrieved August 15, 2021, from https://uk.mathwo rks.com/help/fuzzy/types-of-fuzzy-inference-systems.html
4. Meier R, Nieuwland J, Zbinden A, Hacisalihzade S (1992) Fuzzy logic control of human blood pressure during anesthesia. IEEE, pp12–16. Retrieved August 20, 2021, from https://ieeexp lore.ieee.org/abstract/document/168811
5. Wang J, Lin C, Liu S, Wen Z (2002) Model-based synthetic fuzzy logic controller for indirect blood pressure measurement. IEEE Transactions on Systems, Man and Cybernetics, Part B (Cybernetics) 32(3):306–315. Retrieved August 20, 2021, from https://ieeexplore.ieee.org/abs tract/document/999807
6. Melin P, Miramontes I, Prado-Arechiga G (2018) A hybrid model based on modular neural networks and fuzzy systems for classification of blood pressure and hypertension risk diagnosis. Expert Syst Appl 107:146–164. Retrieved August 25, 2021, from https://doi.org/10.1016/j. eswa.2018.04.023
7. nhs.uk. (n.d.) *Cardiovascular disease*. Retrieved August 25, 2021, from https://www.nhs.uk/ conditions/cardiovascular-disease/
8. www.heart.org. (n.d.) Understanding blood pressure readings. Retrieved August 30, 2021, from https://www.heart.org/en/health-topics/high-blood-pressure/understanding-blood-pressure-readings
9. Bloodpressureuk.org. (n.d.) Blood Pressure UK. Retrieved August 30, 2021, from http://www. bloodpressureuk.org/your-blood-pressure/understanding-your-blood-pressure/what-do-the-numbers-mean/
10. Bhf.org.uk. (n.d.) High blood pressure—symptoms and treatment. Retrieved August 30, 2021, from https://www.bhf.org.uk/informationsupport/risk-factors/high-blood-pressure/symptoms-and-treatment
11. nhs.uk. (n.d.) Low blood pressure (hypotension). Retrieved August 30, 2021, from https:// www.nhs.uk/conditions/low-blood-pressure-hypotension/
12. nhs.uk. (n.d.) High blood pressure (hypertension). Retrieved August 30, 2021, from https:// www.nhs.uk/conditions/high-blood-pressure-hypertension/

An AI-Based Approach to Identifying High Impact Comorbidities in Public Health Management of Diseases

Raymond Moodley

Abstract The impact of comorbidities on the treatment of a primary disease is high-lighted with specific focus given to disease management by public health authorities. With finite resources and several major diseases being strongly linked to preventable comorbidities, public health authorities must often prioritise campaigns to ensure maximum benefit for their citizens. A simple, yet effective AI model is proposed to help prioritise public health campaigns, with a case study involving coronary health disease in the United Kingdom used to illustrate the approach. Results from the case study show that it is possible to use an AI-based approach to rank comorbidities based on their impact on a population and using this, create targeted campaigns to enhance resource utilization and the effectiveness of public health management.

Keywords Comorbidity · Disease management · Artificial intelligence · Public health

1 Introduction

Patients with comorbidities have always presented with an increased risk when treating a primary disease or condition. Comorbidity may be defined as the simultaneous presence of two or more diseases or medical conditions in a patient [5]. The treatment of random comorbidities, defined as diseases or conditions that co-occur in the same patient by pure chance e.g., seasonal allergies and cardiovascular disease (CVD), are less-interesting, as one typically does not impact the other, however, the treatment of non-random comorbidities (defined as diseases or conditions that influence the treatment of the primary disease) is far more complex [11]. This study focusses on non-random comorbidities which is discussed further in Sect. 2.1.

Whilst at an individual level, the management of non-random comorbidities can be very complex; at an aggregate level there are typically some established patterns between several non-random comorbidities and their impact on the primary disease;

R. Moodley (✉)
Institute of Artificial Intelligence, De Montfort University, Leicester, UK
e-mail: raymond.moodley@dmu.ac.uk

thus, lending themselves to public health management interventions [11]. A good example of a such a case may be smoking. A ninety-five-year-old individual that has smoked for most of their adult life and has recently been diagnosed with CVD may not see the direct benefit of quitting, however from an aggregate perspective, smoking is a well-established cause of CVD, with the general public advised to quit [8, 7]. Given that public health management is generally concerned with the wellbeing of a population (be it within a city, region, or country) as opposed to an individual, the aggregate management of diseases or conditions becomes the key focus for public health leaders.

At a global level, prioritising targets for public health campaigns is a significant undertaking as it not only straddles sectors within healthcare, but all other areas of governments including the economy, welfare, and defence [1]. Whilst there are several criteria for prioritising health care campaigns, especially as resources are scarce, a central theme across these criteria is that priority must be given to areas that will result in maximum public gain [1]. Defining the concept of maximum gain is in itself complex, however one universally accepted measure is indeed minimising mortality, i.e., priority should be given to health issues that have the maximum impact on mortality [1].

As a result, public health management typically focusses on campaigns that seek to reduce the impact of highly associated, non-random comorbidities in the management of a primary disease within the population. However, public health leaders have limited resources (financial, infrastructural etc.) and thus must prioritise campaigns. In this regard the focus is typically on selecting campaigns that minimising mortality and morbidity in the largest number of people as possible. Thus, not all co-morbidities can be treated equally, as some are more severe than others. Being able to identify the most severe co-morbidity and selecting campaigns to reduce its impact is a complex, but essential task. As an added complication, decision makers may sometimes be influenced by conflicting agendas, whilst public misinformation can adversely influence the population and shift focus away from high priority areas. The head of Public Health, England noted in [17] that good data can often be lost when stakeholders pursue different agendas, whilst [13] criticised the role of the media in misrepresenting medical studies and/or for extrapolating the results of small-scale studies too widely to create hype and increased readership in their quest for profits. As a result, both studies called for greater ethicality in medical research to create value and instil ongoing public trust. In this regard, the key conclusion drawn from [17] on achieving value from public health data analytics was considered apt: "to find truths from complexity of data, present it in an unambiguous way and explicitly counteract those perceptions which are not based on the facts."

Given the above, artificial intelligence (AI), more specifically data analytics, can play an important role in helping public health leaders select the optimal condition to target, thus speeding up the decision-making process. This chapter presents a data analytics approach to optimising public health campaigns targeting the reduction of non-random co-morbidity conditions in the treatment of primary diseases. A case study involving the management of coronary heart disease (CHD) within the United

Kingdom (UK) is used to illustrate this approach. More specifically, the market target (mt) model first introduced in [14], is used to optimise public health campaigns and focus attention on high impact areas.

2 Background

2.1 Non-random Comorbidities

Non-random comorbidities may be categorised into three broad classes [11]. The first class is Direct co-morbidity in which the primary disease being treated is directly linked to the secondary disease (e.g., stroke and hypertension). Treatment of patients with Direct co-morbidities remains the main thrust of comorbidity disease management, and indeed forms the basis of this chapter. For completeness, the second class is Indirect co-morbidity and is typically defined as where the treatment of the primary disease is impacted by the secondary disease with both diseases having no association. An example of Indirect co-morbidity may be where a patient being treated for cancer has severe anxiety with regards to hospitals and needles. The third class of non-random co-morbidity is that of diseases or conditions with a common cause. This may include diseases or conditions that result from a traumatic event e.g., accidents and natural disasters or common genetics factors. For example, because of a motor vehicle accident, a victim may suffer severe kidney damage as well as third degree burns.

2.2 Coronary Heart Disease (CHD) in the UK

CHD is a subset of CVD and occurs when the arteries of the heart become narrowed or blocked and is thus unable to deliver oxygen rich blood to the heart. Once an artery is blocked, blood supply to the heart muscle is cut-off and the patient experiences a myocardial infarction or commonly referred to as a heart attack [4, 8]. CHD is a leading cause of death and accounted for 16% of world's total deaths in 2019 [18].

Given the above, public health departments are naturally focussed on reducing CHD and as a result turn their attention to managing the conditions that are commonly associated with CHD. Together with smoking, the four, direct conditions (Direct comorbidities) commonly associated with CHD are: (1) Being Overweight or high Body Mass Index (BMI), (2) Hypertension (HBP), (3) Diabetes, and (4) Raised Cholesterol [4, 8]

Over the years, residents of several countries have been exposed to a broad range of public health initiatives that seek to reduce the prevalence of these four commonly associated conditions. In the UK, for example, these include television and radio advertising that ask residents to consider their salt, sugar and fat intake, increased taxation on foods that contain high quantities of sugar, and improved food labelling (e.g., traffic light system in the United Kingdom) to make residents aware, in a simple way, of what they are consuming. In addition, both the UK National Health Service (NHS) and non-governmental organizations like the British Heart Foundation (BHF) spend considerable time and resources on educating the public on heart health [4].

However, it is not uncommon for patients to have two or more of the four conditions, and this coupled with the inconsistent messaging typically leaves patients confused [19]. In addition, campaigns recommend stringent dietary restrictions, and for some patients managing multiple conditions, these can become too restrictive. As a result, patients see these restrictions as diminishing their quality of life and thus become nonchalant and tend to increasingly rely on medication to manage their conditions [7]. Apart from being costly, medication have side effects which exposes the patients to other medical risks, and given that patients do not make significant changes to their lifestyle once on medication, dosages must be increased over time, thus increasing the impact of side effects, and reducing the quality of life of the patient. For example, a common side effect of blood pressure medication is dizziness. Hence, a patient taking blood pressure medication could become dizzy, lose balance, and fall. Falls in elderly patients can be especially dangerous, with many leading to fractures. A severe fracture in an elderly patient can leave them wheelchair-bound for several months, if not indefinitely, thus significantly impacting their quality of life. Thus, it is vitally important to manage conditions without introducing debilitating side effects. One successful treatment approach to disease management is to make small changes to patients' lifestyles or medication. This approach can also be used at the public health level [16].

2.3 The "Small Changes" Philosophy

The notion of making small incremental changes over an extended period, or continuous improvement is used in several sectors. Indeed, in production environments, the concept of Kaizen theory has been well-established [10]. Roughly translated, Kaizen means "change for good" and focusses on continuous improvement, that is, making small, incremental changes over an extended period that results in a big change overall. The principle is that small changes are both easy to make, and easy to adopt. As a result, such change is less likely to be reversed.

This concept has been well-established in disease/ medical condition management as well. For example, [6] concluded that making small and incremental changes in both diet and physical activity improved weight management. Similarly, [7] noted that asking patients to make small, attainable changes that can be adhered to can have a significant and long lasting, positive impact on patient wellbeing.

The natural follow-on question from this is: given all the small changes possible, which small change should be made first and why? The answer to this question is quite intuitive. Make the change that provides the best combination of providing the largest positive impact towards attaining the goal, whilst using the least resources. This concept is not new, and indeed behavioural science research has shown that people are more likely to accept a change and stick with it if it is easy to make and they can see noticeable positive change [2]. From a public health management perspective, this translates into launching public health campaigns that focus on initiatives that have the largest impact on reducing mortality and morbidity from a primary disease whilst minimising the use of resources.

This interplay between positive impact and use of resources is quite complex and thus deciding on change initiatives is not an easy task. Clearly there will be some changes that can be eliminated, e.g., those that provide low impact whilst being costly to implement, and there will be some that provide high impact at low cost which can be adopted immediately, but a significant proportion of changes are likely to require further analysis as they will involve decisions that play impact against resources. In this regard, the use of data analytical decision-making models, like the market target (mt) model introduced in [14] can be very useful.

2.4 The Market Target (mt) Model

The mt model, outlined in Eq. (1), has been shown to be very flexible and support decision-making in several diverse sectors, notably in grocery retail [14] and in education [15]. Mathematically, the mt model is expressed as follows:

$$mt = \frac{P(A)}{P(A, C)} - \frac{P(A)}{minsup} \qquad (1)$$

where $P(A)$ is the "ideal state", $P(A,C)$ is the current state, and $minsup$, is the compromise state, with $0 \le P(A), P(A,C), minsup \le 1$.

Intuitively, mt may be seen as the "effort" required to move from the current state to the "ideal state". Clearly, the larger the mt value, the greater the effort. Thus, by comparing mt values of alternatives, practitioners can understand the "effort" required for each alternative, and thus make an informed decision. The notion of "effort" is not necessarily financial or energy but may also be lives lost or natural resources consumed, or time taken etcetera.

3 Case Study: Using the mt Model to Support Decision-Making in the Public Health Management of CHD in the UK

3.1 Overview

The mt model was applied to public health data related to CHD in the UK, and its relationship with the four direct conditions associated with CHD. The two aims of this case study were: (1) to support the notion of finding truth in complex data and presenting it in an unambiguous way, and (2) to establish whether the mt model can aid in setting public healthcare priorities.

Data for CHD prevalence and mortality for 2017 was obtained from [9, 4]. The data was then analysed using Microsoft Excel. The underlying premise of the analysis was that in general, the population within that age group is considered healthier, in terms of any of the four direct conditions, than the people that died of CHD because of one or a combination of these conditions. For example, the proportion of people that died at age 35 of CHD because of a high BMI, or where high BMI was one of the attributable causes, should be higher than the general population at age 35. If the population is taken as the "ideal state" and the people that died as the "undesirable" or current state, then the mt value can be used as a measure for the deviation from "ideal" for each the four conditions within each age group. Thus, by comparing mt values, the "true" impact of each condition on the overall CHD mortality within that age group can be assessed.

The specific mt parameters are thus as follows: $P(A)$ will be the percent prevalence of the condition within the age group, $minsup$ will also be the percent prevalence, i.e., $minsup = P(A)$, as the compromise state is indeed the "ideal state" in this scenario, and $P(A,C)$ will be the percent of people that died of CHD with that condition. Consequently, the higher the mt value, the more severe the condition is in terms of CHD death. Similarly, a negative mt value will imply that people that die from CHD with that condition present may likely have died because of a direct impact by another cause, or that in general that metabolic condition within that age group, is not highly impactful.

3.2 Results and Discussion

The results of the data analysis conducted on the datasets described in Sect. 3.1 is detailed.

3.3 Deaths by CHD

From Fig. 1, approximately 90% of all CHD deaths that occurred in the UK in 2017 were of people aged over 60 years, with 70% occurring over the age of 75 years. Although CHD deaths remains largely an "older person issue", the contributory effect of CHD to the overall mortality in the over 75 age group has been reduced over time. According to the British Heat Foundation [4], in 2017, CHD contributed to 11% of all deaths in the over 75 age group compared to 13% in 2012. Several reasons have been put forward for this, including improved treatment, and advances in medical interventions [19].

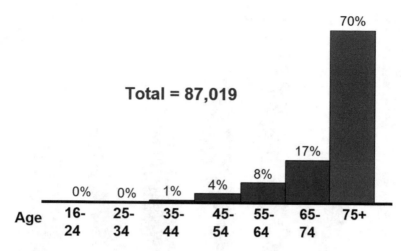

Fig. 1 CHD deaths by age group

3.4 Prevalence Versus Deaths

From Figs. 2, 3, 4 and 5, the four metabolic conditions across the six age groups results in twenty-four potential initiatives for CHD alone. Deciding on whether to prioritise one of the four conditions, or a selection of the twenty-four potential initiatives is a daunting task, let alone deciding across the healthcare spectrum that includes other major diseases like cancer, mental health or liver disease [19]. For example, within CHD, is a cholesterol lowering campaign in under 45 s more impactful than a diabetes campaign in the over 55 s? Inspecting the graphs in Figs. 2, 3, 4 and 5, it is evident that for some conditions, e.g., BMI, which is a proxy for obesity, the prevalence of having a high BMI is larger than in those that died from CHD. In this regard, it could suggest that a high BMI is protective against CHD mortality, which is contradictory to the multitude of public health campaigns that profess a positive correlation between BMI and CHD [8]. Conversely, the prevalence of diabetes is significantly lower, in most cases less than half, than in those that die from CHD, as shown in Fig. 5. Thus, making such choices are not straightforward, even when looking at it from a purely data analytics perspective.

The mt values for each of the twenty-four combinations, as shown in Table 1, were calculated using the values for the mt variables discussed in Sect. 3.1. As noted in Sect. 3.1., the combination with the highest, positive mt value is the most serious, as it shows a significant difference between those that die from CHD and the population at large. From Table 1, diabetes is a significant risk factor across all age groups, while BMI appears to be inversely correlated to CHD mortality for all age groups, especially in the over 75 s. Similarly, high blood pressure and cholesterol appears to be an issue with younger age groups but becomes less of an issue amongst the older age groups. One possible explanation for this is that people in older age groups

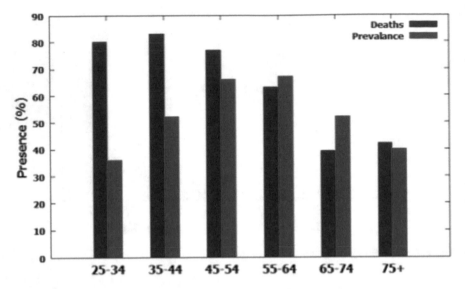

Fig. 2 Deaths versus prevalence—cholesterol

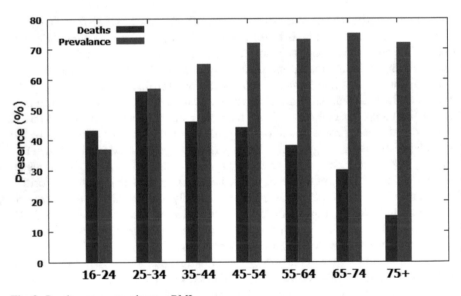

Fig. 3 Deaths versus prevalence—BMI

tend to be on blood pressure and cholesterol-lowering medication, as a result these conditions are better managed.

These results were discussed with the University of Leicester Cardiology Research Team, and it was noted that the BMI results correlate with the obesity paradox principle, where "fatter" people are more likely to survive CHD events than their "thinner"

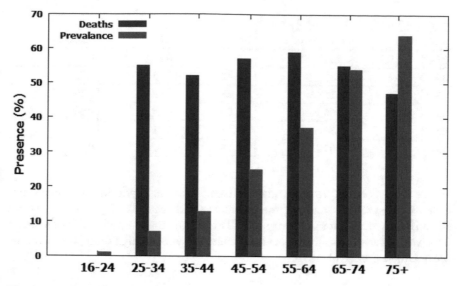

Fig. 4 Deaths versus prevalence—HBP

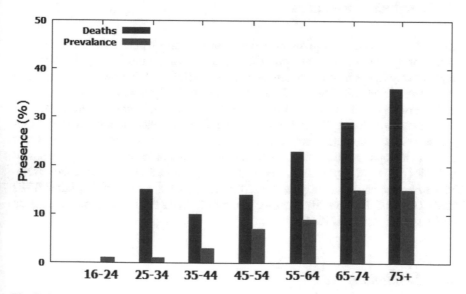

Fig. 5 Deaths versus prevalence—diabetes

counterparts [12, 19]. Similarly, the diabetes results also correlate with current observations, and indeed it is now becoming one of the top causes of premature deaths globally, not only as part of its contribution to CHD, but to other illnesses as well including cancer, organ failure, and circulatory diseases [3].

Table 1 mt values for the metabolic risk factors by age group

Age group	Cholesterol	BMI	HBP	Diabetes
25–34	0.55	−0.02	0.87	0.96
35–44	0.38	−0.42	0.75	0.72
45–54	0.15	−0.65	0.56	0.50
55–64	−0.06	−0.95	0.38	0.62
65–74	−0.34	−1.53	0.01	0.49
75+	0.03	−3.78	−0.36	0.58

The mt model does provide a quantitative mechanism to prioritise initiatives. For example, from Table 1, reducing the prevalence of diabetes and high blood pressure should be the focus across all age groups. This is particularly important for the under 34 s where diabetes has the highest mt value of 0.96, and high blood pressure, the second highest value of 0.87.

4 Concluding Remarks

The mt model was used to support the prioritisation of public health initiatives, and to bring clarity to the data with the aim of presenting the findings in an unambiguous way. Experiments conducted on the UK CHD for 2017 showed that in general diabetes and high blood pressure should be prioritised for public health campaigns. This correlated well with current global mortality rates and trends where cardiovascular disease, including CHD, remains the number one killer globally, with diabetes and high blood pressure being key contributors [3]. The results also showed that contrary to popular belief, people with high BMIs are not necessarily at an increased risk for CHD mortality. Indeed, this is a well-recognised fact amongst the cardiovascular research community, with the obesity paradox, people with higher BMIs having better CHD mortality outcomes than their lower BMI counterparts, being an active area of research [12, 19].

4.1 Limitations

An important limitation in the interpretation of the results is the role of confounding factors, including the impacts of other diseases that people may suffer from concurrently. For example, there is an argument that people aged 75+ may have lived for several years with CHD, and that they would have died earlier had their BMI been higher [19]. Hence 75+ CHD mortality has a high negative correlation with BMI [19]. Similar arguments may be used for high blood pressure and cholesterol. However, it should be noted that the mt model normalises these arguments in that it compares the age groups to their peers, based on prevalence. Thus, it could be asked: if low BMI prevented the earlier onset of CHD mortality, and that high BMI generally enables other confounding conditions, then how is it possible that the general population of 75+ have higher BMIs? Surely, a larger proportion of this age group should have died much earlier because of high BMI-related confounding conditions?

Clearly there is further investigation required to fully address these questions. However, it is evident that this analysis demonstrates the power of the mt model, in that it can be easily applied to global data and through this high-level, data driven approach, it can uncover subtleties, like the obesity paradox, and create a platform for further discussion. In this regard, the conclusion of University of Leicester Cardiology Research Team is apt: "the mt model and conclusions from its analysis could be used to quickly uncover some associations and generate hypotheses for further studies" [19].

References

1. Allin S, Mossialos E, McKee M, Holland WW (2004) Making decisions on public health: a review of eight countries. In: Technical report. WHO Regional Office for Europe, Copenhagen.
2. Amabile T, Kramer S (2011) The progress principle: using small wins to ignite joy, engagement, and creativity at work. Harvard Business Press
3. BBC (2019) What do the people of the world die from? Retrieved October 27, 2021, from https://www.bbc.co.uk/news/health-47371078
4. British Heart Foundation (BHF) (2017) Cardiovascular disease statistics. Retrieved October 27, 2021, from https://www.bhf.org.uk/what-we-do/our-research/heart-statistics/heart-statis tics-publications/cardiovascular-disease-statistics-2017
5. Buddeke J, Bots ML, Van Dis I, Visseren FL, Hollander M, Schellevis FG, Vaartjes I (2019) Comorbidity in patients with cardiovascular disease in primary care: a cohort study with routine healthcare data. Br J Gen Pract 69(683):e398–e406
6. Hills AP, et al (2013) Small changes to diet and physical activity behaviours for weight management. Obesity Facts 6(3):228–238
7. Hooker S, et al (2018) Encouraging health behaviour change: eight evidence-based strategies. Fam Pract Manag 25(2):31–36
8. Imperial College, London (2019) Heart disease deaths nearly halved in uk—but condition remains top killer. Retrieved October 27, 2021, from https://www.imperial.ac.uk/news/191 414/heart-disease-deaths-nearly-halved-uk/
9. Institute for Health Metrics and Evaluation (IHME) (2017) Global burden of disease study 2017. Retrieved October 27, 2021, from http://ghdx.healthdata.org/gbd-2017
10. Iwao S (2017) Revisiting the existing notion of continuous improvement (Kaizen): literature review and field research of Toyota from a perspective of innovation. Evolut Instit Econ Rev 14(1):29–59
11. Kessler RC (2001) Comorbidity. In: Smelser NJ, Baltes PB (eds) International encyclopaedia of the social & behavioural sciences, pergamon. PP 2389–2393
12. Lavie CJ, De Schutter A, Parto P, Jahangir E, Kokkinos P, Ortega F, Arena R, Milani R (2016) Obesity and prevalence of cardiovascular diseases and prognosis—the obesity paradox updated. Prog Cardiovascular Dis 58(5):537–547
13. McCartney M (2016) Media's misrepresentation of science. Retrieved October 27, 2021, from https://www.bmj.com/bmj/section-pdf/914631?path=/bmj/352/8044/Comment.full.pdf
14. Moodley R, Chiclana F, Caraffini F, Carter J (2019) A product-centric data mining algorithm for targeted promotions. J Retail Consum Serv 101940

15. Moodley R, Chiclana F, Carter J, Caraffini F (2020) Using data mining in educational administration: a case study on improving school attendance. Appl Sci 10(9):3116
16. National Health Service (NHS) (2021) High blood pressure—hypertension. Retrieved October 27, 2021, from www.nhs.uk/conditions/high-blood-pressure-hypertension/treatment/
17. Public Health England (PHE) (2015) Making sense of data: challenge and a responsibility. Retrieved October 27, 2021, from https://ukhsa.blog.gov.uk/2015/11/13/making-sense-of-data-a-challenge-and-a-responsibility/
18. World Health Organization (WHO) (2020) The top 10 causes of death. Retrieved October 27, 2021, from https://www.who.int/news-room/fact-sheets/detail/the-top-10-causes-of-death
19. University of Leicester Cardiology Research Team (LCG) (2019) Personal communication with leadership. Personal communication

Risk Detection of Heart Disease

Karina Macakaite and Arjab Singh Khuman⑩

Abstract Cardio Vascular Disease (CVD) is the leading cause of death worldwide and a significant contributor to the rising cost of health care. Due to the growing patient population, existing healthcare systems are becoming increasingly burdened and unable to effectively manage the increased demand for health care services. The purpose of this paper is to demonstrate the design of a fuzzy logic-based system for a patient's detection of heart disease risk at home. The system is implemented in the MATLAB software, using the fuzzy logic toolbox. This paper provides the technical description of the system and evaluates its performance. The dataset from the Framingham Heart Study was used for the system's implementation.

1 Introduction

Worldwide, the mortality rate from various diseases is continuing to rise at an alarming rate. According to the World Health Organization (WHO), cardiovascular disease is one of the deadliest diseases, accounting for millions of deaths every year (CVDs) [1]. Cardiovascular diseases are disorders of heart and blood vessels. Elevated blood pressure, high cholesterol, and obesity can be indicators of a higher risk of heart complications.

Identifying potential life-threatening factors at an early stage would allow for the possibility of avoiding the worst-case scenario in many situations. However, identifying early signs of CVD can be challenging. Factors such as high blood pressure rarely cause symptoms, and it is frequently referred to as the "silent killer" [2]. At times, it's extremely difficult to determine whether a person is at risk of contracting a disease. Each person is unique, and some indicators may be normal for some while

K. Macakaite
School of Computer Science and Informatics, De Montfort University, Leicester, UK
e-mail: P2429404@alumni365.dmu.ac.uk

A. S. Khuman (✉)
School of Computer Science and Informatics, Institute of Artificial Intelligence (IAI), Leicester, UK
e-mail: arjab.khuman@dmu.ac.uk

© The Author(s), under exclusive license to Springer Nature Singapore Pte Ltd. 2022
T. Chen et al. (eds.), *Artificial Intelligence in Healthcare*, Brain Informatics and Health,
https://doi.org/10.1007/978-981-19-5272-2_14

being abnormal for others, which creates lots of ambiguity. Another problem is long waiting times for non-urgent appointments with GP. If there is a risk of CVD, the prolonged waiting period can have a detrimental effect on health if the problem is not identified on time and no action of treatment is taken [3].

Until now, health care services have been designed in such a way that patients could visit a hospital when symptoms of a disease appeared, be diagnosed via various tests and be prescribed a treatment method to eliminate symptoms. Nowadays, it is easier to resolve medical issues, as technological advancements continue to have a positive effect on healthcare. Numerous researchers have developed Artificial Intelligence technologies such as fuzzy logic, artificial neural networks, and genetic algorithms to address problems of extreme uncertainty. In a large number of medical cases, fuzzy logic is used to reduce uncertainty in diagnosis and predict the risk of developing a disease [4].

Fuzzy logic is a kind of logic system which can define realities with more than a true and false statement and its final approach to compute based on the degrees of truth. Additionally, fuzzy logic is capable of dealing with truth values ranging from 0–1, which are referred to as degrees of truth. For instance, by utilizing fuzzy logic, a different logic value can be assigned to each disease, ranging from 0 to 1, based on the symptom's severity.

The purpose of this chapter is to propose the system for self-detection of CVD risk using patient-detectable factors that will aid in understanding current health status of a patient. In order to design a solution for the specific problem, a fuzzy logic-based decision-making system is used.

2   Related Work

In practice, a system which would show the precise results in real life applications like medicine could hardly be found. The boundaries are usually unclear when it comes to the relationship of the symptoms trying to determine the disease. In this case, the fuzzy logic is the ideal option to deal with approximate data like medicine. It is a powerful system for decision-making programmes such as structure classification systems and expert systems. There are numerous medical systems which have already been developed based on the fuzzy set and applied in treatments and diagnosis.

Fuzzy logic expert systems are critical in medical examinations because they produce an accurate evaluation report based on the medical data provided to the system. These types of systems enable rapid and simple medical examinations. Additionally, this beneficial in situations where medical professionals are not present. These systems produce results based on the knowledge they have accumulated from experts and authorities in their fields [5].

In the article titled "A fuzzy logic-based warning system for patient's classification" the authors demonstrate the implemented fuzzy logic-based health warning system. They have tried to design and implement the equivalent health warning system to The Modified Early Warning Score (MEWS) which was developed to assist hospital staff. Their collected data, about patient condition, vital signs, was classified into 1 to 15 risk groups. Depending on which classification the patient belongs to, the hospital personnel will be able to determine the procedure. The proposed fuzzy system was tested and compared with the results of the MEWS system. The outcome of the system based on fuzzy logic was as precise as the existing system. This research showed that the fuzzy approach can work from approximate values [6].

N. Allahverdi gave examples of fuzzy logic applications in medical areas. One of these applications was for the determination of disease risk. The fuzzy expert system has been designed to determine the risk of coronary heart disease and possible treatment method. Inputs were based on the people lifestyle and health characteristics, and the output value was the risk of the disease. This system calculated the total risk and depending on some factors the system provided an output, which was recommending the appropriate treatment, if it is needed. This case also showed that such systems can be useful for doctors to make a decision on treatments [7].

Also, other authors that were designing a fuzzy system to predict the diagnoses of the heart disease, were using similar parameters such as blood pressure, blood sugar, cholesterol, electrocardiography and other.

A. Zabeen, A. Utsav and K. Lal have presented the heart disease detection system with 80% accuracy. They have used seven inputs and one output processed with 50 distinct rules. They also did a comparison with a neural network system, which had less accuracy [8].

Another system was presented by V. Madaan and A. Goyal with 85% efficiency using eight inputs and one output, with 162 rules to cover all possibilities of symptoms which contributes to heart diseases. The input ranges and rules were validated by human experts before getting the final results [9].

Kasbe and Pippal [10] developed a system by taking a total of 86 fuzzy rules using ten inputs and one output. They have used all possible input variables with distinct combinations to calculate the corresponding output. After testing, their proposed system has achieved 93.33% accuracy. They state that this system's quality is based on the proper combination of the rules.

3 System Overview

Sometimes people are not aware of their health condition, as some diseases can be asymptomatic and can increase a risk of progressing further without them knowing about it. The sooner they are informed of the situation, the greater possibility that they will receive appropriate treatment and avoid complications.

The proposed system in this chapter is designed to assist people in determining the risk of heart disease prior to consulting with a physician. It is specifically targeting people above 18 as it requires a self-examination and contacting the doctor if needed.

After conducting the research, there were numerous of tests found which could help to detect the risk of CVD. However, some of tests require advanced medical equipment or qualified medical specialist to do lab tests and diagnostic procedures.

The system is designed using a fuzzy logic approach, and as a result, it requires appropriate inputs, which means that an average person could perform a test at home without the assistance of a medical professional. This would be beneficial because they would be able to get tested from the comfort of their own homes and would be more aware of their health condition as well.

The following are the factors that were found to be the most suitable for detecting cardiovascular disease risk and that could also be found or performed at home:

- Body mass index (BMI)
- Blood pressure (BP)
- Heart rate
- Cholesterol

Each input will be assigned to a category of a fuzzy set based on evidence from medical guidelines. By providing these inputs, the system is able to determine which of the defined rules should be executed and then return an output which is assigned to the result indicating the risk of CVD. There are five possible results:

1. Healthy
2. Mild risk
3. Elevated risk
4. High risk
5. Very High risk

Each of these results will give an instruction or recommendation to patients, what should they do next.

The system was implemented in MATLAB software using Mamdani fuzzy inference system. MATLAB has fuzzy toolbox which was used to represent the fuzzy sets graphically. It used the Framingham Heart Study dataset, which contains all of the input values that were required for the selected inputs, in order to improve accuracy.

4 System Design and Configuration

Four inputs were selected to produce an output which will predict the risk of the heart disease. Although BMI and BP are also sub systems as these systems require additional variables to get the result which will be used in the main risk detection system (see Fig. 1).

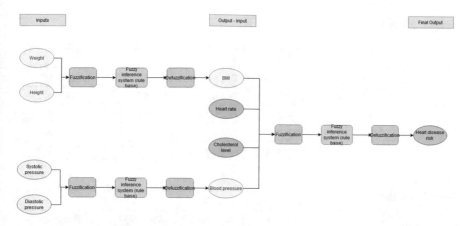

Fig. 1 Risk detection system

4.1 System Inputs

4.1.1 BMI

According to the medical article titled "The Impact of Obesity on the Cardiovascular System" [11], obesity is one of the main factors that contributes to heart disease. As a result, the body mass index (BMI) was chosen as one of the system's inputs when determining whether a person's weight is healthy for their height. This input will be further broken down into two inputs, as it requires the weight and height of the user and will result in the creation of a subsystem. The calculation of BMI can be seen in Eq. 1.

$$BMI = \frac{weight}{height\,(in\,meters)^2} \tag{1}$$

The average weight and height vary by continent [12]. Hence, based on the world data chart of average size and weight by continent, five fuzzy sets for weight and five for height were created (see Tables 1 and 2).

Initially, it was designed with a larger weight range and a smaller height range with less fuzzy sets, but due to the range difference, the results were inaccurate. This led to the adjustment of the range and the number equalisation of fuzzy sets. For both inputs the most left and right fuzzy sets were trapezoidal MF. The middle three fuzzy sets all presented in triangular MF, where the apex (the middle number of parameter values) is the average of particular fuzzy set range. All sets overlap to show gradual change from one to another.

The taller a person is, the more weight they need to maintain a healthy weight. For example, if a person is 160 cm tall and weighs 35 kg, it indicates that weight is unhealthy and it fall into the category of underweight, as the BMI is less than 18.5

Table 1 Weight

Weight [35 110] (kg)

Fuzzy set	Membership function	Parameter values	Range (kg)
Very light	Trapezoidal	[35 35 40 50]	(35–50)
Light	Triangular	[40 47.5 55]	(40–55)
Average	Triangular	[50 64.5 79]	(50–79)
Heavy	Triangular	[73 84 95]	(73–95)
Very heavy	Trapezoidal	[90 98 110 110]	(90–110)

Table 2 Height

Height [135 205] (cm)

Fuzzy set	Membership function	Parameter values	Range (cm)
Very short	Trapezoidal	[135 135 140 145]	(135–145)
Short	Triangular	[140 150 160]	(140–160)
Medium	Triangular	[155 167.5 180]	(155–180)
Tall	Triangular	[175 185 195]	(175–195)
Very tall	Trapezoidal	[190 195 205 205]	(190–205)

(see Table 3). If height is 160 cm and weight is 48 kg, it belongs, to 'healthy' fuzzy set, as the BMI is 18.8 (see Table 3). If the BMI is 18.8 and falls within the 'healthy' category, it is still considered a risky weight, as it is closer to the borderline, and it is very easy to lose weight and revert to the 'underweight' fuzzy set of the BMI variable. To be considered a member of the 'healthy' fuzzy set, the weight should be roughly in the middle.

The BMI output will be used as an input in the main system, which will determine the risk of heart disease.

Table 3 BMI

BMI [8 55]

Fuzzy set	Membership function	Parameter values	Range
Underweight	Trapezoidal	[8 8 17 19.5]	< 18.5
Healthy	Triangular	[17 22 27]	18.5 -24.9
Overweight	Triangular	[23 28 33]	25.0–29.9
Obese	Trapezoidal	[29 32 55 55]	> 30.0

4.1.2 Rules and Defuzzification Method

Simultaneous design of fuzzy sets and rules aided in the system's efficiency. It has been 80 rules in the beginning. However, the majority of them made no sense, and the results were the completely inaccurate. Later rules were created by comparing one of the weight fuzzy sets to each of the height fuzzy sets using the BMI matrix table. In this case, it was clear where these values fit into the BMI category. Following configuration, the total number of rules were 36.

Twenty training data values were used to evaluate the system's performance. When the results of each defuzzification method were compared, it was determined that the most accurate method was 'bisector,' which achieved 100% accuracy.

4.1.3 High Blood Pressure

High blood pressure, or hypertension, is a major risk factor for heart attacks, as it can damage blood vessels when it is too high. Hypertension can be asymptomatic, and can be developed, if it stays unnoticed, therefore it is very important to check the blood pressure regularly.

Blood pressure consists of two numbers. The first is systolic pressure, which is responsible for the heart contracting and pumping oxygen-rich blood to the organs. The second is diastolic, which is always less than systolic because it ensures that the heart muscle rests following contraction. That is why blood pressure will be divided into two inputs in order to obtain the final blood pressure reading, which will serve as the input for the final system output.

The Tables 4 and 5 show the actual ranges of systolic and diastolic pressures, which were expanded based on Joanna C. Silva's medical article [13]. The expanded values are displayed in the column titled 'parameter values.'

The highest membership degree is presented in the center of the fuzzy set range, and then slowly decreases and overlaps with another fuzzy set. This is why triangular MF was the most suitable to present 'normal', 'elevated' and 'high' fuzzy sets. The most left and right fuzzy sets are trapezoid MF.

Table 4 Systolic pressure

Systolic pressure			
Fuzzy set	Actual range	Membership function	Parameter values
Low	<90	Trapezoidal	[70 70 85 90]
Normal	90–120	Triangular	[80 105 130]
Elevated	120–130	Triangular	[110 125 140]
High	130–140	Triangular	[120 135 150]
Very high	>140	Trapezoidal	[135 140 160 160]

Table 5 Diastolic pressure

Diastolic pressure			
Fuzzy set	Actual range	Membership function	Parameter values
Low	<60	Trapezoidal	[40 40 55 60]
Normal	60–80	Triangular	[50 70 90]
High	80–90	Triangular	[70 85 100]
Very high	>90	Trapezoidal	[80 90 120 120]

Table 6 Blood pressure

BP [1 10]			
Fuzzy set	Membership function	Parameter values	Systolic/diastolic
Normal	Trapezoidal	[1 1 2 3]	Everything below 120/80
Elevated	Triangular	[2 3.5 5]	Between 120/40–129/80
High	Triangular	[4 5.5 7]	Between 130/80–139/89
Very high	Trapezoidal	[6.5 7 10 10]	Above 140/90

The final Blood Pressure (BP) range is illustrated in Table 6. Low blood pressure was not taken into consideration in this system because it does not have a significant impact on the development of heart disease. In most cases, it is even desirable when the blood pressure is low. The range was chosen between 1 and 10 to make it easier to visualise the blood pressure level. The smallest numbers indicate normal blood pressure, while the largest numbers indicate severe hypertension, which can result in heart attacks. Triangular MF was used for elevated and high fuzzy sets, as the apex has the highest membership degree. Due to the fact that this fuzzy set is at its peak, value is mostly true when degree is 1. The closer it is getting to another fuzzy set, the more membership degree of that fuzzy set decreases and overlaps with other fuzzy set. Trapezoid MF was used for normal and very high fuzzy sets.

The final result of both systolic and diastolic blood pressures is presented clearly in the matrix table in Fig. 2.

4.1.4 Rules and Defuzzification Method

The Blood Pressure system's rules were created using the same matrix table of systolic and diastolic pressures. Twenty logical rules were created. To perform defuzzification, the "centroid" was selected as it is where all of the membership's highest degrees are found in the fuzzy set. The 'LOM' or 'SOM' would be unsuitable here because they would return either the largest or smallest maximum crisp value.

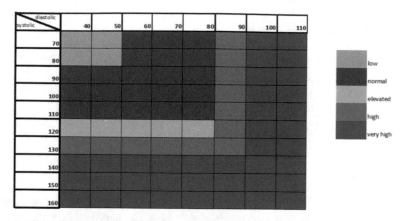

Fig. 2 Systolic and Diastolic matrix table

4.1.5 Heart Rate

Another input is resting heart rate. The heart rate is measured in a calm and relaxed state. In this condition, heart does not have to pump a large amount of the blood in our body, therefore it is easy to see any abnormalities that are out of healthy heartbeat range.

A normal resting heart rate is between 60–100 beats per minute (bpm). However, it can vary due to a variety of reasons. It can depend on the person's physical condition. People who are physically active usually have lower heart rate and maintain a steady heartbeat, as with each heartbeat it pumps greater amount of blood.

A heart rate higher than 100 can be sometimes due to the stress or other illness. Although, if rapid heart rate consistently occurs in resting condition, it should not be ignored and immediately treated. The increased heartbeat could disrupt normal heart function and lead to serious complications.

The Table 7 illustrates the resting heart rate of a person with a 'low', 'normal', or 'high' heart rate. The first column displays the normal heart rate range. Everything below 60 is considered low, while everything above 100 is considered high. However, 'normal' fuzzy set will overlap with 'low' and 'high' fuzzy sets. As regard to the facts about physical active people and increased heart rate due to the stress can be considered sometimes as normal, if not consistent [14]. That is why the range for the 'normal' fuzzy set was broadened and the triangular MF type was used, as the perfect heart rate is located in the middle of the fuzzy set. For the 'low' and 'high' fuzzy sets, trapezoidal MF were used.

Table 7 Heart rate

Heart rate [20 160]				
Normal heart rate	Fuzzy set	Range for my system	Membership function	Parameter values
60–100	Low	<60	Trapezoidal	[20 20 40 60]
	Normal	30–110	Triangular	[30 70 110]
	High	<90	Trapezoidal	[100 110 160 160]

4.1.6   Cholesterol

High cholesterol can lead to heart attacks and strokes. It usually does not have any signs or symptoms, so it is imperative to check the cholesterol level regularly. It was chosen as an input because it can be done at home using the finger prick test, which collects a small amount of blood.

In previously created systems mostly three values of cholesterol were used which are Low Density Lipoprotein (LDL), High Density Lipoproteins (HDL) and triglycerides. In this case, the total amount of cholesterol was used, which includes all of these values, as most home tests measure only total cholesterol. It is measured in milligrams per decilitre (mg/dL).

Low cholesterol was excluded, as according to medical article written by R. Goldman it does not have a big impact on the heart diseases, usually the lower cholesterol the better, however the high levels are causing the problems [15].

Table 8 illustrates fuzzy sets of 'normal', 'borderline high' and 'very high'. On the second column, the range based on medical guidelines is shown. For 'normal' fuzzy, trapezoidal MF type was used, everything below 200 will be considered as 'normal'. For 'very high' MF trapezoidal was also used, however the range starts from 220 mg/dL and goes above. MF for 'borderline high', is triangular type, and ranges between 170 mg/dL and 239 mg/dL.

Table 8 Cholesterol levels

Cholesterol levels [100 280]			
Fuzzy set	Actual range of cholesterol levels	Membership function	Parameter values
Normal	<200 mg/dL	Trapezoidal	[100 100 180 200]
Borderline high	200–239 mg/dL	Triangular	[170 204 239]
Very high	>240 mg/dL	Trapezoidal	[220 240 280 280]

Table 9 Final risk output

Risk level [−1 4]		
Fuzzy set	Membership function	Parameter values
Healthy	Trapezoidal	[−1 −1 −0.1 0.8]
Mild	Triangular	[0 0.8 2]
Elevated	Triangular	[1 1.8 3]
High	Triangular	[2 2.8 3.5]
Very high	Trapezoidal	[3 3.1 4 4]

4.2   System Output

4.2.1   Prediction of the Risk Level

The output of the main system is the Risk level detector of any heart diseases. Table 9 presents five fuzzy sets, which are 'healthy', 'mild','elevated','high' and 'very high'. If value is in the healthy range that means that there is nothing to worry about and just maintain healthy lifestyle. Mild range shows the slight risk of the disease, but it is not urgent to see a doctor, however it is still recommended. The elevated fuzzy set means that it is recommended to book an appointment to see specialist and get medical advice. If the value is within 'high' range, it is recommended to not hesitate and see doctor as soon as possible, and 'very high' risk means is urgent to get the treatment and these patients should be prioritized to see a doctor as soon as possible.

4.2.2   Rules and Defuzzification Method of Final System

The main system used all defined inputs: Cholesterol level, heart rate, BMI, and Blood pressure. As mentioned earlier, BMI and BP inputs are the outputs from their subsystem. To create rules for this system it had been started from the simplest case where the output is 'healthy' or "very high". If all inputs are normal/low/healthy, the output is always healthy. If all of the inputs are high/very high/obese, the output will indicate that risk as very high. If any of the inputs are in high range, that means the output will be elevated. If there more than two in high range, then the output will be 'high'. In total, 41 rules were created. Defuzzification method was 'centroid', as it used mostly the triangular MFs, where apex is the center of the defined range.

5   System Performance

Throughout the system's development, it was trained using 20 chosen data values from the Framingham Heart study dataset. For the testing part, another 20 randomly selected data values were used, to see the efficiency of the system. Each subsystem was tested separately before running the final system which detects the risk of CVD. It was important to make sure that each subsystem has high output accuracy, as this is used as an input for the main system. It has been extensively tested with each of the inputs in order to achieve the desired results. A small change in the range of a single fuzzy set could have a significant impact on the overall performance of the system.

Following several tests on the BMI subsystem, the most effective defuzzification method was Bisector, which achieved a 75% accuracy rate. Blood pressure subsystem had 100% accuracy using 'centroid', 'mom' and 'bisector' methods while conducting some testing. With all inputs prepared, the risk detection system has been tested with all possible defuzzification methods. Considering that BMI subsystem is less accurate, the results were still satisfying as it has almost 100% accuracy.

6 Critical Evaluation

Evaluating the performance of the risk detection system was performed well. The system was accurate. However, it cannot be completely reliable as BMI subsystem has some errors.

It was expected that the BMI subsystem would operate more precisely, as it was built on a matrix table containing all possible BMI outcomes. As the system was developed and trained on 20 dataset values, it could be one of the reasons why the system had some inaccuracies, even when it had 100% of accuracy. However, when it was tested with another 20 different values, it produced a number of errors. A sufficient training dataset would result in a better results and more efficient system. Another issue was that the BMI subsystem was designed for all adults, and the range was based on the average height and weight of adults on each continent. It would be more efficient to design a system for a single continent or country, as the average height and weight would be more precise.

Blood pressure subsystem performance has been more accurate, even when the subsystem was designed similarly to the BMI subsystem. Correspondingly, it was trained on 20 input data and tested on 20 dataset values. However, the results were correct both times. The only distinction between the two subsystems was that the BP subsystem's fuzzy sets and ranges were based on medical guidelines. As they are already correct, all that was required was to expand the range of fuzzy sets so that they could overlap. Regarding the other fuzzy sets, cholesterol, and heart rate, they were similar to BP as the number of fuzzy sets and their range were defined according to medical guidelines.

The system still needs to be greatly improved. As a result, it is currently unsuitable for use in real-world applications. The system could be improved by adding the age and gender of the patient, which would help to improve the performance of BMI system. It would produce more accurate results, as it would be more precise in classifying an individual's healthy weight. In addition, the risk detection system for heart disease could make use of input such as a family history of heart disease. If one of the family members has health problems, there is a possibility that disease will develop. As a result, this factor would also contribute to system accuracy improvement.

7 Conclusion

Fuzzy logic can be used in a variety of applications, and it is especially useful in today's healthcare. It can greatly simplify the work of medical professionals by designing a correct system with the appropriate knowledgebase that will make decisions and provide results based on that knowledge.

This chapter's specific system was created Mamdani fuzzy system, which detects the risk of heart disease based on four inputs: cholesterol, heart rate, BMI, and blood pressure. The goal of designed system was to help become more aware of their health condition. Majority of the fuzzy sets and ranges were defined using medical guidelines where it says exactly what range is 'healthy' or 'normal' for patients. As a result, both the blood pressure subsystem and the risk detection system performed well. The BMI subsystem was defined using fuzzy sets that were based on the average height and weight of all people on the planet. Because every range of the fuzzy set was approximate, the system's performance was lower when compared to the BP subsystem and the Risk detection system, for example.

In order to achieve the desired performance, it is necessary to conduct extensive testing with the appropriate number of fuzzy sets and logically defined ranges of each input. The use of the incorrect fuzzy set range or the incorrect rules number can cause the system to perform poorly and produce results that are completely misleading.

References

1. WHO 2017 World health organization. https://www.who.int/en/news-room/fact-sheets/detail/cardiovascular-diseases-(cvds) Last Accessed 23 11 2020
2. Centers for disease control and prevention (2019) Know your risk for heart disease. https://www.cdc.gov/heartdisease/risk_factors.htm Last Accessed 11 09 2021
3. Thorlby R, Gardner T, Turton C (2019) NHS performance and waiting times. https://www.health.org.uk/publications/long-reads/nhs-performance-and-waiting-times Last Accessed 12 09 2021
4. Ahmadi H et al (2018) Diseases diagnosis using fuzzy logic methods: A systematic and meta-analysis review. Comput Methods Programs Biomed 161:145–172
5. Rana M, Sedamkar R (2013) Design of expert system for medical diagnosis using fuzzy logic. Int J Sci Eng Res 4(6)
6. AI-Dmour JA, Sagahyroon A, AI-Ali A, Abusnana S (2017) A fuzzy logic–based warning system for patients classification. Health Inform J 25(3):1004–1024
7. Allahverdi N (2014) Design of fuzzy expert systems and its applications in some medical areas. Int J Appl Math Electron Comput
8. Zabeen A, Utsav A, Lal K (2018) Detection of Heart Disease Applying Fuzzy Logics and Its Comparison with Neural Networks. IEEE
9. Madaan V, Goyal A (2018) X-Cardio: fuzzy inference system to diagnose heart diseases. IEEE

10. Kasbe T, Pippal RS (2017) Design of heart disease diagnosis system using fuzzy logic. IEEE
11. Csige I, Ujvarosy D (2018) The impact of obesity on the cardiovascular system. J Diabetes Res
12. World data (2019) Average sizes of men and women. https://www.worlddata.info/average-bod
    yheight.php Last Accessed 05 12 2020
13. Silva JC (2018) What are diastole and systole in blood pressure?. https://www.medicalnewst
    oday.com/articles/321447 Last Accessed 3 12 2020
14. Shaikh J (2020) What is a good heart rate for my age?. https://www.medicinenet.com/
    what_is_a_good_heart_rate_for_my_age/article.htm Last Accessed 01 12 2020
15. Goldman R (2020) The recommended cholesterol levels by age. https://www.healthline.com/
    health/high-cholesterol/levels-by-age LastAccessed 1 12 2020

AI for Diabetes

A Case Study of Diabetes Diagnosis Using a Neuro-Fuzzy System

Reginald Russell, Tianhua Chen, and Richard Hill

Abstract Diabetes is a complex disorder that can lead to numerous severe complications. Early diagnosis and treatment significantly contributes to a better quality of life for patients and can protect against associated complications. This chapter proposes the application of an Adaptive Neuro-fuzzy Inference System (ANFIS), with system parameters optimised by Genetic Algorithm (GA) and Particle Swarm Optimisation (PSO). A comparative experimental study is conducted with application upon the UCI Early-Stage Diabetes Risk Prediction dataset, demonstrating effectiveness of the neuro-fuzzy system in diagnosing diabetes.

Keywords Diabetes · Fuzzy system · Neuro-fuzzy · ANFIS

1 Introduction

Diabetes mellitus is a disease affecting the human metabolism. This complex disorder is associated with prolonged hyperglycemia, due to defective insulin production or response within the human body. Initial symptoms are characterized by increased urination, thirst and appetite. Without treatment, diabetes can result in a cascade of systemic complications, such as, diabetic ketoacidosis, hyperosmolar hyperglycemic state, glucose toxicity, and even death. Prolonged conditions include heart or kidney disease, stroke, nerve, vision, or cognitive impairment [31, 32].

Of the various forms of diabetes, Type 1 and Type 2 are the most common. Type 1, or juvenile diabetes, is a condition where the pancreas is unable to produce sufficient insulin due to a beta cell deficiency. Type 2, or adult-onset diabetes, is a condition where the body does not exhibit the proper response to insulin, leading to insulin deficiencies over time. Type 2 diabetes is linked to obesity and is considered preventable. With early diagnosis, symptoms are easily mitigated via prescribed medication, diet and lifestyle changes.

R. Russell · T. Chen (✉) · R. Hill
School of Computing and Engineering, University of Huddersfield, Huddersfield, UK
e-mail: T.Chen@hud.ac.uk

© The Author(s), under exclusive license to Springer Nature Singapore Pte Ltd. 2022
T. Chen et al. (eds.), *Artificial Intelligence in Healthcare*, Brain Informatics and Health,
https://doi.org/10.1007/978-981-19-5272-2_15

Because the common symptoms of diabetes are often associated with other illnesses, many patients suffering from obesity or other diseases with a symptomatic profile similar to diabetes may not be aware of their condition, until as much as 10 years after onset [32]. Early diagnosis of diabetes is, therefore, paramount. Recent advances in artificial intelligence (AI), along with rapidly generated electronic data have resulted in the development of intelligent systems in numerous disciplines [34], including the health and medicine sector [2, 3, 13, 24–26]. Such intelligent systems, when trained on historical patient data, can be used to establish a predictive model of factors, symptoms and indicators associated with a specific disease, for instance, the early diagnosis of diabetes.

Among the techniques that have been employed in medical settings, resulting in an immediate effect on the well-being of patients, fuzzy rule-based systems (FRBS) [5] expressed through a collection of IF–THEN conditional statements are well-known for interpretability through their approximate reasoning framework designed to mimic human reasoning and support non-technical experts, such as clinicians, to comprehend and interrogate any machine-drawn conclusions. Constructed from fuzzy sets that permit partial matching, the use of a fuzzy system also facilitates handling of the uncertainty and imprecision that may arise from inaccurate test results, or ambiguity in the verbal description of symptoms, thus, further enhancing the underlying system's diagnostic capability.

In working towards establishing an intelligent model for early detection of diabetes, this paper proposes the popular Adaptive Neuro-fuzzy Inference System (ANFIS) [11], with optimization of system parameters adjusted by a Genetic Algorithm (GA) and Particle Swarm Optimisation (PSO), validated by the commonly used UCI Early-Stage Diabetes Risk Prediction dataset (Dataset) [23].

The remainder of this paper is organized as follows. Section II reviews the related work of recent fuzzy systems as applied to diabetes diagnosis. Section III presents details of the ANFIS framework as well as GA and PSO. Section IV presents and discusses the experimental study. Section V concludes the paper and identifies ideas for further development.

2 Literature Review

FRBSs have been applied to numerous medical sectors to generate predictive outcomes and resolve diagnosis problems [4]. A 2006 study [19] applied FRBS to detect diabetes using principal component analysis (PCA) for feature reduction, and an adaptive neuro-fuzzy inference system (ANFIS) to reason and make decisions for patient classifications. Combined with tenfold cross validation (CV), 89.47% accuracy was achieved. Similarly, [4] used a decision tree initialized ANFIS-based fuzzy system for diabetes diagnosis; while in 2010, [6] used if–then fuzzy rules in combination with ant colony optimization to diagnose diabetes. Classification demonstrated 79.48% accuracy, which improved in subsequent iterations using ant pheromone values as a control to reinforce the rule.

In 2011, [14] presented FRBS to diagnose diabetes with a semantic decision support agent and a 5-layer, fuzzy ontology-based model. The 5 fuzzy layers of the ontology included: (1) knowledge, (2) group relation, (3) group domain, (4) personal relation, and (5) fuzzy personal domain. Concepts were built up over the knowledge domain, along with the creation of concept relations. Classification accuracy ranged from 77.3–91.2%. In 2015, [7] also developed a fuzzy ontology for diabetes prediction. A fuzzy logic algorithm with a trapezoidal waveform for membership function was implemented. Inconsistent data was eliminated via min–max normalization, then knowledge was extracted with an ontology graph showing abstract symptomatic relationships to form the basis for a high accuracy, low complexity model.

Some studies have applied case-Based Reasoning (CBR), to address diabetic diagnosis. For example, [17] used FRBS for managing Type 2 diabetes, pairing rule and case-based reasoning. In conjunction, fuzzification addressed factor interdependencies (age, gender, and BMI) for personalized diabetes management. Triangular and trapezoidal membership functions facilitated classification and rule generation. However, output was rendered only as general recommendations. More recently, [1] combined CBR and FRBS to predict diabetes by evaluating similar cases using a k-nearest neighbors algorithm, facilitated by a fuzzified decision tree, resulting in a highest accuracy of 90% (using blood sugar/average blood sugar).

In 2011, [12] created a scaled FRBS decision system for the early detection of possible diabetes using triangular membership functions based on low, medium, and high class-based numbers, achieving 85% accuracy. Another paper, [28] designed a similar rule-based system which was tested and validated against the medical diagnosis of 30 various diabetic patients. A 2018 study, [16] developed a 5-step FRBS for early diagnosis of diabetes, consisting of: (1) domain problem, (2) fuzzification, (3) fuzzy rules, (4) defuzzification, and (5) evaluation. 96% accuracy was achieved (48 out of 50 correct diagnoses).

A 2016 study, [22] combined FRBS, fuzzification and FireflyBat optimization for diabetes diagnosis. Feature reduction and a locality preserving projection algorithm helped to navigate the search space without losing accuracy. In 2015, [15] developed a fuzzy hierarchical model for early diabetes detection. The model's 3 variables included the initial inputs, temporary fuzzy input values, and the predictive output. Crisp values were fuzzified using a 5-step inference process, each with 9 rules working together to determine the fuzzy and predictive output, ending with crisp values.

In contrast, [21] combined fuzzy modeling with a neural network for diabetic diagnostics of new symptoms. Fuzzy membership functions and a backpropagation algorithm were used to classify patients into 2 categories, Type 2 diabetes or non-diabetic using a neural network in real time. Accuracy was achieved at 82.9% for training and 83.3% for testing. In a subsequent paper, [20] focused on the uncertain hazard boundary of negative risk factors for diabetes. Association rules were used to identify attribute patterns and correspondence by measuring support percentages and confidence levels. The fuzzy association rules were constructed by pairing patterns with their matching class labels, resulting in a highest confidence level of 1.

The recent literature clearly suggests that although there has been much progress using FRBS for predictive diagnosis, particularly with diabetes, still more is needed. Some of the best results have been obtained when FRBS was combined with other methodologies. For instance, fuzzy logic paired with neural networks or other optimization techniques have demonstrated effectiveness for accuracy and minimizing ambiguity. However, there is no one classification method that can encompass all of the various diabetic symptoms without diluting its relevance or accuracy.

As a result, many of the studies reviewed generally focused on specific features or goals in their models, leaving other aspects unaddressed. Certain demographics were also overlooked as some studies focused solely on gender, specific symptoms, diabetes type, or age groups. Moreover, most models could only predict singular diabetic outcomes. Multiple diabetic disease types could not be identified or classified. Future FRBS models will continue to combine methodologies to obtain better accuracy and overcome these limitations, using adaptive neural networks combined with fuzzy or other optimizing algorithms. Our work, following on the popular trend as reviewed, aims to establish a case study demonstrating the effectiveness of fuzzy systems in support of diabetes diagnosis.

3 Methods

Owing to the proven effectiveness of the Adaptive Neuro Fuzzy Inference System's (ANFIS) ability, in numerous applications [4], to harness the computational power of an Artificial Neural Network (ANN) and a Fuzzy Inference System's (FIS) ability to imitate human reasoning, this paper proposes to apply the ANFIS framework to the diagnosis of diabetes, which is further enhanced by the exploration of two powerful evolutionary algorithms, i.e., the Genetic Algorithm (GA) and Particle Swarm Optimisation (PSO), that will be employed to optimize parameters embedded within ANFIS. The following reviews the technical details of these methods.

1. *Adaptive Neuro Fuzzy Inference System (ANFIS)*

Takagi–Sugeno ANFIS is configured with inputs, outputs, and weights that correspond to FIS-type measurements, in a 5-layered structure [29, 33]. Assuming two fuzzy rules, inputs (x, y), and output (z), ANFIS can be visualized by the graphical structures depicted below in Figs. 1 and 2 [11].

   Rule 1. If x is A_1 and y is B_1, then $f_1 = p_1 x + q_1 y + r_1$.
   Rule 2. If x is A_2 and y is B_2, then $f_2 = p_2 x + q_2 y + r_2$.
   The individual layers can be described accordingly:

Layer 1, Fuzzification. Nodes are square and adaptive, fuzzifying inputs from x and y for membership function output.

$$O_i^1 = \mu_{Ai}(x),$$

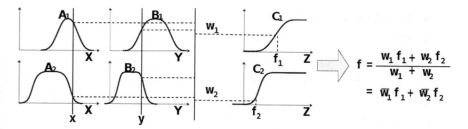

Fig. 1 Example FIS structure

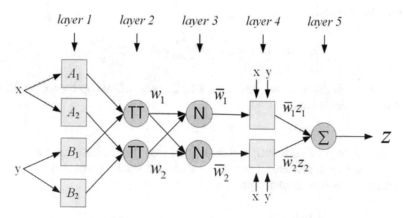

Fig. 2 Equivalent ANFIS structure

where,

x = input, to node i.

A_i = word label related to node function.

O^l_i = node membership function.

$\mu_{Ai}(x)$ = Gaussian, bell-shaped, or other membership function.

Layer 2, Product Multiplier. All nodes are circular, labeled Π, and fixed, functioning as signal and corresponding rule strength multipliers for weight, ω_i, output.

$$\omega_i = \mu_{Ai}(x) \times \mu_{Bi}(x), i = 1, 2$$

Layer 3, Normalization. Nodes are labeled N, remain circular and fixed, calculating rule strength ratios and normalizing weights.

$$\bar{\omega}_i = \frac{\omega_i}{\omega_1 + \omega_2}, i = 1, 2$$

Layer 4, Defuzzification. Adaptive layer with parameters for first order rule consequents.

$$O_i^4 = \overline{\omega}f_i = \overline{\omega}(p_i x + q_i y + r_i),$$

where,

$\overline{\omega}_i = $ output,

$(p_i, q_i, r_i) = $ the set of consequent parameters.

Layer 5, Output Finalization. Singular node, circular and fixed, aggregates signals and finalizes output [11].

$$O_i^5 = overall\ output = \sum_i \overline{\omega}_i f_i = \frac{\sum_i \omega_i f_i}{\sum_i \omega_i}.$$

Overall, the nodes in layer 1 and 4 are adaptive and will be optimized by the GA and PSO as reviewed below.

2. Genetic Algorithm (GA)

GA implements population-based optimization that mimics biological differentiation and selection to achieve its results. GA populates with particles that represent potential chromosome or phenotype solutions.

$$M\ individuals,\ Pop\ (g) = \{x_1(g), \ldots, x_M(g)\}$$

Through various iterations, these chromosomes evolve into potential chromosome-like solutions, until the required criteria (population number or processing time) are met resulting in an optimum solution [9, 10].

3. *Particle Swarm Optimization (PSO)*

By simulating the socialization of a flock of birds, the PSO algorithm uses a fitness function to search for the best values of the optimal particles in each iteration. One best solution is each particle's current *pbest*, the best personal solution attained so far by the particle.

$$pbest_i = F(\vec{x}(t))$$
$$\vec{x}_{pbest_i} = \vec{x}_i(t)$$

Another best solution is *gbest,* the best global solution achieved so far by any member of the swarm.

$$gbest_i = F(\vec{x}(t))$$
$$\vec{x}_{gbest} = \vec{x}_i(t)$$

PSO's update rule imparts memory and social ability, enabling each particle to remember its own historical *pbest* so far, and share that information with other particles [27]. Degrees of trust can be established to increase community or isolation, influencing each particle's velocity or position [8, 18].

$$\vec{v}_i(t) = \vec{v}_i(t-1) + \rho_1\left(\vec{x}_{pbest_i} - \vec{x}_i(t)\right) + \rho_2\left(\vec{x}_{gbest} - \vec{x}_i(t)\right)$$

where,
random variables $= \rho_1$ and ρ_2.
$\rho_1 = r_1 C_1$ and $\rho_2 = r_2 C_2$, C is a constant[1] with $r_1, r_2 \sim U\,(0,1)$.
cognitive component $= \rho_1 = \left(\vec{x}_{pbest_i} - \vec{x}_i(t)\right)$.
social component $= \rho_2\left(\vec{x}_{gbest} - \vec{x}_i(t)\right)$.

4 Experimentation

A. *Understanding the Dataset*

The Dataset was obtained from the National Institute of Diabetes and Digestive and Kidney Diseases with 768 observations, a mix of positive and negative diagnoses for diabetes, along with 8 clinical variables and 1 target. It was originally used in a study to predict diabetes in Pima Indian women. Observations were 21 years of age or older, of Pima Indian heritage, and residing in Phoenix, Arizona, USA.

Of the Dataset's 768 diabetic observations, there were 268 positives and 500 negatives, along with 8 clinical variables: (1) past pregnancies, (2) 2-h oral glucose levels (mg/dl), (3) diastolic blood pressure (mm Hg), (4) triceps skin-fold thickness (mm), (5) insulin levels (mu U/ml), (6) body mass index (BMI, kg/m2), (7) diabetes pedigree function (DPF), and 8) Age. Also, the sole target (Outcome), was a binary variable used to classify the testing result (0, negative: 1, positive) see Table 1 [23].

B. *Data Pre-processing*

Preprocessing of the data included normalization to fix variable values between 0 to 1, reducing data bias. Separate datasets were created for the inputs/target and transposed to fit a row, rather than column, orientation. No missing data, values, or N/As were found.

C. *Model Development*
(1) *ANFIS*

The model was developed using MATLAB, version R2020b (Matlab). Data was split 70/30 for training and testing over a network topology of 8 inputs, 1 output, and 1

---

[1] r is a random variable with a standard uniform distribution between 0 and 1.

Table 1 Pima Indian diabetes data statistics

Variable	Label	Mean	Std D.	Min/Max
X1	Pregnancies	3.8	3.4	1/17
X2	Glucose	120.9	32	56/197
X3	Blood pressure	69.1	19.4	24/110
X4	Skin thickness	20.5	16	7/52
X5	Insulin	79.8	115.2	15/846
X6	BMI	32	7.9	18.2/57.3
X7	Diabetes Pedigree Function (DPF)	0.5	0.3	0.085/2.32
X8	Age	33.2	11.8	21/81

hidden layer with 10 FIS rules. In Matlab, Gaussian membership functions and fuzzy c-means subtractive clustering were used to form the base structure [30]. After an initial PCA, input variables were reduced from 8 to 6, and then further reduced to only 5.

The model structure using 6 variables is depicted below for illustrative purposes (Fig. 3).

(2) *GA Algorithm*

Binary GA was implemented with roulette wheel selection, crossover, and mutation. After implementation of the ANFIS structure, ANFIS was trained on its antecedent and conclusion parameters with GA to optimize layers 1 and 4, for Gaussian membership functions (MF) and coefficients for first order consequent, respectively.

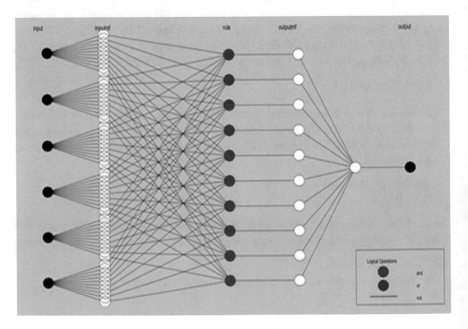

Fig. 3 Illustrated ANFIS implementation (6 variables)

During the training process, MFs were transformed using the antecedent parameters and the conclusion parameters to form genetic phenotypes or chromosomes, discrete bits of 0's and 1's, equal in length to the number of original inputs, which functioned as binary chromosomes where 1 selected for the attribute and 0 did not [9, 10].

GA initiated with a random population, using several operators, designed to find a solution to the objective function. Selection simulated genetic survival of the fittest. Crossover emulated the natural mating process for genetic diffusion and expression. Mutation produced more diversity and prevented the global search from stalling in local minima. Fitness of potential solutions, or chromosomes, was measured by the mean squared error and its standard deviation (MSE/RMSE) to evaluate the model's prediction residuals, $f(x)$ fitted for each potential solution [9, 10].

$$L_{fit} = \frac{1}{n} \sum_{i=1}^{n} (f_i - t_i)^2$$

$t =$ the vector of training targets.
$n =$ the instances in the training data.

The trend shown in Table 4 shows decreasing cost and MSE/RMSE results as the iterations increase with the lowest cost (0.7838) reached at 500 iterations without PCA (and 0.7912 with PCA). The parameters used for training ANFIS with GA and the various iterations are given in Table 2, below.

The parameters and the various iterations for GA are given in Table 2, below.

The process for GA was as follows:

(1) Population generated.
(2) Particles assigned random values.
(3) Population selection and sorting.

Table 2 GA parameters

Parameters	Value		
Iterations	100	300	500
Population	25	50	50
Chromosome length	8	8	8
MaxGen	100	300	500
MaxStallGen	100	300	500
Selection method	Roulette wheel		
Selection pressure	8	8	8
Crossover fraction	0.4	0.4	0.4
Crossover offspring	2	2	2
Mutation percentage	0.7	0.7	0.7
Mutation rate	0.15	0.15	0.15

(4)   Fitness function applied.

Main Loop:

(5)   Iteration started.
(6)   Crossover based on predetermined probability (0.4).
(7)   Creation and evaluation of new offspring.
(8)   Mutation based on predetermined probability (0.7).
(9)   Fitness function evaluated newly merged population.
(10) Termination if requirements met.
(11) If not, return to step 4.

(3)   *PSO Algorithm*

In addition to using GA for optimising ANFIS, PSO was also used to adapt the antecedent and conclusion parameters of ANFIS to optimize layers 1 and 4, for Gaussian membership functions (MF) and coefficients for first order consequent, respectively.

During PSO training, each PSO particle maintained its own cognitive and social ability and represented a unique potential solution based on its position in the search space. At each iteration, every particle knew its own personal best, *pbest*, and the *gbest* of the swarm. The aim of each particle, at each iteration, was to use its current speed/distance to move from *pbest* to *gbest*. The mean square error, and its standard deviation (MSE/RMSE), was used to evaluate the algorithm's performance. The trend shown in Table 5 shows decreasing cost and MSE/RMSE results as the iterations increase with the lowest cost (0.6799) reached at 500 iterations. The parameters used for training ANFIS with PSO and the various iterations are given in Table 3, below [8, 9, 27].

The process for PSO was as follows:

(1)   Swarm generated.
(2)   Particles randomly positioned.
(3)   Particle velocity initialized.
(4)   Fitness function evaluated positions and quality of solutions.
(5)   Each particle's *pbest* position updated.
(6)   *gbest* updated.

Table 3 PSO parameters

Parameters	Value		
Iterations	100	300	500
Population	25	50	50
Inertia weight	1	1	1
Damping factor	0.99	0.99	0.99
Personal training coefficient c1	1	1	1
General training coefficient c2	2	2	2

Table 4 ANFIS-GA testing results

ANFIS-GA testing/training iterations

100			300	500
BestCost	w/o PCA	0.7948	0.8078	0.7838
	w/ PCA	0.8415	0.8006	0.7912
MSE	w/o PCA	0.7990/0.6318	0.6454/0.6526	0.8035/0.6143
	w/ PCA	0.7053/0.7081	0.7974/0.6409	0.7503/0.6260
RMSE	w/o PCA	0.8939/0.7948	0.8034/0.8078	0.8963/0.7838
	w/ PCA	0.8398/0.8415	0.8930/0.8006	0.8662/0.7912
Error Mean	w/o PCA	0.0036/0.0153	0.0082/−0.0252	−0.0136/−0.0116
	w/ PCA	0.0037/0.0078	−0.0438/0.0205	−0.0684/−0.0371
Error St. D.	w/o PCA	0.8958/0.7954	0.8051/0.8082	0.8982/0.7844
	w/ PCA	0.8516/0.8422	0.8938/0.8010	0.8653/0.7910

Table 5 ANFIS-PSO testing results

ANFIS-PSO testing/training iterations

		100	300	500
BestCost	w/o PCA	0.8139	0.6808	0.6799
	w/ PCA, NB, SVM	0.8159	0.7350	0.7353
MSE	w/o PCA	0.6778/0.6625	0.8624/0.4635	0.8820/0.4623
	w/ PCA, NB, SVM	0.7197/0.6658	0.8859/0.5403	1.0697/0.5408
RMSE	w/o PCA	0.8232/0.8139	0.9286/0.6808	0.9391/0.6799
	w/ PCA, NB, SVM	0.8483/0.8159	0.9412/0.7350	1.0343/0.7353
Error Mean	w/o PCA	−0.1247/−0.0210	0.2126/−0.0122	0.0342/0.0007
	w/ PCA, NB, SVM	0.0346/0.0304	0.0903/−0.0104	−0.1185/−0.0190
Error St. D.	w/o PCA	0.8155/0.8144	0.9060/0.6813	0.9405/0.6805
	w/ PCA, NB, SVM	0.8494/0.8161	0.9389/0.7356	1.0297/0.7358

Main Loop:

(7) Velocity and position updated/limits applied.
(8) Velocity mirror effect applied.
(9) Positions and quality of solutions evaluated.
(10) Particle *pbest* updated.
(11) *gbest* updated.
(12) Determine if fitness function requirements met.
(13) If not, return to step 7.

(4) *PCA*

PCA was used for feature selection and as an evaluative tool. Eigenvalues were calculated with visualizations, including variance/percentage of variance, and distributions to better understand variable importance.

The top 3 PCA scores were Pregnancies (PC1 @ 29%), Glucose (PC2 @ 20%), then a sharp drop with BloodPressure (PC3 @ 13%). These top 3 PCA scores explained roughly 52% of the data variance see Fig. 4.

PC1-PC6 described roughly 87% of the total variance. PC7 (DPF) and PC8 (Age) explained only 7%, see Fig. 5 below.

After some additional analysis, PCA was further modified to remove PC6 and additional optimization was applied, using only PC1-PC5 to describe 90% of the data variance.

(5) *Optimization*

Matlab's ANFIS hybrid training algorithm was used for initial optimization. Training and testing epoch iterations were 100, 300, and 500 for two different versions of the model, with/without PCA: (1) ANFIS-GA, and (2) ANFIS-PSO.

The best result was obtained using the ANFIS-PSO/PCA model. Initially, this model was implemented with 8 variables. PCA analysis was used to decrease the

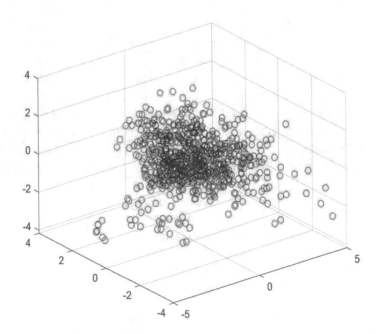

Fig. 4 Scatterplot of the top 3 variables

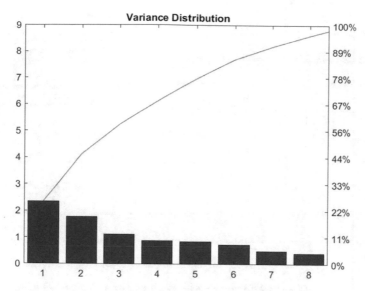

Fig. 5 Variance distribution

number of variables from 8 to 6. PSO was then used to train the model. Upon further PCA, the model was implemented with just 5 predictive variables (PC1—PC5). Additional optimization techniques were implemented using Naïve Bayes (NB), and Support Vector Machines (SVM) to produce results superior to ANFIS-GA/PCA.

(6) *Comparative Study with Naïve Bayes and Support Vector Machine Optimization*

ANFIS-PSO/PCA's superior performance employed tenfold CV, and NB optimized with SVM. Accuracy of 77.3% was achieved. NB achieved a minimum classification error (MCE) and bestpoint of 0.2525 after about 7 iterations. At this point, PCA was modified and only the first 5 variables were retained to explain 90% of data variance. After the added optimization with SVM, the MCE was further reduced: (1) initially to 0.229, then (2) 0.228, and (3) 0.224 after 46 iterations, as illustrated by the Figs. 6 and 7 below.

The CM shows the number of observations considered (768). Of that number, 443 (88.6%) were classified correctly as negative (depicted as lower bound, −0.73164) and 151 (56.3%) were classified correctly as positive (depicted as upper bound, 1.365).

However, 57 (11.4%) were false positives (negative but incorrectly classified as positive) and 117 (43.7%) were false negatives (positive but incorrectly classified as negative). The true positive rate (TPR) for negative diagnosis was 88.6 and 56.3% for positive diagnosis. The false negative rate (FNR) was 11.4% for negative diagnosis and 43.7% for positive diagnosis, as shown by Figs. 8 and 9.

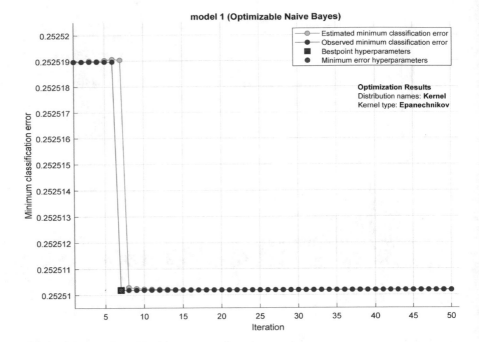

Fig. 6 NB optimization

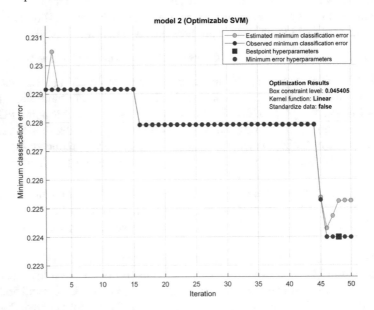

Fig. 7 SVM optimization

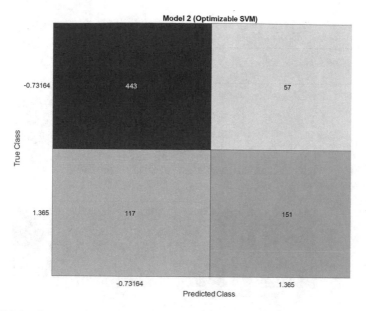

Fig. 8 CM showing class observations

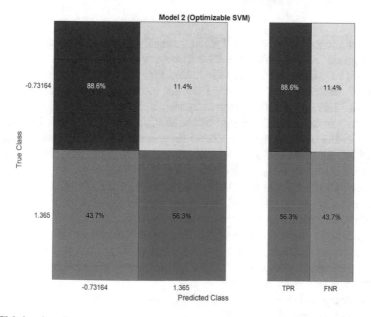

Fig. 9 CM showing class percentages

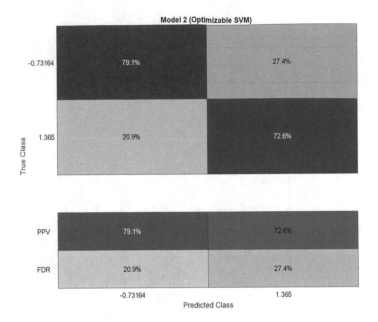

Fig. 10 CM showing PPV and FDR

The positive predictive value (PPV) indicates the percentage of correct classifications per predicted class, while the false discovery rate (FDR) shows the percentage of incorrect classifications per predicted class. PPV for correct diagnosis of negatives was 79.1% and 72.6% for positives. FDR for incorrect diagnosis of negatives was 20.9% and 27.4% for positives, shown by Fig. 10 below.

The CM's findings are reinforced by the ROC, illustrated in Figs. 11 and 12. The ROC shows the true positive rate (TPR) for negative diagnosis was 88.6 (89) and 56.3% (56%) for positive diagnosis. The false negative rate (FNR) was 11.4% (11%) for negative diagnosis and 43.7% (44%) for positive diagnosis.

The parallel coordinates plot (PCP) also confirms the CM's findings, illustrating the prediction response and the data distribution for each of the variables. Row_5 (Insulin) shows a wide standard deviation in correct/incorrect classifications for negative diagnosis. In contrast with row_2 (Glucose) which shows a high concentration of incorrect classifications for positive diagnosis see Figs. 13 and 14.

Figures 15 and 16 compare the output (black) versus the expected results (red) at 500 iterations.

The training and test results for ANFIS, using GA and PSO, are shown in the following tables for each iteration.

Reduction of features had the effect of producing a similar result, with less cost, less time, and less features but with lower accuracy. Accuracy could likely be improved by increasing the number of hidden neurons, or the training and testing iterations.

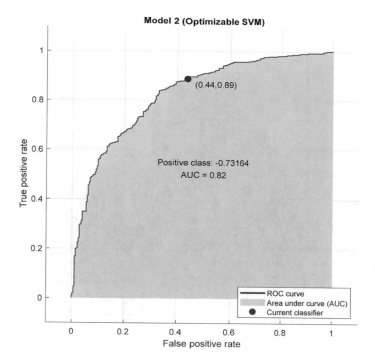

Fig. 11 ROC for negative diagnosis

Further optimization using PCA, NB, and SVM, along with CM, and ROC produced consistent results. However, they were not superior to the original best cost or accuracy.

5 Conclusion

With the objective of establishing a fuzzy rule-based system for early detection of diabetes, this paper applied the powerful neuro-fuzzy ANFIS framework. Through a comparative study optimizing ANFIS with GA and PSO, as well as with/without PCA as a pre-processing step, the best accuracy achieved was 77.3%, which is comparable to recent literature. Most of the errors that occurred were from false negative classifications, with actual positives being diagnosed as negatives. Notwithstanding this, we have established that ANFIS-PSO's best cost has outperformed the ANFIS-GA based approach. Future studies will now consider evaluating the hyper parameter tuning of GA/PSO on ANFIS. Particularly, the effect of swarm socialization and cognition on velocity or positioning.

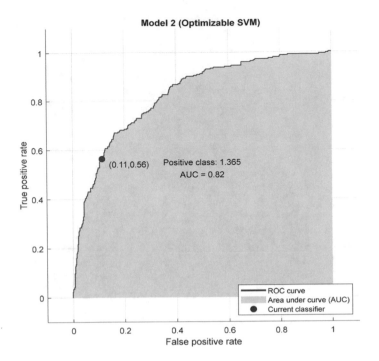

Fig. 12 ROC for positive diagnosis

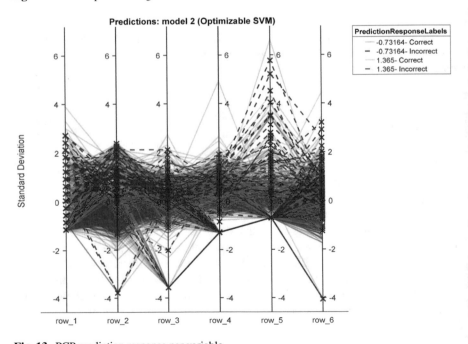

Fig. 13 PCP prediction response per variable

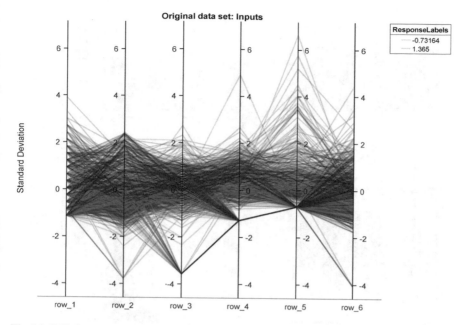

Fig. 14 PCP data per variable

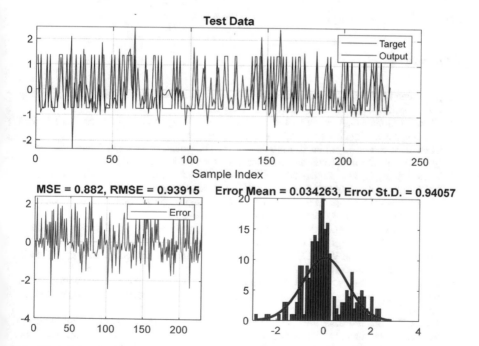

Fig. 15 ANFIS-PSO testing results

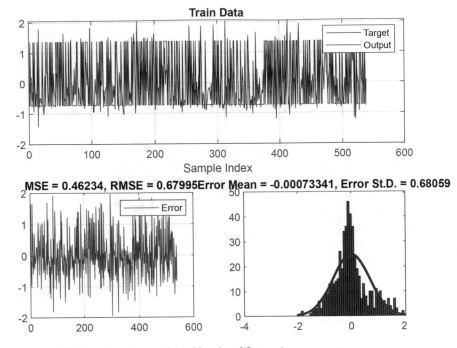

Fig. 16 ANFIS-PSO testing results (with reduced features)

References

1. Benamina M, Atmani B, Benbelkacem S (2018) Diabetes diagnosis by case-based reasoning and fuzzy logic. Int J Interact Multim Artif Intell 5:72–80
2. Chen T, Antoniou G, Adamou M, Tachmazidis I, Su P (2021) Automatic diagnosis of attention deficit hyperactivity disorder using machine learning. Appl Artif Intell 1–13
3. Chen T, Keravnou-Papailiou E, Antoniou G (2021) Medical analytics for healthcare intelligence–recent advances and future directions. Artif Intell Med 112:102009
4. Chen T, Shang C, Su P, Keravnou-Papailiou E, Zhao Y, Antoniou G, Shen Q (2020) A decision tree-initialised neuro-fuzzy approach for clinical decision support. Artif Intell Med 111:101986
5. Chen T, Shang C, Yang J, Li F, Shen Q (2020) A new approach for transformation-based fuzzy rule interpolation. IEEE Trans Fuzzy Syst 28(12):3330–3344
6. Ganji M, Abadeh MS (2010) Using fuzzy ant colony optimization for diagnosis of diabetes disease. In: Proceedings of ICEE 2010, pp 11–13
7. Gomathi C, Rajamani V, Jeya K (2018) Prediction of diabetes using fuzzy ontology approach. Int J Eng Res Technol (IJERT) TITCON, 3
8. Ghomsheh VS, Shoorehdeli MA, Teshnehlab M (2007) Training anfis structure with modified pso algorithm. In: Proceedings of the 15th mediterranean conference on control and automation. pp 1–6
9. Hassan R, Cohanim B, de Weck O (2005) A comparison of particle swarm optimization and the genetic algorithm. In: Proceedings of the 46th AIAA/ASME/ASCE/AHS/ASC structures, structural dynamics and materials conference austin, Texas, AIAA 2005–1897
10. Haznedar B, Kalinli A (2016) Training anfis using genetic algorithm for dynamic systems identification. Int J Intell Syst Appl Eng 4:44–47

11. Jang J (1993) Anfis: adaptive-network-based fuzzy inference system. IEEE Trans Syst Man Cybern 23:665–685
12. Kalpana M, Kumar AVS (2011) Fuzzy expert system for diabetes using fuzzy verdict mechanism. Int J Adv Netw Appl 3:11–28
13. Knox SA, Chen T, Su P, Antoniou G (2021) A parallel machine learning framework for detecting alzheimer's disease. In: Proceedings of the international conference on brain informatics. Springer, pp. 423–432
14. Lee C, Wang M (2001) A fuzzy expert system for diabetes decision support application. IEEE Trans Syst Man Cybern Part B (Cybernetics) 41:139-153
15. Lukmanto RB, Irwansyah E (2015) The early detection of diabetes mellitus (dm) using fuzzy hierarchical model. Procedia Comput Sci 59:312–319
16. Niswati Z, Mustika FA, Paramita A (2018) Fuzzy logic implementation for diagnosis of diabetes mellitus disease at Puskesmas in east Jakarta. J Phys Conf Ser
17. Nnamoko N, Arshad F, England D, Vora J (2013) Fuzzy expert system for type 2 diabetes mellitus (T2DM) management using dual inference mechanism. In: Proceedings of the AAAI spring symposium: data driven wellness
18. Perez R, Behdinan K (2007) Particle swarm approach for structural design optimization. Comput Struct 85:1579–1588
19. Polat K, Günes S (2007) An expert system approach based on principal component analysis and adaptive neuro-fuzzy inference system to diagnosis of diabetes disease. Digit Signal Process 17:702–710
20. Rajeswari A, Sidhika MS, Kalaivani M, Deisy C (2018) Prediction of prediabetes using fuzzy logic based association classification In: Proceedings of the second international conference on inventive communication and computational technologies (ICICCT), pp. 782–787
21. Rajeswari K, Vaithiyanathan V (2011) Fuzzy based modeling for diabetic diagnostic decision support using artificial neural network. Int J Comput Sci Netw Secur 11:126–130
22. Reddy GT, Khare N (2016) Ffbat-optimized rule based fuzzy logic classifier for diabetes. Int J Eng Res Afr 24:137–152
23. Smith JW, Everhart JE, Dickson WC, Knowler WC, Johannes RS (1988) Using the adap learning algorithm to forecast the onset of diabetes mellitus. In: Proceedings of the annual symposium on computer application in medical care, american medical informatics association. pp 261
24. Stirling J, Chen T, Bucholc M (202) Diagnosing alzheimer's disease using a self-organising fuzzy classifier. In: Proceedings of the Fuzzy logic: recent applications and developments. Springer,
25. Su P, Chen T, Xie J, Ma B, Qi H, Liu J, Zhao Y (2020) A density and reliability guided aggregation for the assessment of vessels and nerve fibres tortuosity. IEEE Access 8:139 199–139 211
26. Su P, Chen T, Xie J, Zheng Y, Qi H, Borroni D, Zhao Y, Liu J (2020) Corneal nerve tortuosity grading via ordered weighted averaging-based feature extraction. Med Phys
27. Sulla-Torres JA, Luna-Luza G, Ccama-Yana D, Gallegos-Valdivia J, Cossio-Bolaños M (2020) Neuro-fuzzy system with particle swarm optimization for classification of physical fitness in school children. In Int J Adv Comput Sci Appl 11:505–512
28. Tabibi ST, Zaki TS, Ataeepoor Y (2013) Developing an expert system for diabetics treatment advices. Int J of Hosp Res 2:155–162
29. Thirugnanam M, Kumar P, Srivatsan S, Nerlesh CR (2012) Improving the prediction rate of diabetes diagnosis using fuzzy, neural network, case based (fnc) approach. Procedia Eng 38:1709–1718
30. Uzuner S (2016) Comparison of artificial neural networks (ann) and adaptive neuro-fuzzy inference system (anfis) models in simulating polygalacturonase production. BioResources 11:8676–8685
31. Varma KV, Rao AA, Lakshmi TSM, Rao PN (2014) A computational intelligence approach for a better diagnosis of diabetic patients. Comput Electr Eng 40:5

32. World Health Organization (WHO), Diabetes fact sheet n°312 (2013). https://www.who.int/news-room/fact-sheets/detail/diabetes
33. Yildirim Y, Bayramoğlu M (2006) Adaptive neuro-fuzzy based modelling for prediction of air pollution daily levels in city of Zonguldak. Chemosphere 63:1575–1582
34. Zhang H, Chen C, Chen T, Wang Z, Chen Y (2021) Mixed aggregation functions for outliers detection. J Intell Fuzzy Syst, 1–14

A Fuzzy Logic Risk Assessment System for Type 2 Diabetes

Jared Anthony Marsh and Arjab Singh Khuman©

Abstract This chapter details the design and evolution of a Mamdani fuzzy logic system to allow users to assess their own risk of developing type 2 diabetes. From the research behind the system to its design, conception and testing to refine the system's accuracy. The system allows users to enter details about their lifestyle and their vital statistics such as height and weight to determine an approximate risk level of developing type 2 diabetes so they can make healthier and more mindful lifestyle choices. Choosing to make better choices will improve their quality of life and save healthcare providers or themselves a vast amount of money in the long run, depending on whether it is a national healthcare service or private provider. This system is not medically tested, and usage of this system without rigorous medical testing and alterations based on that testing is not advised.

1 Introduction

At first glance, two responses to this system could be, "We have doctors and health systems to diagnose a user's risk for conditions, so why could a computer system be useful?" Furthermore, "Why would a user even want to be able to assess their risk of getting type 2 diabetes?" Both are easily answerable. Firstly, doctors and healthcare providers are vital to society. Thanks to the ongoing coronavirus pandemic, they are incredibly overworked at the time of writing. Lessening their workloads is of crucial importance to keep society functioning. As well as this, in healthcare systems where people must spend large sums of money to use it; if people are made aware they are at a higher risk of developing a condition and change their habits to reduce that risk, it will mean they spend less money on healthcare in the future too.

J. A. Marsh · A. S. Khuman (✉)
School of Computer Science and Informatics, De Montfort University, Leicester, UK
e-mail: arjab.khuman@dmu.ac.uk

J. A. Marsh
e-mail: P2430436@alumni365.dmu.ac.uk

© The Author(s), under exclusive license to Springer Nature Singapore Pte Ltd. 2022
T. Chen et al. (eds.), *Artificial Intelligence in Healthcare*, Brain Informatics and Health,
https://doi.org/10.1007/978-981-19-5272-2_16

To put the expenditures and workload for type 2 diabetes into perspective, according to Hex et al., in 2012, the NHS spent approximately £9.8bn on the direct costs of diabetes in the period 2010/11, £8.8bn (89.8%) of that on type 2 diabetes specifically. Hex et al. then used data from the Office of National Statistics to estimate the rise in diabetes-related costs for the NHS in 2035/6. They estimated that the total direct cost would be £16.9bn and £15.1bn (89.35%) for type 2 diabetes [9]. Moreover, for its economic effects on a larger scale, the American Diabetes Association estimated that in 2017, the total direct cost of diabetes in America was $237bn (~£170.3bn). Also, people with diagnosed diabetes' care accounted for 1 in every 4 dollars spent on healthcare and that the average person annually would incur ~$9600 (~£6899) in medical expenses directly caused by diabetes [2]. Of course, the split between type 1 and type 2 was not present in those findings, but the NHS spending mentioned above shows that type 2 takes up a much more significant proportion of that spending.

According to the World Health Organization, the good thing is that people in the early stages of diabetes can postpone or even avoid diabetes complications in their entirety by making healthier lifestyle choices [20]. Diabetes UK and other organisations are currently discussing new findings and research that some people can put their type 2 diabetes into remission, mainly by losing weight [6].

This delaying or avoidance of developing type 2 diabetes is where this system will be helpful. If someone can determine their approximate risk for diabetes, that can push them to make healthier lifestyle choices. Those choices not only could save them or their health system a vast sum of money per year, but they will also be on the lookout for symptoms and meet with their physician if they are experiencing them. This is because, like any significant illness, catching type 2 diabetes in its early stages means it is easier to treat and prevent.

MATLAB and its fuzzy logic toolkit were vital throughout the development of this system. The ease of use and comprehensive feature set of both enabled rapid development of the system, accurate benchmarking and debugging of errors. Another helpful feature was easy reading and manipulation of XLS files which significantly improved the testing workflow.

2   Related Research

2.1   What is Fuzzy Logic, and How Does It Work?

Traditional Boolean logic, true or false, 1 or 0, is how logical systems usually work. Something is either true or false, and there is no in-between [10–12]. This Boolean logic is perfect if a system needs to assess whether one number is greater than another or if two values are equal. However, for a system that needs to see if things are partially true, such as if a person is somewhat tall or if a car is going slightly fast, a different type of logic is needed that can handle these partial truths.

Fuzzy logic fills this gap. It uses partial classification, which means any statement has some degree of truth. In fuzzy logic, all values have some degree of membership or truth, 100% (1) membership, 0% (0) membership, or anywhere between [10–12]. This means that fuzzy logic is easier to understand and is more flexible because it is based on natural language and how we think [10–12]. This natural and easy to understand logic is obvious when looking at a fuzzy system's rules. Fuzzy rules are written in an if–then manner. For instance, if a car is going very fast and the road is very wet, then a crash is very likely [10–12].

For the description of how fuzzy systems work, the following example system will be used, and the terminology explained:

Inputs: Car speed (mph), road water coverage (%).

Input fuzzy sets: Car is slow, car is fast, road is dry, road is wet.

Output: Chance of crash (%).

Output fuzzy sets: Crash is unlikely, Crash is likely, Crash is very likely.

Rules:

- If car is slow and road is dry, then crash is unlikely.
- If car is slow and road is wet, then crash is likely (to a lesser degree).
- If car is fast and road is dry, then crash is likely (to a lesser degree).
- If car is fast and road is wet, then crash is very likely.

Fuzzy systems start by taking in crisp inputs. In this example, it takes a speed of 70 mph and a road water coverage of 10%. The system then uses these inputs to determine their degree of membership (truth) to each of their fuzzy sets using mathematical membership functions. This step is known as fuzzification [10–12]. For speed in the example system, it will evaluate to a high truth value for 'car is fast' but a much lower truth value for the 'car is slow' set, 0.7 for fast and 0.05 for slow, for instance.

If a rule has multiple inputs, the next step is to apply a fuzzy operator to each rule and the appropriate fuzzy sets to get a single value for the rule's truth. This operation is like Boolean logic, combining multiple statements with AND or OR to get a resultant truth value. The operator used corresponds to the wording in the rule. If 'and' is in the rule, the AND operator's chosen method is applied [10–12].

After determining the rule's truth value, every rule has a weighting which is usually 1. This weighting affects the rule's relative 'strength' compared to other rules and is multiplied by the result of the previous step. This weighted truth value is then applied to the fuzzy output set from the rule, such as 'crash is likely' from the example system. It uses the system's set implication method to alter its membership function based on the weighted truth. Furthermore, this implication step repeats for every appropriate rule [10–12].

As described in the fuzzification step, any input value can apply to multiple fuzzy sets, so every rule that contains each suitable combination is used in the implication step, which generates multiple membership functions for the output, in this case, the chance of a crash. The penultimate step, known as aggregation, uses the system's aggregation method to build a total membership function for the fuzzy output set as a whole. From chance of crash unlikely to very likely in the example system [10–12].

The final step, called defuzzification, uses the aggregated fuzzy membership function and transforms that into the final crisp value, in the example's case, the percentage chance of a crash. This is done usually using one of five in-built methods when using MATLAB [10–12].

2.2 How Can Fuzzy Logic Be Applied to the Healthcare Field?

Fuzzy logic has numerous applications in almost any field where traditional Boolean logic is currently used for systems that deal with questions that need an almost human level of reasoning behind it. The healthcare field is full of systems just like this, and there has been considerable research and examples across this sector.

Allahverdi, in 2014, surveyed a range of designs for fuzzy systems across the healthcare and medical sectors, some of which are more in-depth and fully featured than others but all of which can be adapted to different needs or conditions. The one system of interest is a system to determine disease risk based on vital statistics, which is described in a significant amount of detail, including an example rule grid, membership function expressions and even an interface. However, the interface will not be beneficial to this system's design. Moreover, they explain that fuzzy logic is helpful for healthcare because medical diagnosis is very complex due to many factors, making Boolean logic much more challenging to use [1].

Diagnosis is one of the main foci for fuzzy logic for that reason, the number of factors. Fuzzy logic is easily scalable; adding to a system with just a new membership function and rules can be done quickly. This means it is much easier than adding all the different logical cases in a more traditional system. Awotunde, Matiluko, Fatai developed a system to accurately diagnose a person's malaria severity based on their symptoms. They chose malaria because it is very prevalent across Africa, so determining its severity is extremely useful. According to their investigation, fuzzy logic will reduce a doctor's workload on an initial consultation and issues with hospital consultations. Adapting the system to various other diseases based on prevalence in a specific location will benefit public health worldwide [3]. A less specialised but more comprehensive use case system created by Dagar, Jatain and Guar uses fuzzy logic and a range of symptoms to determine which out of six possible diseases a person is most likely to have. The system is useful because the chosen conditions, prevalent in India, have overlapping symptoms. To remove that ambiguity, choosing fuzzy logic and its human-like reasoning was the decision they made, and it was the right one. This fuzzy reasoning leads to a tested and accurate likelihood of each condition, meaning a faster and more accurate diagnostic assumption before any clinical testing [5].

Another key focus, one that is of particular importance for this system, is risk assessment. Thanks to how fuzzy logic dispels ambiguity with its reasoning, it is much easier to determine risk from several completely different factors. Yunda, Pacheco and Millan created a web-based tool using fuzzy logic to evaluate a person's risk of acquiring or worsening cardiovascular disease. They did this by asking for a user's age, blood pressure, BMI and other statistics. Then using test data and medical knowledge, determine an accurate risk level that will speed up any assumptions and decisions healthcare professionals make. The overall design can be easily augmented for any other disease or illness. Their main reason for choosing fuzzy logic was to, and there is a pattern emerging here, deal with the ambiguity in the risk classification. The human body will often react similarly in different conditions, and fuzzy logic can help differentiate them. Also, adjusting different symptom's membership functions instead of arbitrary numbers means a much easier to adjust system [21]. A very relevant system for the system this chapter is developing is a system designed by Shahjalal et al., which measures someone's risk from a diabetic attack, mainly written to help insurance underwriters. However, the reason behind its development is not what is useful; it is some of the factors used in it and how similar they may be to risk factors for this chapter's system. If there is a prize for guessing why they used fuzzy logic, using the previous reasoning of other systems would almost get that prize, they chose fuzzy logic due to its handling of imprecise or otherwise known as ambiguous data [17].

2.3 How Does Fuzzy Logic Improve This System?

Overall, fuzzy logic improves this system by allowing its design to be like how humans process information. If these things are somewhat true or false, then this is the result as opposed to these things both must be 100% true or false for this to get a result. This design is vital because it makes the system much easier not only to develop, as it is much more intuitive but also accurate due to this human-like reasoning. Like all the previously mentioned research and designs of related systems, it removes ambiguity more than a classic Boolean logic-driven application to get that more accurate result.

It will also increase the range of inputs that could be entered instead of picking from a selection of ranges when inputting into the system. For instance, entering more specific input values is now possible, and once refined, the system will produce accurate evaluations of those inputs. Accuracy is critical when it comes to people's health and well-being. That, coupled with the reasoning method above, is why fuzzy logic is a much better choice than Boolean logic.

3   Final System Overview

See Fig. 1.

3.1   Description

The final system design is a modular system divided into three subsystems. Firstly, a standalone user-submitted subsystem known as the patient subsystem that uses a user's vital statistics to generate a risk level. There is a separate patient subsystem for both males and females as there are different risk factors and criteria for both sexes.

There are also two optional subsystems. A doctor subsystem that uses clinical test results that patients cannot perform readily, such as cholesterol and blood sugar tests, to determine a clinically accurate risk. If needed, this subsystem could also be a standalone system and obtain these results from a database in an actual application. Furthermore, a total risk subsystem combines the doctor and patient subsystems to build an overall risk level that is even more accurate as users can make errors, bend the truth about certain lifestyle aspects, and tests doctors perform cannot.

This modular and optional subsystem design shows how a system like this could exist in the real world. Patients could get a risk level on their own or have blood test results saved on a database that combines with their entered information to determine an even more accurate risk level. Moreover, the patient and doctor subsystems can be extended for any other disease and risk factors to save healthcare systems and patients even more money by reducing the number of people developing such expensive diseases.

3.2   Patient/User Risk Inference Subsystem

See Fig. 2.

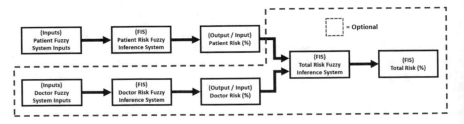

Fig. 1 Final system overview diagram

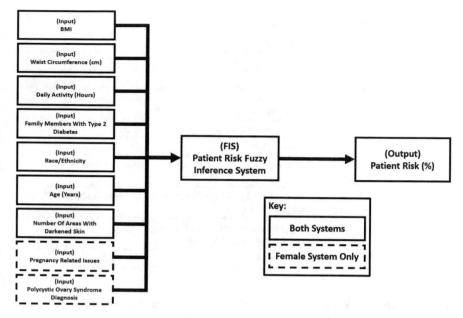

Fig. 2 Patient/user risk subsystem diagram

3.2.1 Description

The patient/user risk assessment subsystem uses user entered inputs such as their waist circumference, age, and BMI to determine their risk of developing type 2 diabetes as a percentage. One hundred percent meaning an incredibly high risk, and zero percent meaning an extremely low risk. There is both a male and female patient subsystem as each sex has different risks and criteria. To determine the appropriate risk profile, an actual application would need to ask what the user's sex was at birth. Extending this subsystem for different risks or conditions is simple, only altering the rules and membership functions to match the new system's requirements.

3.2.2 Inputs and Justifications

See Table 1.

The Mayo Clinic has a comprehensive list of type 2 diabetes risk factors which inspired the input names and some of the range values for the patient subsystem [13]. Some factors in that list do not have specific ranges or values, so they were obtained from common sense based on this system's requirements or other sources.

Weight was the first factor on the list, stating that overweight or obese people have a higher type 2 diabetes risk, but weight alone does not determine if someone is overweight for their height. Hence BMI was chosen to substitute it. According to the NHS, the average BMI ranges are less than 18.5 means underweight, 18.5–24.9

Table 1 Patient/User subsystem inputs/ranges

Variable	Range
Input—BMI	8–50
Input—Waist circumference	55–200 cm
Input—Daily activity	0–8 h
Input—Family members with type 2 diabetes	0 members–6 members
Input—Race/Ethnicity	0–2
Input—Age	18 years–120 years
Input—Number of areas with darkened skin	0 areas–3 areas
Input (Female Only)—Pregnancy related issues	0 issues–2 specified issues
Input (Female Only)—Polycystic ovary syndrome diagnosis	0 (no)–1 (yes)
Output—Patient risk	0–100%

is healthy, 25–29.9 is overweight, and 30–39.9 is classified as obese [15] The final system followed these ranges. However, less than 24.9 was classified as low risk, with overweight as high risk and obese as a very high risk. In the final system, a 10 BMI buffer below 18 and above 40 ensures that a vast group of people can use the system, and if the range needs to be modified later, it can be easily.

Waist circumference ranges for diabetes risk are different for males and females. A waist circumference above 101.6 cm increases the risk for males, and it is 88.9 cm for females [13]. The British Heart Foundation provides a concrete set of ranges for both diabetes and heart disease. For males, below 94 cm is low risk, 94–102 is high risk, and above 102 cm is very high risk. For females, below 80 cm is low risk, 80–88 cm is high risk, and above 88 cm is very high risk [4]. The final system's lower and upper limits of waist circumference are 55 cm, commonly known as size zero, up to 200 cm to be as inclusive as possible.

Daily activity is the average number of hours per day the patient/user spends exercising over a week, as a more sedentary lifestyle means a higher type 2 diabetes risk [13]. According to the UK Chief Medical Officers in 2019, every adult should accumulate at least 2.5 h of exercise every week and the more activity, the better [18]. The range of 0–8 h per day may seem like an extensive range. However, athletes may exercise far longer than everybody else, so the range is larger to be more inclusive. Of course, if this range or its membership intervals need adjusting, it is straightforward to do so.

The number of close family members with type 2 diabetes also increases someone's risk of developing it. According to the National Institute for Health and Care Excellence, the more family members have it, the higher the risk [14]. The maximum range for this is set to six family members to be fully inclusive as having above six members in a person's immediate family is rare, especially them all having diabetes.

Race and Ethnicity plays a role as well. Black, Hispanic, Native American, Asian or Pacific Islanders are more likely to develop type 2 diabetes than White people [13]. The range 0–2 in this input has 0 meaning a White individual, 1 means a mixed-race/biracial individual with one White parent, and 2 is an individual that is Black, Hispanic, Native American, Asian or Pacific Islander.

The reason for a separate biracial option is that a biracial child may have an increased risk, depending on the genetic traits passed down from their parents. For instance, according to WebMD, Asian people tend to have more body fat at the same height and weight as White people and carry more of it in their belly, making them more resistant to insulin [19]. The biracial input level can be removed if it is proven that biracial children are not affected by their higher risk parent's genetic trait. However, there was little available research on the topic relating to diabetes specifically.

Age is another crucial factor, with Mayo Clinic outlining that risk increases as people age and when over the age of 45, the risk is especially high [13]. Therefore, the age range of 18–120 will cover every adult, excluding the world's oldest people who probably do not need their diabetes risk checked. Unfortunately, they are probably struggling a lot more medically. Of course, increasing the range if future generations live longer is easy.

The number of darker skin areas, known medically as acanthosis nigricans, display insulin resistance and are a symptom of prediabetes [13]. They usually appear in skin folds such as the neck, armpits and groin areas, so this system has a range of no areas affected to three different areas affected with increasing risk for each area.

Building the female patient subsystem was necessary due to their differing range of waist circumferences, pregnancy-related risk factors and polycystic ovary syndrome, which only affect people born as females. There are two main issues with pregnancy, according to Mayo Clinic. Developing gestational diabetes during pregnancy or giving birth to a baby heavier than 4 kg, so one issue would be an increased risk, and both issues would be an even higher risk [13]. Polycystic ovary syndrome (PCOS) also raises the risk, so the input is set to allow the user to say they have that diagnosis or not, hence the 0–1 range [13].

3.3 Doctor Risk Inference Subsystem (Optional)

See Fig. 3.

3.3.1 Description

The doctor risk assessment subsystem uses doctor-provided test results or measurements for the patient to determine a more accurate diabetes risk level as clinical tests do not lie. In contrast, patients/users tend to bend the truth about their activity levels, as an example, negatively affecting the system's accuracy. As well as this, clinical

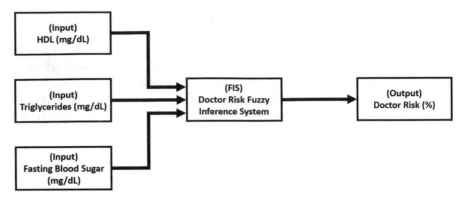

Fig. 3 Doctor risk subsystem diagram

tests may not be possible for patients/users to administer, so having recent test results stored in a database would be far more accessible. Whilst not being a requirement for this system to perform a type 2 diabetes risk assessment, clinical tests as mentioned improve accuracy, which is why this subsystem is optional but encouraged. There is a female doctor subsystem as well, only due to HDL cholesterol level interval differences. Extending this subsystem for different risks or conditions is easy, just like the patient subsystem.

3.3.2   Inputs and Justifications

See Table 2.

According to Mayo Clinic, an increased risk of developing type 2 diabetes comes from the factors mentioned in the patient subsystem and a low HDL cholesterol level, high levels of triglycerides, and a prediabetic blood sugar level [13].

Healthline provides acceptable, high and low values for both the HDL and triglyceride levels to assist in specifying the exact range of those inputs. HDL levels are low if it is less than 40 mg/dL for men and less than 50 mg/dL for women, acceptable between 40–60 mg/dL for men and 50–60 mg/dL for women and are at ideal levels when above 60 mg/dL for both sexes. Triglyceride levels are ideal when less than 100 mg/dL, good when less than 149 mg/dL, borderline between 150–199 mg/dL and high above 200 mg/dL. Healthline also mentions that 500 mg/dL is very high for triglycerides, so going above that to 750 mg/dL accounts for very high levels [8].

Table 2 Doctor subsystem inputs/ranges

Variable	Range
Input—HDL	0 mg/dL–120 mg/dL
Input—Triglycerides	0 mg/dL–750 mg/dL
Input—Fasting blood sugar	70 mg/dL–250 mg/dL
Output—Doctor risk	0%–100%

For blood sugar values, diabetes.co.uk has the appropriate blood sugar levels for a random blood test, when fasting and 2 h after eating. The fasting blood levels were chosen as doctors usually ask patients to fast before taking a blood test, so these results are the most likely type to be used. A normal blood sugar level is below 100 mg/dL, a prediabetic level is between 100–125 mg/dL, and a diabetic level is 200 mg/dL or more. 250 mg/dL was chosen as an end of the range to give some headroom above 200 mg/dL. However, if a patient's blood sugar is that high, they will probably already have a diabetes diagnosis [7].

3.4 Total Risk Inference Subsystem (Requires Other Subsystems)

See Fig. 4.

3.4.1 Description

The total risk assessment subsystem uses the patient and doctor subsystem results as inputs and combines them to build a total risk percentage. Only when using both the doctor and patient subsystems is this subsystem used, as each of the other subsystems can work as standalone systems. Altering this subsystem would only be needed if the number of membership conditions changes in the outputs of the other two subsystems.

3.4.2 Inputs and Justifications

See Table 3.

This subsystem, if both the other subsystems are present, receives their outputs as its inputs. Hence the ranges and membership intervals for its input variables match

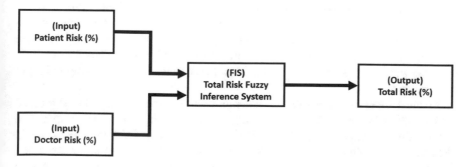

Fig. 4 Total risk subsystem diagram

Table 3 Total subsystem inputs/ranges

Variable (%)	Range (%)
Input—Patient risk	0–100
Input—Doctor risk	0–100
Output—Total risk	0–100

the output variables of the subsystems. This aids to the modularity of this system as any subsystem with a percentage output can easily replace either the doctor or patient subsystems. The output of this system is a total risk percentage. 0% does not mean the user will never get type 2 diabetes; just relative to the general population, it is improbable. This percentage can be shown to the user in an actual application to kickstart their lifestyle changes to lower their risk percentage. However, altering genetic factors is impossible, so everyone will have a lower risk limit, which will differ on a case-by-case basis.

4 Design Evolution and Evaluation

4.1 Initial System

The initial design has rules that cover every possible input combination meaning there are well over fifty thousand of them in total due to the number of inputs for the female patient subsystem and the number of membership functions for each input. The output of the doctor and patient subsystems is determined by adding up the membership function numbers in the input membership combinations and then using that score to determine the correct output membership function. For instance, there are twenty possible scores in the male patient subsystem, so each of its five output membership functions has four possible scores assigned to them. The female patient subsystem, however, has twenty-three possible scores, so there are two groups of four scores and three groups of five, where the groups of five are for the higher risk levels as it is more likely that a user will have at least an average risk of developing a condition in relation to the general population where genetic factors play a role.

The only difference in output calculation is in the total risk subsystem, where the rule's output is determined by averaging the two input membership function numbers. Only rounding up the output number if it is odd to ensure consistency with the other two subsystems, ensuring the higher risk levels have more assigned input combinations.

All the doctor and patient subsystem's inputs are based on the previously discussed ranges and guidelines. Their outputs and most of their inputs have trapezoidal membership functions at the start and end intervals to smooth/plateau membership distribution at the bounds of each input. This smoothing is because more minor input changes do not make as large of an impact on an input's start and ending membership intervals. Using a triangular membership function would not make sense as that is a linear distribution. The other intervals in those inputs used triangular membership functions as a change in input will make a much more drastic change in membership, so the linearity of triangular membership functions is much better suited than the smoother Gaussian function or trapezoidal function with its plateau. In other inputs, such as whether a female patient/user has a polycystic ovary syndrome diagnosis, the membership functions are all triangular as there will only be specific possible answers/points and not a wide range of results with overlap.

4.2 Test Data and Data Generation

The testing data consists of two tests for minimum and maximum risk values for all subsystems to ensure they give 0 and 100% relative risk as an output, as they should be possible output values and are key boundary cases. Furthermore, there are ten tests each for the two patient subsystems with their appropriate doctor subsystem. These tests use randomly generated input values instead of hand-picked values to ensure no bias and mimic the nearly random inputs that the general population could enter. These values are then compared to the expected output range of each subsystem and will pass if it falls within that expected range.

Generating the test values required a random number generator that was as truly random as possible. This need for pure randomness is where RANDOM.ORG comes in. RANDOM.ORG generates "True random numbers… generated from atmospheric noise… which for many purposes is better than the pseudo-random number algorithms typically used in computer programs" [16]. Therefore, these numbers will be unpredictable and more like the uniqueness of individual users submitting their information (Table 4).

Table 4 Testing data for patient and doctor subsystems

Test Values	Patient Test Inputs									Doctor Test Inputs		
	BMI	Waist Circ.	Daily Activity	Family Members	Race / Ethnicity	Age	Darkened Skin Areas	Pregnancy Issues	PCOS Diagnosis	HDL	Triglycerides	Fasting Blood Sugar
Min Risk Male	8	55	8	0	0	18	0			120	0	70
Max Risk Male	50	200	0	6	2	120	3			0	750	250
Male #1	34.5	102.2	5.6	5	2	31	2			88.4	310.4	231.3
Male #2	27.7	196.8	5.5	4	0	19	0			48.7	628.1	144.7
Male #3	37.4	90.6	6.1	3	2	32	3			17	461	121.4
Male #4	42.8	77.7	1.5	2	1	89	0			79	449.4	74
Male #5	24.4	129.4	7.5	1	2	34	1			91.5	275.6	147.9
Male #6	21.1	58.7	5.1	4	1	47	2			52.7	444.4	92.5
Male #7	16.5	148.1	3.7	3	1	109	3			27.4	98.2	121.9
Male #8	13.7	122.5	1.2	5	0	98	1			23.9	341.9	151.1
Male #9	24.9	60.6	4.5	3	1	37	1			11.1	95.4	106.9
Male #10	16.5	116.8	2	2	1	20	0			22.3	61.2	74.5
Min Risk Female	8	55	8	0	0	18	0	0	0	120	0	70
Max Risk Female	50	200	0	6	2	120	3	2	1	0	750	250
Female #1	30.9	165.4	2.1	0	2	20	3	1	1	21.7	724.8	200.6
Female #2	27.6	147.9	0.4	5	1	47	2	1	1	32.5	13.1	151.4
Female #3	19.8	124.3	4.6	6	0	80	3	0	0	17	582.9	177.2
Female #4	9.1	95.9	2	1	2	45	2	2	0	38.7	213.1	157.3
Female #5	11.4	137.2	5.6	6	0	114	1	1	0	44.5	311.9	92.3
Female #6	12.8	151.1	2.6	2	1	51	0	2	1	66.4	44.9	197.4
Female #7	35	102.9	2.7	4	2	65	2	1	0	111.5	708.7	138.1
Female #8	15.2	100.2	3	4	1	27	1	0	0	57.9	243.8	110.4
Female #9	22.8	94	3	3	0	33	3	2	0	96.7	236.8	91
Female #10	23.7	59.3	2	0	1	34	2	2	1	50.2	174.1	72.8

Table 5 Original boundary test results for patient/doctor subsystems

Test Results	Expected Min (%)	Expected Max (%)	Centroid	Bisector	MoM	SoM	LoM
Min Risk Male	0	0	FALSE	FALSE	FALSE	TRUE	FALSE
Max Risk Male	100	100	FALSE	FALSE	FALSE	FALSE	TRUE
Min Risk Female	0	0	FALSE	FALSE	FALSE	TRUE	FALSE
Max Risk Female	100	100	FALSE	FALSE	FALSE	FALSE	TRUE

Table 6 Boundary test results after making start and end intervals Gaussian membership functions

Test Results	Expected Min (%)	Expected Max (%)	Centroid	Bisector	MoM	SoM	LoM
Min Risk Male	0	0	FALSE	FALSE	TRUE	TRUE	TRUE
Max Risk Male	100	100	FALSE	FALSE	TRUE	TRUE	TRUE
Min Risk Female	0	0	FALSE	FALSE	TRUE	TRUE	TRUE
Max Risk Female	100	100	FALSE	FALSE	TRUE	TRUE	TRUE

4.3   Test and Test Results Summary

4.3.1   #1—Checking that the Subsystems Pass the Boundary Cases

The first test ensures that the initial system passes the boundary cases before choosing any methods and tuning any of the rules. It should pass, there is sound logic to its design, and on evaluating the test data, it… does not pass them in either the doctor or patient subsystems, so there is no hope for it passing in the total subsystem as it uses the other two as inputs.

The first thought is that all the defuzzification methods work on the resultant fuzzy set, and at both ends of the subsystem outputs, there are trapezoidal membership functions. Trapezoidal membership functions have a plateau, meaning there is no single point at 0 or 100%. Therefore, to correct this, changing the subsystem outputs and the total subsystem inputs to have a Gaussian membership function at both boundaries is needed. The Gaussian functions chosen for them were a gauss function with a standard deviation of 10 to maintain a similar level of overlap as the trapezoidal functions and a smoother distribution but with a single point at both 0 and 100%, which resulted in the tests passing for three defuzzification methods (Tables 5 and 6).

4.3.2   #2—Choosing a Defuzzification Method for Each Subsystem

After ensuring the boundary cases pass, it is time to decide on a defuzzification method for each subsystem, which turns the resultant fuzzy set into an output value, a relative risk percentage. This choice is not necessarily about choosing the most accurate defuzzification method according to the test results. It is about choosing the method with the results that fit best with the testing data. To deal with the overlap of the resultant fuzzy sets, the original expected ranges had a 2.5% reduction on their minimum value and a 2.5% addition to their maximum to allow for any slight overlaps in membership. This overlap results from the sheer number of rules firing, making a resultant output function less likely to be within the original expected range.

As the centroid and bisector methods do not pass the boundary cases, as seen in Table 5, only MoM, SoM and LoM are suitable choices for this system. When testing just these methods, MoM was the only one that returned 100% accuracy across all three subsystems. However, all its resultant values showed repetition (multiple 100, 50, 75 and 25% results) due to how MoM works. MoM returns the middle of the tallest plateau in the resultant membership function. As multiple results will have similar output functions, MoM is a vast generalisation of the truth, which is unsuitable for a health risk system, so discounting MoM is the only option. This leaves only SoM and LoM as viable options, and their results are as follows (Tables 7, 8 and 9).

The results show that both SoM and LoM have one test that fails to pass testing within the patient subsystem. The doctor subsystem completely passes, and the SoM and LoM inputs into the total subsystem produce two combinations with 100% accuracy. It is always better to overestimate the risk than to underestimate it regarding health and particularly risk assessments. Underestimation could lead to a nonchalance in a patient/user and anger if they developed a condition such as type 2 diabetes thinking it was improbable. This overestimation and the fact that SoM results are too low in some tests, such as 11% for male #5 and 16% for male #10, is why LoM is the best defuzzification method. SoM produces values that could give users a

Table 7 Patient subsystem SoM/LoM test results

System Outputs	Outputs		Patient Risk Results			
	SoM	LoM	Expected Min (%)	Expected Max (%)	SoM	LoM
Min Risk Male	0	0	0	0	TRUE	TRUE
Max Risk Male	100	100	100	100	TRUE	TRUE
Male #1	36	89	60	90	FALSE	TRUE
Male #2	44	56	35	65	TRUE	TRUE
Male #3	62	88	60	90	TRUE	TRUE
Male #4	64	86	60	90	TRUE	TRUE
Male #5	11	64	10	40	TRUE	FALSE
Male #6	41	59	35	65	TRUE	TRUE
Male #7	63	87	60	90	TRUE	TRUE
Male #8	39	61	35	65	TRUE	TRUE
Male #9	39	61	35	65	TRUE	TRUE
Male #10	16	34	10	40	TRUE	TRUE
Min Risk Female	0	0	0	0	TRUE	TRUE
Max Risk Female	100	100	100	100	TRUE	TRUE
Female #1	68	82	60	90	TRUE	TRUE
Female #2	65	85	60	90	TRUE	TRUE
Female #3	60	90	60	90	TRUE	TRUE
Female #4	38	62	35	65	TRUE	TRUE
Female #5	37	63	35	65	TRUE	TRUE
Female #6	41	59	35	65	TRUE	TRUE
Female #7	61	89	60	90	TRUE	TRUE
Female #8	43	57	35	65	TRUE	TRUE
Female #9	70	80	60	90	TRUE	TRUE
Female #10	42	58	35	65	TRUE	TRUE
			% In Expected Range		95.83%	95.83%

Table 8 Doctor subsystem SoM/LoM test results

| | Outputs | | Doctor Risk Results | | | |
System Outputs	SoM	LoM	Expected Min (%)	Expected Max (%)	SoM	LoM
Min Risk Male	0	0	0	0	TRUE	TRUE
Max Risk Male	100	100	100	100	TRUE	TRUE
Male #1	65	85	60	90	TRUE	TRUE
Male #2	65	85	60	90	TRUE	TRUE
Male #3	65	85	60	90	TRUE	TRUE
Male #4	37	63	35	65	TRUE	TRUE
Male #5	39	61	35	65	TRUE	TRUE
Male #6	39	61	35	65	TRUE	TRUE
Male #7	39	61	35	65	TRUE	TRUE
Male #8	63	87	60	90	TRUE	TRUE
Male #9	45	55	35	65	TRUE	TRUE
Male #10	14	36	10	40	TRUE	TRUE
Min Risk Female	0	0	0	0	TRUE	TRUE
Max Risk Female	100	100	100	100	TRUE	TRUE
Female #1	91	100	85	100	TRUE	TRUE
Female #2	13	37	10	40	TRUE	TRUE
Female #3	89	100	85	100	TRUE	TRUE
Female #4	36	64	35	65	TRUE	TRUE
Female #5	39	61	35	65	TRUE	TRUE
Female #6	42	58	35	65	TRUE	TRUE
Female #7	67	83	60	90	TRUE	TRUE
Female #8	41	59	35	65	TRUE	TRUE
Female #9	15	35	10	40	TRUE	TRUE
Female #10	49	51	35	65	TRUE	TRUE
			% In Expected Range		100.00%	100.00%

Table 9 Total risk subsystem SoM/LoM test results

| | Outputs | | | | Expected Range | | Total Risk Results | | | |
| | SoM Inputs | | LoM Inputs | | | | SoM Inputs | | LoM Inputs | |
System Outputs	SoM	LoM	SoM	LoM	Expected Min (%)	Expected Max (%)	SoM	LoM	SoM	LoM
Min Risk Male	0	0	0	0	0	0	TRUE	TRUE	TRUE	TRUE
Max Risk Male	100	100	100	100	100	100	TRUE	TRUE	TRUE	TRUE
Male #1	39	61	89	100	60	90	FALSE	TRUE	TRUE	FALSE
Male #2	65	85	65	85	60	90	TRUE	TRUE	TRUE	TRUE
Male #3	63	87	88	100	60	90	TRUE	TRUE	TRUE	FALSE
Male #4	38	62	63	87	60	90	FALSE	TRUE	TRUE	TRUE
Male #5	14	36	64	86	35	65	FALSE	TRUE	TRUE	FALSE
Male #6	39	61	39	61	35	65	TRUE	TRUE	TRUE	TRUE
Male #7	63	87	63	87	60	90	TRUE	TRUE	TRUE	TRUE
Male #8	63	87	63	87	60	90	TRUE	TRUE	TRUE	TRUE
Male #9	39	61	39	61	35	65	TRUE	TRUE	TRUE	TRUE
Male #10	14	36	14	36	10	40	TRUE	TRUE	TRUE	TRUE
Min Risk Female	0	0	0	0	0	0	TRUE	TRUE	TRUE	TRUE
Max Risk Female	100	100	100	100	100	100	TRUE	TRUE	TRUE	TRUE
Female #1	91	100	92	100	85	100	TRUE	TRUE	TRUE	TRUE
Female #2	38	62	38	62	35	65	TRUE	TRUE	TRUE	TRUE
Female #3	64	86	90	100	85	100	FALSE	TRUE	TRUE	TRUE
Female #4	38	62	63	87	35	65	TRUE	TRUE	TRUE	FALSE
Female #5	38	62	63	87	35	65	TRUE	TRUE	TRUE	FALSE
Female #6	41	59	41	59	35	65	TRUE	TRUE	TRUE	TRUE
Female #7	64	86	89	100	60	90	TRUE	TRUE	TRUE	FALSE
Female #8	41	59	41	59	35	65	TRUE	TRUE	TRUE	TRUE
Female #9	40	60	40	60	35	65	TRUE	TRUE	TRUE	TRUE
Female #10	42	58	42	58	35	65	TRUE	TRUE	TRUE	TRUE
					% In Expected Range		83.33%	100.00%	100.00%	75.00%

false sense of security in their low risk. In contrast, LoM produces probably a slight overestimation but a fair value based on the input data.

For the total risk subsystem with LoM inputs, the only valid and 100% accurate option is to use SoM as the defuzzification method. Using LoM with LoM inputs causes multiple 100% relative risks and very few lower risk values that do not make sense given the input data.

There is, however, a failing patient test for the LoM method, male #5. As well as an outlying result in the total subsystem for male #10, who has a 14% risk, different to similar user's total risk results. Both are probably not a malfunction of the system, rather a malfunction of the testing method. The expected values in the testing come from calculating the patient and doctor subsystem scores manually and by using the total subsystem's rules, choosing the correct output membership range. This estimation is perfect if the input data is not close to overlapping points in membership functions. The overlap and the massive number of rules, 9,216 for the male patients and 55,296 for female patients, can skew the output function. Therefore, the actual resultant output score can be ± 1 the estimated output score ($\sim \pm 25\%$). This difference is expected behaviour in fuzzy systems that the testing methodology did not account for and therefore is a failure of the testing, so to be fair on the system, discounting these 'failed' tests was the only viable option.

4.3.3 #3—Testing a Smaller Set of Membership Intervals and Ruleset

Finally, it is time to see if the system can maintain its accuracy with fewer input membership intervals and fewer rules. Not discounting the previously mentioned outlier and failed tests due to the testing system means a patient subsystem accuracy of 95.83%, a doctor accuracy of 100% and a total risk accuracy of 100%. If they are discounted, however, the accuracy is 100% across all three subsystems. This test should reveal a definite increase in performance. However, that performance increase may not be worth it if it loses a substantial amount of accuracy, especially when it comes to people's health.

The main subsystems that need to have a membership interval and rule reduction are the two patient subsystems. A total of 64,512 rules between them is excessive but currently necessary for the number of membership intervals. Therefore, after removing any unnecessary intervals, the system needs to be tested using the same methodology, even with its flaw in expected outputs, to maintain consistency.

It was possible, after reducing the BMI, age and activity inputs down to just three membership functions to reduce the male subsystem's ruleset to 3,888 rules. Furthermore, making identical reductions to the female patient subsystem lowered its rule count to 23,328. That is a 57.8% decrease in rules for both patient subsystems, with only 27,216 between the two patient subsystems now.

The results in Tables 10 and 11 may look disappointing, to begin with, with the patient and total subsystems having a reduction in accuracy to 91.67%. However, both subsystem's outputs are out of their expected ranges by 1%, based on the previous discussion that there will be overlapping rules in the subsystems. The expected results

Table 10 Patient subsystem reduced ruleset test results

Patient Risk Subsystem	Outputs	Expected Min (%)	Expected Max (%)	Results
Min Risk Male	0	0	0	TRUE
Max Risk Male	100	100	100	TRUE
Male #1	89	60	90	TRUE
Male #2	61	35	65	TRUE
Male #3	85	60	90	TRUE
Male #4	86	60	90	TRUE
Male #5	64	35	65	TRUE
Male #6	65	35	65	TRUE
Male #7	87	60	90	TRUE
Male #8	86	60	90	TRUE
Male #9	66	35	65	FALSE
Male #10	33	10	40	TRUE
Min Risk Female	0	0	0	TRUE
Max Risk Female	100	100	100	TRUE
Female #1	57	35	65	TRUE
Female #2	90	60	90	TRUE
Female #3	66	35	65	FALSE
Female #4	62	35	65	TRUE
Female #5	63	35	65	TRUE
Female #6	64	35	65	TRUE
Female #7	89	60	90	TRUE
Female #8	32	10	40	TRUE
Female #9	80	60	90	TRUE
Female #10	58	35	65	TRUE
			% In Expected Range	91.67%

can be out of range by ± 1 score ($\sim \pm 25\%$ risk) due to the testing not accounting for this overlap. 1% out of range is insignificant. Therefore, the reduced ruleset system will become the final design.

4.4 Final System

To recap, the final system, after testing and refining the initial system, is 100% accurate and has a 57.8% decrease in rules in two subsystems. Therefore, reducing addrule function calls and reducing the time input evaluation takes as it must compare the inputs to fewer rules. The system is, in fact, ~55.18% or 55.33 s faster obtained from the average of 3 runs. Each subsystem now uses a gaussian membership function at the start and end intervals of their outputs instead of a trapezoidal one to allow for 0 and 100% relative risk results whilst maintaining a smooth distribution at either end. The rule base of this system could be optimised further by testing against real patient data or studies into the amount each risk factor affects diabetes development so the rule weights can be adjusted accordingly.

Table 11 Total risk subsystem reduced ruleset test results

Total Risk Subsystem	Outputs	Expected Min (%)	Expected Max (%)	Results
Min Risk Male	0	0	0	TRUE
Max Risk Male	100	100	100	TRUE
Male #1	89	60	90	TRUE
Male #2	64	60	90	TRUE
Male #3	65	60	90	TRUE
Male #4	63	60	90	TRUE
Male #5	64	35	65	TRUE
Male #6	64	35	65	TRUE
Male #7	63	60	90	TRUE
Male #8	63	60	90	TRUE
Male #9	66	35	65	FALSE
Male #10	14	10	40	TRUE
Min Risk Female	0	0	0	TRUE
Max Risk Female	100	100	100	TRUE
Female #1	68	60	90	TRUE
Female #2	63	35	65	TRUE
Female #3	91	60	90	FALSE
Female #4	63	35	65	TRUE
Female #5	63	35	65	TRUE
Female #6	64	35	65	TRUE
Female #7	89	60	90	TRUE
Female #8	41	35	65	TRUE
Female #9	40	35	65	TRUE
Female #10	42	35	65	TRUE
			% In Expected Range	91.67%

5 Reflection

5.1 Testing

Testing is the main issue that arose with this system's development, and at first glance, it appeared the system was at fault. However, fuzzy systems combine all partially true rules to generate the resultant membership function in its aggregation step. This means that if inputs are at boundaries between their membership functions, the number of rules that will generate the resultant membership is much larger than if all the input values were at the peaks of their respective membership functions. Therefore, the resultant output membership may shift closer to a different expected range than what was manually calculated by the scoring system in testing. This difference is why testing and being observant of actual test results is critical, as improving the system cannot happen without understanding the results and the testing methodology. Why did these outputs not fit? What could have caused that? Without that understanding, it is easy to blame the system when the testing itself has this flaw, which is why discounting the 'failed' tests was possible. This testing method was carried forward to ensure consistency as the first two test sets used the same method, and changing it for the third set would be unfair.

A combination of the following procedures is necessary to improve the testing for further development: Testing with real patient data, calculating rule weight based on different risk factors' effects, and allowing for a much larger range of possible results on inputs at boundaries. These would ensure a more rigorous test of the system and a lot less time spent justifying false-negative test results.

5.2   Effects of Different Risk Factors

Of course, like any medical condition, different risk factors may carry different levels of effectiveness in terms of how much they increase the risk of developing the condition. The list of type 2 diabetes risk factors compiled by the UK based National Institute for Health and Care Excellence contains statistics such as "Obesity accounts for 80–85% of the overall risk for developing type 2 diabetes." As well as "People with a family history of diabetes are 2–6 times more likely to have diabetes...." If obesity accounts for 80% of the overall risk, that leaves 20% to divide amongst the other risk factors, so understanding the actual percentage risk associated with each factor is extremely difficult [14]. Moreover, studying how much each factor affects the risk relative to one another is not easy because some factors such as lack of activity and obesity can be interlinked. Fuzzy systems, however, would benefit a lot from this information so rule weightings can be adjusted so that the more dangerous risks have a higher weighting and more of an impact than the less dangerous ones.

5.3   System Performance and Possible Improvements

The system, including all three subsystems and, in particular, the standalone patient subsystem, perform with 100% accuracy if the false negative tests are discounted due to testing issues. It does what it was designed to do. Users can enter their information and be given a relative risk of developing type 2 diabetes. If needed, their doctors can submit blood test results to combine with the user's input to determine a more accurate risk percentage.

To improve the system's execution time more than the current ruleset reduction already has, the ruleset could be reduced further by reducing the number of membership functions in other inputs or outputs or removing rules that do not make utterly sound sense. For instance, non-sensical rules such as a user with a low BMI and high activity levels with a massive waist circumference which is not a typical combination. The reason that rules such as that remain in the system is that this current system is an example of what fuzzy logic can achieve and has been built to take in any input within its given input ranges, not just typical scenarios but atypical ones. To optimise the ruleset further, the fuzzy system could be trained on real patient data that a healthcare professional has decided is either high, low or medium risk to build up its ruleset. However, the current set more than complies with the system's requirements.

6 Conclusion

Overall, this system completes its required task. A user can input their vital statistics such as their BMI, waist circumference and age to receive an approximate risk percentage of developing type 2 diabetes. This risk percentage can also be made more accurate by having test results from a doctor or healthcare professional.

Thanks to the modular design of this system, the patient/user and doctor subsystems can both be used as standalone systems or combined with the total risk subsystem to achieve a result. This design also means the system or subsystems can be modified to have other risk factors or clinical test results as inputs for other diseases. An example of this is malaria which would be incredibly useful in areas where malaria is particularly prevalent as it would save doctors valuable time in diagnosing their patients.

There may have been two false-negative test results, but the testing was consistent and unbiased throughout. If anything, those false negatives resulted from the tests being too strict for a fuzzy system. Therefore, there is a high level of confidence that the system is a strong example of a fuzzy risk assessment system. However, review and modification by healthcare professionals is advised because the developer of this system does not have the medical qualifications or license necessary to state that with certainty.

The only possible improvements would be to use real patient data as test values and liaising with doctors and other healthcare professionals to build a system that could be genuinely used in the real world. Though this chapter and system help move that dream into a reality and show just how useful fuzzy logic can be in the healthcare field to save not only a healthcare provider's time and money but also a patient's.

References

1. Allahverdi N (2014) Design of fuzzy expert systems and its applications in some medical areas. Int J Appl Math Electron Comput 2(1):1–8
2. American Diabetes Association (2018) Economic costs of diabetes in the U.S. in 2017. Diabetes Care 41:917–928
3. Awotunde JB, Matiluko OE, Fatai OW (2014) Medical diagnosis system using fuzzy logic. African J Comput ICT 7:99–106
4. British Heart Foundation (2021) Measuring your waist-Heart Matters I BHF. https://www.bhf.org.uk/informationsupport/heart-matters-magazine/medical/measuring-your-waist Accessed 31 July 2021
5. Dagar P, Jatain A, Gaur D (2015) Medical diagnosis system using fuzzy logic toolboX. Int Conf Comput Commun Automat 1(1):193–197

6. Diabetes UK (2021) What is diabetes remission and how does it work? | Diabetes UK. https://www.diabetes.org.uk/guide-to-diabetes/managing-your-diabetes/treating-your-dia betes/type2-diabetes-remission. Accessed 26 July 2021
7. Diabetes.co.uk (2019) Normal and diabetic blood sugar level ranges-blood sugar levels for diabetes. https://www.diabetes.co.uk/diabetes_care/blood-sugar-level-ranges.html. Accessed 30 July 2021
8. Healthline (2021) Cholesterol levels: by age, LDL, HDL, and more. https://www.healthline.com/health/high-cholesterol/levels-by-age. Accessed 30 July 2021
9. Hex N et al (2012) Estimating the current and future costs of Type 1 and Type 2 diabetes in the UK, including direct health costs and indirect societal and productivity costs. Diabet Med 29:855–862
10. Mathworks (2021) Foundations of fuzzy logic. https://uk.mathworks.com/help/fuzzy/founda tions-of-fuzzy-logic.html. Accessed 27 July 2021
11. Mathworks (2021) Fuzzy inference process. https://uk.mathworks.com/help/fuzzy/fuzzy-inf erence-process.html. Accessed 27 July 2021
12. Mathworks (2021) What is fuzzy logic? https://uk.mathworks.com/help/fuzzy/what-is-fuzzy-logic.html. Accessed 27 July 2021
13. Mayo Clinic (2021) Type 2 diabetes-symptoms and causes-mayo clinic. https://www.mayocl inic.org/diseases-conditions/type-2-diabetes/symptoms-causes/syc-20351193. Accessed 30 July 2021
14. National Institute for Health and Care Excellence (2021) Risk factors | Background information | Diabetes - type 2 | CKS | NICE. https://cks.nice.org.uk/topics/diabetes-type-2/background-information/risk-factors/. Accessed 30 July 2021
15. NHS (2019) What is the body mass index (BMI)?-NHS. https://www.nhs.uk/common-health-questions/lifestyle/what-is-the-body-mass-index-bmi/. Accessed 30 July 2021
16. RANDOM.ORG (1998) RANDOM.ORG-True random number service. https://www.random.org/. Accessed 30 July 2021].
17. Shahjalal M et al (2016) Measuring risk of diabetic: a fuzzy logic approach. Progress Nonlinear Dyn Chaos 4:23–33
18. UK Chief Medical Officers (2019) UK chief medical officers' physical activity guidelines. https://assets.publishing.service.gov.uk/government/uploads/system/uploads/attachment_d ata/file/832868/uk-chief-medical-officers-physical-activity-guidelines.pdf. Accessed 31 July 2021
19. WebMD (2021) Type 2 diabetes: how race plays a part. https://www.webmd.com/diabetes/type-two-diabetes-race. Accessed 31 July 2021
20. World Health Organization (2021) Diabetes. https://www.who.int/news-room/fact-sheets/det ail/diabetes. Accessed 26 July 2021
21. Yunda L, Pacheco D, Millan J (2015) A web-based fuzzy inference system based tool for cardiovascular disease risk assessment. NOVA 13:7–16

Printed in the United States
by Baker & Taylor Publisher Services